Spending Wisely

Buying Health Services for the Poor

Spending Wisely

Buying Health Services for the Poor

Edited by

Alexander S. Preker and John C. Langenbrunner

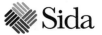

**SWEDISH INTERNATIONAL
DEVELOPMENT COOPERATION
AGENCY**

Stockholm

Canadian
International
Development
Agency

Agence
canadienne de
développement
international

Gatineau, Quebec

THE WORLD BANK

Washington, D.C.

© 2005 The International Bank for Reconstruction and Development / The World Bank
1818 H Street, NW
Washington, DC 20433
Telephone 202-473-1000
Internet www.worldbank.org
E-mail feedback@worldbank.org

1 2 3 4 08 07 06 05

ISBN 0-8213-5918-5
eISBN 0-8213-5919-3

Library of Congress Cataloging-in-Publication Data

Spending wisely : buying health services for the poor / Alexander S. Preker, John Langenbruner.
    p. cm.
  Includes bibliographical references and index.
  ISBN 0-8213-5918-5
  1. Poor—Medical care—Finance. 2. Poor—Medical care—Economic aspects. I. Preker, Alexander S., 1951– II. Langenbruner, John, 1951–

RA418.5.P6S67 2005
338.4'33621—dc22

Contents

TABLES

BOX

FIGURES

Acknowledgments

The editors are grateful for the inspiration provided by the following individuals who pioneered earlier work on resource allocation and purchasing in developing countries: Brian Able-Smith, Howard Barnum, Robert Evans, William Hsiao, Jerry LaForgia, John Øevretveit, Helen Saxenian, George Schieber, and Jeffrey Hammer.

The editors thank Hon. Dr. Kwaku Afriyie, former Minister of Health, Ghana, for his insights on practical application of strategic purchasing to a low-income context.

The following individuals provided valuable reviews of the early drafts of the volume: Michael Joseph Borowitz, Jan Bultman, Mukesh Chawla, Rena Eichler, Varun Gauri, Pablo Gottret, Loraine Hawkins, William Jack, Joe Kutzin, Akiko Maeda, Philip Musgrove, William Savedov, Agnes Soucat, Adam Wagstaff, and Abdo Yazbeck.

Important access was provided to parallel and ongoing research undertaken by the World Health Organization, the European Observatory, and close collaboration with Josep Figueras, Elke Jakubowski, Elias Mossialos, Jean Perrot, and Ray Robinson on resource allocation and purchasing in Central and Eastern Europe.

Valuable insights were provided by regional reviews of resource allocation and purchasing carried out by Enis Baris, John Fiedler, Daniel Kress, Jack Langenbrunner, Benjamin Loevinson, Akiko Maeda, Tonia Marek, Philipp Schnabl, and Edit Velenyi and country case studies undertaken by Enis Baris, Sarbani Chakraborty, Philip G. Cotterill, Maria Hofmarcher, Kees Klostermans, Joe Kutzin, Xingzhu Liu, Anne Mills, Eva Orosz, and Oscar Picazo.

Others who contributed in various ways to reviews and inputs to the volume include Laszlo Balkanyi, Mark Bassett, Karl Carol, Cheryl Cashin, Robert Dredge, Maureen Lewis, Matthias Lundberg, Tatyana Makarova, Sheila O'Dougherty, Mead Over, Andreas Seiter, Agnes Soucat, Dennis Streveler, Zhenya Symushkin, Robert Taylor, Marko Vujicic, and Olga Zus

The editors are grateful to the Governments of Sweden, Canada, and the United States for providing direct or indirect financial support, through the Canadian International Development Agency (CIDA), the Swedish International Development Cooperation Agency (SIDA), and the U.S. Agency for International Development (USAID), for the research and leadership in the field of health care reform.

Acronyms and Abbreviations

ABC	Activity-based costing
AN-DRGs	Australian National Diagnosis-Related Groups
BNHI	Bureau of National Health Insurance, Taiwan (China)
BINP	Integrated Nutrition Project
CABG	Coronary artery bypass graft
CBD	Community-based distribution
CHST	Canada Health and Social Transfer
CPR	Contraceptive prevalence rate
CRHCC	Central Florida Health Care Coalition
DHS	Demographic and health-survey
DOT's	Directly observed therapy short course
DRC	Depreciated replacement cost
EDL	Essential Drugs List
EOC	Essential obstetric care
EU	European Union
FFS	Fee for service
FONASA	Fondo Nacional de Salud, Chile
FSU	Former Soviet Union
GFHR	Global Forum for Health Research
HALE	Health-adjusted life expectancy
HC	Historic cost
HMO	Health care management organization

HPAR   Health promotion accountability region

ICD   International Classification of Diseases

ICU   Intensive care unit

IDO   Integrated delivery organization

ILO   International lending organization

IMCI   Integrated management of childhood illnesses

IMR   Infant mortality rate

INCLEN   International Clinical Epidemiology Network

LSMS   Living Standards Measurement Survey

MHI   Mandatory Health Insurance, Russia

MCH   Maternal and child health (care)

MEA   Modern equivalent asset

MSA   Medical savings account

NBCH   National Business Coalition for Health, United States

NGO   Nongovernmental organization

NHS   National Health Service, United Kingdom

NRV   Net realizable value

ORT   Oral rehydration treatment

PBGH   Pacific Business Group on Health

PC   Provider consortium

PCA   Principal component analysis

PRSP   Poverty Reduction Strategy Paper

QUALYs   Quality Adjusted Life Years

PRP   Performance-related pay

RAP   Resource allocation and purchasing

R&D   Research and development

RBRVS   Resource based relative value scale

RFI   Standardized health plan Request for Information

SWAp   Sector Wide Approach Prevention of Maternal Mortality

TBA   Traditional birth attendant

Under-5   Children under five years of age

UPHCP   Urban Primary Health Care Project

Introduction

Alexander S. Preker and John C. Langenbrunner

Promoting health and confronting disease challenges requires action across a range of activities in the health system: making improvements in the policy-making and stewardship role of governments; obtaining better access to human resources, drugs, medical equipment, and consumables; and encouraging a greater and deeper engagement of both public and private providers of services.

Great progress has been made in recent years in securing better access and financial protection against the cost of illness through collective financing of health care. Managing scarce resources and health care effectively and efficiently is an important part of the story. Experience has shown that without clear spending policies and effective payment mechanisms, the poor and other disadvantaged people often get left out.

The shift from the passive budgeting of in-house staff within the public sector to strategic purchasing or contracting of services from nongovernmental providers—that is, outsourcing—has been at the center of a lively debate on collective financing of health care during recent years. The premise underlying the change is that it is necessary to separate the functions of financing from the production of services to improve public sector performance and accountability.

This publication—*Spending Wisely: Buying Health Services for the Poor*—is the latest in a series of World Bank books on getting better value for money spent on health care. The book reviews how knowledge gained from recent experience of strategic purchasing in other sectors of the economy is now being extended effectively to the health sector in many developing countries. Many of the contributing authors demonstrate how the interest of the poor would often be better served through the fundamental shift in the way public money is spent on health services.

The book is divided into six parts, which cover the conceptual framework, transformation of strategic purchasing so that it is pro-poor, purchase of health services, purchase of inputs, the supply/demand/market behavior of purchasers, and legal and regulatory issues. The following summaries provide a roadmap for the book.

PART I: THE CONCEPTUAL FRAMEWORK

The chapters in part 1 present a conceptual framework that will help the uninitiated reader get familiar with the basic concepts and language used in strategic purchasing of health services for the poor. It highlights the need for policy makers to ask five fundamental questions: for whom to buy, what to buy, from whom to buy, how to pay, and at what price? In coming to grips with these questions, different authors throughout the book emphasize the important role of organizational, institutional, and management issues to the performance of public spending on health care.

In chapter 1, "Managing Scarcity through Strategic Purchasing of Health Care," Alexander S. Preker provides a rationale for collective spending on health care. He argues that the increased complexity of health care that has occurred over time has made it impossible for individuals to buy health care in the same way that they might buy groceries or other consumer goods. Furthermore, the cost of catastrophic care requires some form of insurance mechanism to avoid impoverishment when illness strikes. For this reason, most developed countries no longer rely on direct user charges to finance expensive health care. Many developing countries are slowly moving in the same direction, although at very low income levels direct fees still predominate.

At first sight, the relationship between the principal (patient) and the agent (purchaser) that has evolved under collective financing of health care helps resolve the problem of individuals having to deal with complex health systems. Similarly, associated pooling of resources helps spread risks across larger population groups.

In reality, things are not that simple because purchasers serve as multiplicitous agents for several different powerful principals, not just as agents for patients and their interests. Three important agency relationships are predominant: the relationship between the purchaser and health care providers (doctors, nurses, allied health care workers), the relationship between the purchaser and various institutional actors (policy makers, regulators, insurance and other funding agencies), and the relationship between the purchaser and health care organizations (hospitals, clinics, ambulatory services).

The interests of these stakeholders differ widely. For example, tension often arises between health care providers that act on behalf of individual patients and policy makers and institutions that focus more on national and population-level issues. The purchaser may be pressured by health care providers to finance the most recent and best-quality care for its patient. At the same time, the institutional actors in the ministry of health may be more concerned about aggregate health outcomes while those in the ministry of finance may be more concerned about the overall fiscal affordability of the health sector. This leads to an irreconcilable situation for the purchaser, which has to act as an agent on behalf of two or more principals, each of which has a very different agenda.

The greater the overlap in interest, the more likely the purchaser will have an authorizing environment that is consistent with the needs and expectations of the patients it serves. When the overlap is small, there is a great risk that both the poor and patients are left out.

From these observations, Preker concludes that, although strategic purchasing of health care provides many advantages, too often decisions are made based on technical criteria that ignore the interest of patient and the poor. One way to address this problem is by always making patients the objectives' focus, by giving patients voice in priority setting and other aspects of the health care they receive, and by providing them with a choice among purchasing agents so that the agents never forget whom they really serve. This tension between the policy interests of health systems and the individual interests of patients is a constant theme throughout the book. These concepts are taken up again by the other authors whose chapters appear in part 1.

In chapter 2, "For Whom to Buy? Are Free Government Health Services the Best Way to Reach the Poor?," Davidson R. Gwatkin makes a compelling case for including a pro-poor focus under the strategic framework of resource allocation and purchasing (RAP). Without it the poor are often left out. As highlighted by the author, equity is frequently used as a justification for government involvement in the health sector. In many countries, this has led to policies that promote universal access to free, government-operated health services. The chapter explores in greater detail the advantages and disadvantages of this approach in meeting the needs of disadvantaged population groups such as the poor and those affected by illness or disease.

Although universal access to a national health service has worked well in addressing the health needs of the poor in higher-income countries, the author challenges the wisdom of this approach in low-income countries. Unrestricted assess to government-operated health services in severely resource-constrained countries usually leads to a de facto reduction in the range of services available to the everyone, including the poor; it may also result in a pro-rich rather than pro-poor allocation of scarce resources. Since richer households can afford to "buy" the excluded services from nongovernmental providers, universal access often leads to a two-tier system even if this is precisely the type of situation that the policy sought to avoid. Far from promoting equity, universal access thus may even work against the poor.

Although there are no perfect solutions to this problem, Gwatkin suggests two alternative approaches that may be better at addressing the interests of the poor. The first approach is to direct government expenditure directly to the poor (that is, targeted demand-side subsidies). This could be achieved at the household level, targeting vulnerable population groups such as children, single mothers, and the elderly—or regions where the poor live. The second approach is to finance programs that address the most common health conditions of the poor or services used by the poor (that is, targeted supply-side subsidies).

In chapter 3, "What to Buy? Revisiting Priority Setting in Health Care," Katharina Hauck, Peter C. Smith, and Maria Goddard emphasize the importance of priority setting in achieving desired outcomes in severely resource-constrained environments. An approach that is often advocated in the health sector is to measure the impact of various interventions on health outcomes and calculate their associated costs. Cost-effectiveness league tables are now available on many of the most common health care interventions used in the health sector of developing countries.

Advocates of the cost-effectiveness approach to priority setting often encourage policy makers to assign a higher priority to interventions that are effective at a low cost. This approach, unfortunately, encourages interventions that address frequent and less serious conditions that most people—even the poor—could afford to pay for themselves; at the same time, it discourages public subsidies for higher-cost interventions that are effective in addressing rarer and more serious health conditions that few households can afford, not just the poor. Setting priorities based on cost effectiveness approach therefore undermines the insurance function, which is needed to protect households against the impoverishing effects of illness.

Furthermore, different societies have different value systems and therefore different ideas about what should be maximized. For example, health sector interventions contribute to the improvement not only of health outcomes, but also of educational attainment, poverty objectives, labor market productivity, and other dimensions of social welfare. But the RAP priorities that would maximize overall health outcomes are different from that which would maximize financial protection, equity, educational attainment, and labor market objectives.

The authors also highlight six major technical constraints of cost-effectiveness: (1) the analysis can be undertaken from a variety of perspectives leading to different rankings; (2) studies carried out in one context may not be generalizable to other settings (those involving nonlinear cost curves and relative prices, for instance); (3) the nature of the target population can affect the cost-effectiveness of interventions (for example, the poor are often much harder and costly to reach than higher-income groups); (4) there is considerable variance in the underlying parameters used in evaluations, which can influence outcomes; (5) evaluation studies are usually done before the medical technologies in question are fully integrated into the health care system, which may influence both their cost and effectiveness; and (6) there are important interactions among different programs, which influences the final cost and effectiveness.

In practice, policymakers do not widely use the results of economic evaluation in the final decisions on setting priorities for public spending. Based on these and other limitations, Hauck, Smith, and Goddard suggest that there is a need for a fundamental reassessment of the role of cost-effectiveness analysis in priority setting in the health sector. They recommend that policymakers also focus on the political economy, as well as organizational, institutional, and other noneconomic factors.

In chapter 4, "From Whom to Buy? Selecting Providers" Fernando Montenegro Torres and Cristian Baeza argue that purchasers should be more strategic in selecting the providers they finance with public funds. The authors recommend that purchasers actively select providers based on the providers' ability to offer services within a desired timeframe, quality range, and price range, rather than their privileged status as part of the publicly owned network of health services.

The authors point out that the greater the complexity of the desired intervention or service, the greater the need to purchase services from integrated delivery systems and not purchase inputs (drugs, equipment, supplies, and so on) or contract with individual providers. In the absence of a functioning delivery system, purchasers may be forced to micromanage by contracting individual services and services in a worst-case scenario, but this should be only a transitory phase while providers develop their capacity to deliver integrated services.

For a purchaser to "match" intervention with the appropriate providers, some basic conditions must be met. First, the purchaser must be entitled institutionally, legally, and administratively to be selective and therefore to take part in the decisions regarding the selection of providers. Second, there must be a variety of providers offering comparable products. Finally, the purchaser and the providers must be able to establish a purchasing-providing relationship within the regulatory and legal environment in which the purchaser carries out its decisions.

Montenegro Torres and Baeza focus on three criteria for selecting a provider and establishing a successful relationship with the purchaser. This includes identification of the goods and services that have to be purchased and "matching" this list with available providers, an assessment of the capability and eligibility of these providers, and selection of the chosen provider through a transparent and competitive process.

In chapter 5, "How to Pay? Understanding and Using Payment Incentives," John C. Langenbrunner and Xingzhu Liu examine the important role that provider payment mechanisms and incentives play in achieving the policy objectives of strategic RAP. In most countries, the mechanism used to pay health care providers is unfortunately highly politicized, with policy options often influenced more by ideology than reason. The authors suggest that under strategic purchasing, payment mechanisms should be tailored to desired policy objectives rather than driven by the vested interests of powerful stakeholders. The chapter provides an objective review of different mechanisms, highlighting known advantages and limitations, in the hope that this will allow policy makers to take rational decision on alternatives.

Under resource allocation and purchasing arrangements, payments to health care providers can be divided into three broad categories: direct payment to providers by the patient; direct payment to providers by the patient, but with later full or partial reimbursement; and direct payment to providers through collective financing arrangements, with only a limited copayment or informal charge paid by the patient. Direct payment by the patient sends the consumer a clear signal about the price of the service. However, poor patients or patients receiving expensive care for major illnesses may not have the disposable income to cover this payment. Even full or partial reimbursement later may not be able to bridge the period between paying for the service and receiving a full or partial reimbursement. When providers are reimbursed primarily through collective financing arrangements rather than by patients, the payment incentives and mechanism used, rather than prices and demand, create the behavioral environment for suppliers of services.

Langenbrunner and Liu conclude that owing to information asymmetry, neither consumers nor producers have full information about preferences, prices, or the market in which they operate. The level, mix, and quality of care can often be ascertained only after the fact. And actual health outcomes often depend on factors other than the health services consumed. Although doctors behave as agents for their patients, even they often do not know the full impact of the interventions that they are recommending. Both consumer and provider behavior are therefore important for better outcomes. Purchasers thus have an opportunity to shape the behavior of these key actors through payment incentives and prices.

In chapter 6, "At What Price? Affordable and Realistic Fees," Hugh Waters and Peter Sotir Hussey review methodologies and international experience related to costing and pricing health services, under market forces and under managed competition. Several factors affect the prices purchasers pay for health services, in addition to supply, demand, and market forces. These factors include the method of provider payment; availability of information on costs, volumes, outcomes, and patient and provider characteristics; methods used to calculate providers' costs; and characteristics of purchasers and providers, including the regulatory environment, provider autonomy, negotiating power, and the degree of competition.

The authors summarize methods for setting levels of payment under different provider payment mechanisms. In developing countries, line items and global budgets in the public sector and user fees in the private sector remain the most common reimbursement methods. Increasingly, however, reforms are introducing mixed payment systems that have greater information demands. The most common payment types used in high-income countries include capitation, payments per case or diagnosis, and fee-for-service. To minimize incentives for under- or overutilization, prices that purchasers pay for health services should be related to the unit costs of the relevant activities. However, establishing the true unit cost of health services is complicated by a number of factors, such as the need to attribute indirect costs and depreciation (for which data are often not readily available). Furthermore, the organizational characteristics of health care providers and their relationships with purchasers strongly influence the choice among payment mechanisms and the way prices for health services are determined. Pertinent characteristics include provider autonomy, provider negotiating power, and the degree of competition.

Waters and Hussey conclude that there are several mechanisms for setting prices and improving the performance of health care systems through provider payment reforms. Options include selective and differential pricing to protect the poor and meeting other policy objectives. Often one of the main constraints is data limitations on costs, volumes, and patient behavior characteristics.

PART II: MAKING STRATEGIC PURCHASING PRO-POOR

Part 2 of the volume includes three chapters that explore in greater depth the challenge of making strategic purchasing pro-poor. The recent *World Development Report 2004* on Making Services Work for Poor People highlighted that the poor often do not benefit from the public services that are supposed to address their needs. It proposed two ways to address this problem: empowering poor people to voice their concerns and monitor service providers, and strengthening the incentives for service providers to serve the poor. The chapters in part 2 build on these concepts.

In chapter 7, "The Equity Dimensions of Purchasing, " Paolo Carlo Belli examines in greater detail the impact of resource allocation and purchasing reforms on equity. . The review, which covers two decades, indicates that there are huge differentials in health expenditure per capita between richer and poorer countries, and that within individual countries, the utilization of health services is strongly pro-rich, despite the fact that the poor bear a disproportionate share of morbidity and mortality.

The author makes the following recommendations in terms of the policy options for strategic resource allocation and selective purchasing of pro-poor health services: design pro-poor geographic resource allocation formulas; favor spending on health services that respond to the health care needs of the poor and on services used most frequently by the poor; improve value for money by ensuring that pro-poor health services are efficient and of high quality; and introduce complementary pro-poor financing reforms in revenue collection and risk pooling.

At the same time, it is becoming clear that RAP reforms are but a small piece in a large puzzle—there is more to improving access and quality of services than allocating resources sensibly. Often other fundamental pieces of the puzzle— such as the role of clients' associations and representative groups, or the quality of medical training—have been neglected, putting excessive weight on single RAP components such as payment system reform. This imbalance has at times doomed reforms.

Belli concludes that RAP reforms are likely to generate trade-offs. By achieving certain aims such as efficiency gains, some purchasing reforms may at the same time move the health system farther away from achieving other objectives such as equity and quality. Policy makers who are able to anticipate these trade-offs can introduce mitigating measures that reinforce the positive and offset the negative impact of such purchasing reforms.

In chapter 8, "Reversing the Law of Inverse Care," Finn Diderichsen observes that although poor people shoulder the greatest burden of disease, they receive a smaller share of health care resources than do healthy and better-off people. In other words, health care resources are distributed inversely in relation to need. The author observes that this relationship holds true from country to country and within countries across socioeconomic groups.

If, following principles of *horizontal* equity (that is, equal treatment for equals), policy makers want to allocate health care resources according to need, a large part of health care budgets will have to be shifted from the richer to the poorer quintiles. If, in addition, policy makers want to reduce inequalities in health status between rich and poor, they have to look closely at the *vertical* aspects of equity (that is, providing preferential treatment for deprived groups) by allocating health care resources so that the poor achieve more rapid improvements in their health status than do richer groups. This distinction between horizontal and vertical aspects of health equity is thus closely linked to two different issues in health policy: how to reduce inequities in access to health care and inequities in health status.

Diderichsen reminds the reader that the equitable and efficient allocation of funds to public services among potentially competing institutions or populations should be a basic function of government at every level. Yet, resources are often allocated according to past trends rather than an objective reassessment of the underlying needs that the resources are trying to address. Strategic RAP offers an opportunity to depart from such historical budgets that perpetuate inequity and mal-distribution of scarce resources.

In chapter 9, "Risk Pooling and Purchasing," Peter C. Smith and Sophie N. Witter review the role of revenue pooling and risk sharing in resource allocation and purchasing. While an individual's expenditure on most basic necessities is largely predictable, that same individual's expenditure on health care is intrinsically uncertain and largely unknowable, both in magnitude and timing. The underlying mechanisms used to pool revenues and share risks across population groups are therefore critical to achieving equity and poverty objectives, even when RAP arrangements are pro-poor.

The authors observe that under collective financing of health care, there is no reason that an individual's own financial contribution to the revenue pool should be related to health risks, health care utilization, and spending patterns. Rather, it is policy makers who determine the extent to which an individual's financial contribution depends on his or her financial means, his or her utilization of health services, and other factors. By "uncoupling" revenues and expenditures in this way, policy makers wield a powerful instrument to achieve both redistributional and health equity goals.

Smith and Witter emphasize that to achieve equity and poverty objectives, RAP mechanisms must be closely coordinated with the insurance function of health care financing. For example, payment mechanisms that allocate prospective budgets to health care provider units that are too small, fragment what might otherwise be a large risk pool, thereby destroying the financial protection that should have been conferred by health insurance. Likewise, copayments collected by health care providers can undo the benefits of premium subsidies for the poor. Prospective budgets allocated to small contracted units are particularly vulnerable to this effect if hard budget cuts are strictly enforced. The general practice fund holder arrangement in the United Kingdom in the 1990s provided a good example of this problem.

PART III: PURCHASING HEALTH SERVICES

Parts 3 and 4 review resource allocation and purchasing mechanisms used to pay, respectively, for health services (public health, ambulatory care, and hospitals) and major inputs (labor, pharmaceuticals, capital, and knowledge, that is, research). During recent years there has been a shift in focus from purchasing inputs to purchasing outputs and even outcomes. The more outcome-based the RAP arrangement, the more likely that it will succeed in achieving underlying efficiency and equity objectives.

One dilemma faced by policy makers is the tension that exists between the scope or size of the entity purchased and the integrity of the underlying insurance function. As seen in previous chapters, when the unit purchased is small (such as in the case of labor, small clinics, or individual hospitals), the payment incentives tend to have a more direct impact on the behavior of the service provider. At the same time—especially when prospective payment mechanisms are used—the insurance function (revenue pool) is fractured, leaving both patients and providers exposed to the risk of expenditure variance. Expenditure ceilings combined with reinsurance can be used to mitigate this negative effect.

On the other hand, when the entity purchased is large (networks of hospitals, ambulatory care providers, or regional/provincial/state health services), the insurance function is usually more likely to be preserved but the payment incentive is much more blunt and indirect. Using geographic allocations to decentralized purchasers can mitigate this negative effect.

In chapter 10, "Paying for Public Health Services: Financing and Utilization," Xingzhu Liu and Sheila O'Dougherty review the role of resource allocation and purchasing in public health. Population-based health promotion and prevention activities often have a large impact on overall health outcomes and large externalities (communicable diseases and secondary inhalation of smoke). Since the benefits of such services occur months or sometimes years after they are delivered, there is often little consumer demand for them. Typically such services are underutilized and underfinanced compared with curative services that are used to treat acute illness.

There is widespread agreement in both theory and practice that some types of public health services that are public goods with large externalities must be publicly financed and coupled with aggressive outreach and communication strategies if they are to be delivered effectively. Otherwise they do not reach their target audience. These include universal public health services such as policy development and enforcement, public health information systems, treatment of polluted water, prevention of air pollution, health education programs through the media, and vector elimination programs for the prevention of infectious diseases. These services are both publicly financed and provided through publicly owned provision systems, although some are contracted out to the private sector.

Liu and O'Dougherty review various options for paying public health providers. The payment system should send a message to the providers to deliver the right kind and volume of public health services and to promote socially desirable outcomes (such as stopping secondhand smoke and spread of communicable diseases). Whereas fee-for-service payments are often considered undesirable in the case of payment for clinical services owing to the overservicing by providers (that is, supplier-induced demand), such payment mechanisms may actually be preferable in the case of public health services where consumer demand is negligible without an active encouragement from providers. The authors conclude that whatever payment methods are used, providers of public health services should be fairly paid. Payment should reflect providers' performance and be on par with the income of other health professionals.

In chapter 11, "Buying Results: Contracting for Primary Health Care Delivery," Benjamin Loevinsohn and April Harding review the evidence on the purchasing of basic health services from nongovernmental and private providers. To achieve the health-related Millennium Development Goals (MDGs), there is a need to increase access by the poor to efficient and high-quality basic health services. Nearly 6 out of 10 child deaths in developing countries could be prevented through better access to a few effective and low-cost interventions. Even when there is a shortage of resources in the publicly owned health care system, providers that offer such services already exist in the nongovernmental and private sector. In most countries the public sector could purchase significant additional basic health care services from the nongovernmental and private sector.

Despite these facts, debate on this topic is heated. Purchasing health services from nongovernmental providers is often stigmatized as a form of privatization and is interpreted as a sign of government abdication of responsibilities in the health sector. Another view is that purchaser-provider splits such as contracting are neoliberal and technocratic reforms, driven by market-oriented "new public sector management" models that focus excessively on efficiency gains at the expense of equity.

Loevinsohn and Harding challenge this view, maintaining that emerging evidence shows that purchasing health services from nongovernmental and private providers can be done in such a manner that it is not only efficient but also pro-poor and of relatively high quality. Purchasers involved in contracting health services in this way are usually motivated by practical concerns, not ideology. Most of these types of reform arise either from an absence of government services or from frustration with the poor quality and coverage of government services, especially for poor people. Advocates of contracting usually express a desire for increased government financing so that services in the community can be expanded and improved. They want to see governments engage with private providers, which already deliver the bulk of curative services in developing countries, to improve quality of care, access, and coordination for the poor and others who need such services.

In chapter 12, "Purchasing Hospital Services: Key Questions for Policymakers," Eric de Roodenbeke reviews the role of RAP in the hospital sector. The hospital sector is often the most expensive part of the health system, and public hospitals are a place of last recourse for patients with serious illness and the poor who may not be able to afford access elsewhere. Hospitals also often participate in providing some population-based essential public health services and training for doctors, nurses, and allied health care workers.

As in the case of ambulatory care services, hospital care can either be produced in-house by government-owned providers or purchased from nongovernmental and private providers. During recent years many countries have tried to transfer responsibility and decision rights over hospital care to local governments, semiautonomous or corporatized hospital boards, and even private providers. As in the primary care sector these reforms are often highly politicized. Such arrangements are not only workable but can also confer a number of advantages in terms of stronger governance and increased responsiveness by the hospital to its constituent clients. This is particularly true when the changes in ownership are coupled with payment incentives under which money follows the patients, who have a choice in where they seek care. This gives patients a strong voice and forces the hospitals to be more sensitive to their needs and demands. It is not a question of whether or not the public sector can purchase hospital care or outsource certain in-patient services to nongovernmental or private providers. Many countries (developed and developing) are already doing that competently. Rather, the real question is how to change the system when policy makers feel that such change is desirable.

De Roodenbeke reviews various payment mechanisms for reimbursing hospital care, each of which has its own unique advantages and disadvantages. Some are better at responding to productivity objectives (fee-for-service, diagnostic-related groups, and other output-based mechanisms). Others are better at controlling costs (global budgets and capitated payments). Increasingly countries are experimenting with both as a way to achieve several objectives—productivity, efficiency, equity, poverty protection, and quality. Whatever the mechanism chosen, there will always be some advantage and some disadvantage. Once policy makers understand that there is no perfect system, they are more likely to have realistic expectations and be able to anticipate and deal with some of the negative aspects.

PART IV: PURCHASING INPUTS

In chapter 13, "Paying for Health Care Labor," Pascal Zurn and Orvill Adams provide a brief introduction to role of resource allocation and purchasing in human resources in health. Labor holds a unique position in the health sector in that it is a critical input to the production process of clinics, hospitals, ministries of health, and health insurance funds. And at the same time it is a unit of production itself, such as in the case of the solo practitioner or pharmacist in his or her small pharmacy, and often a part of management. Labor may be purchased directly by a health insurance fund or it may be financed indirectly when hired by health care organizations that are contracted by the insurer. The boundaries among inputs, production processes, outputs, and management therefore often become blurred in the case of labor.

Labor costs are one of the main cost drivers in the health sector. Small changes in the size or income levels of the workforce can have a pronounced impact on the overall cost of the health system itself. Yet management control over labor costs is often not fully integrated into the service unit that is responsible for the budget. Often health care workers remain civil servants and are paid out of centrally controlled funds long after other financing reforms have delegated such responsibilities to local service providers such as hospitals or clinics. This significantly reduces the decision rights of and control by local service providers' labor. A main advantage of purchasing health services from non-governmental and private providers is that it allows circumventing the labor constraint in the public sector. Furthermore, in many countries, a large share of the health labor force works outside the publicly run national health services. Taking advantage of the valuable human resources that are available in the non-governmental and private sector is particularly critical in countries where there are serious productivity problems and staff shortages in the public sector.

Zurn and Adams remind the reader that the performance of health care services often depends directly on the availability of appropriately skilled staff and their underlying motivation to work. Therefore payment mechanisms can have a powerful impact on the health labor market. Typically, output-based payment mechanisms increase productivity, while salaries and global prospective payment mechanisms restrain productivity and may fracture the risk pool, thereby passing the financial risk of illness back to the patient and the doctor. Unpopular policies can lead to serious labor unrest and disruption in the provision of services to patients. Yet reforming payment incentives and other aspects of the health labor force—such as civil service reform, resource allocation, and purchasing of labor, and employment practices—are highly sensitive politically and may have large fiscal implications.

In chapter 14, "Purchasing Pharmaceuticals," Ulrika Enemark, Anita Alban, Enrique C. Seoane-Vazquez, and Andreas Seiter observe that drug expenditures account for a large share of total healthcare costs in developing countries. Most drugs are being paid for directly by patients out of pocket, which is often a significant financial burden for the poor. Another major source of financing for drugs is government budgets. Unfortunately, severe funding constraints in the public sector often translate into shortages in the supply of drugs, once again affecting the poor because they rely heavily on such providers for their treatment.

The authors highlight that policy options for making resource allocation and purchasing of drugs more pro-poor include subsidized exemption schemes, patient cards or vouchers, and subsidized health insurance. To secure the financial sustainability of subsidized drug plans, it is critical that such programs be accompanied by adherence to guidelines on the rational use of drugs. This can be done by limiting choice through essential drug lists and standard treatment guidelines, creating incentives for rational prescribing, and educating professionals and consumers.

As in the case of labor, pharmaceuticals may be purchased directly by a health insurance fund (that is, in the form of a pharmaceutical benefit scheme) or financed indirectly as part of the overall health benefit plan (that is, included in the plan). Whereas there are considerable advantages in bulk purchasing of pharmaceuticals in terms of price negotiations and quality assurance, payment systems are usually more efficient when they are decentralized and controlled by smaller units. Some countries have found ways to allow health insurers to control some aspects of purchasing pharmaceuticals—through outsourcing/contracting and regional partnerships, for example—while ensuring that prices are kept low through bulk purchasing of more essential medications.

Enemark et al. conclude that the optimal RAP arrangements for drugs in developing countries are those that take into account these demand- and supply-side factors. The best purchasing strategies are those that develop a balance between custom demand (represented, for example, by the community or a member-owned insurance scheme) and provider interests. Since such systems tend to be dynamic—which means users and providers may develop ways to exploit the system—the system should have a built-in mechanism for incremental adjustment over time.

In chapter 15, "Paying for Capital," Jon Sussex and Sandra Sosa-Rubi summarize the principles of effective, efficient, and equitable capital financing and capital charging in health care systems. Although capital charging is still not used extensively internationally, a few low- and middle-income countries have started to use the approach—and have had some success. No country has reversed the policy. The authors propose a set of policy options for putting principles known in western countries into practice in low- and middle-income countries.

When capital assets are subsidized by governments or donated by aid organizations, health care providers have an incentive to overdemand capital investments initially and undermaintain them subsequently. There is also no penalty for underusing assets once procured. Wrongly located or inappropriate facilities, only partially used and poorly maintained, are the result. Such facilities provide a poor standard of care, divert resources away from where they could be used more effectively, and damage staff morale, thus weakening services further. Most health care systems, therefore, have room for improving efficiency in the use of physical capital— particularly buildings and equipment. Efficiency incentives are often weaker in the processes by which capital is allocated and paid for than in those for use of labor, medicines, and other inputs.

Sussex and Sosa-Rubi conclude that finance for investment in the physical capital of health care provision may be available from government, international organizations, and the private sector. Whatever the source of finance, the application of capital charging for publicly owned health care providers is a practical and worthwhile measure that has potential benefits. These benefits include making managers aware of the costs of capital, improving the efficiency with which capital is used and ensuring an appropriate mix of capital and labor, enabling comparison of costs between providers, and establishing a basis for fair competition between public and private sector providers.

A range of options exist for the precise form that capital charging may take. The balance of pros and cons among these options suggests the following approach in most cases: apply to existing as well as new assets; use real, not just notional, capital charges but allow a transitional period; use a constant annuity rather than a declining time profile of charges over an asset's life; and value assets on a depreciated replacement cost basis.

In chapter 16, "Paying for Knowledge and Research," Dean T. Jamison discusses issues related to the acquisition of knowledge as an important part of RAP in the health sector. Most of the issues discussed in chapter 1 concerning the agency role and organizational, institutional, and management aspects of RAP are relevant to research and development.

Jamison reminds the reader that the 20th century has witnessed a global transformation in human health. Chile's experience illustrates the magnitude of this transformation. By the mid-1990s Chile's per capita income had reached about US$4,000 (adjusted for purchasing power), and Chilean women had achieved a life expectancy of 79 years. A century ago, in 1900, today's high-income countries also had income levels around $4,000—and, therefore, had resources sufficient to provide their populations with adequate food, water, shelter, and sanitation. Yet, for them, female life expectancy at the time was perhaps 30 years less than it is in Chile today.

Why has health improved so dramatically after controlling for income, and hence availability of commodities, such as food, that are essential for health? While there can be no unambiguous answer to this question, Jamison concludes that advances in scientific knowledge and its application have contributed both to creating powerful interventions and in guiding behavior. Acquisition and utilization of health research and development or its products becomes, then, an essential part of an effective spending on health services that benefit the poor.

In chapter 17, "Using Resource Profiles," Anders Anell presents data and resource profiles from selected low- and middle-income African and Latin American countries in an effort to illustrate the importance of a multidimensional approach to the measurement and monitoring of health care resources.

Health care delivery entails combining many resource inputs to provide a mix of services that will satisfy overall objectives and priorities. This sounds simple, but it is not—for a number of reasons. First, providers have to respond to an extraordinary array of immediate health problems. Second, health care relies heavily on human resources, and the quality of care ultimately depends on individuals' skills, training, and motivation. Therefore investments in facilities and equipment have to be balanced against investments in human capital—education and training. Third, the financial resources that pay for health care are often collected and pooled by a third party not directly involved in providing care. This third party could be a ministry or central board of health, a provincial government, a not-for-profit sickness fund, or a commercial insurance company. While approaches vary considerably, they all depend on the third party to act as a "good agent" on behalf of individuals in buying services from various providers. Fourth, good health has become close to a right in modern society, raising the question, with ever expanding possibilities to treat and prevent bad health, "How should priorities be set and implemented?"

Anell concludes by reminding the reader that health care delivery in low-income countries is confronted by a nearly bottomless pit of health problems and extreme shortages of physicians, trained nurses, medicines, and equipment. The importance of balancing and promoting efficient use of available resources is clear. So too are the negative consequences—in terms of life years lost—if this objective is not met. In practice, however, problems of inefficiency seem to be more pronounced in low-income countries. Working morale is often low because of inadequate pay and poor working conditions. Facilities and equipment are often not fully operational since capital investments and recurrent costs are poorly balanced. Institutions that promote accountability for overall objectives and transparency of actual resource allocations are usually weak. It is in this context that more strategic resource allocation and purchasing mechanisms could make a significant contribution. Continuing business as usual along historical spending patterns is not likely to meet the health care delivery challenge in most countries.

PART V: SUPPLY, DEMAND, AND MARKETS

The chapters in part 5 present two sides of an active and unresolved debate—how many purchasers lead to the best performance in resource allocation and purchasing. Most countries today have health insurance systems that protect their populations against the financial risks of illness and to help them obtain appropriate medical and preventive care. All health insurance systems have mechanisms for collecting and pooling revenues, spreading risk, and purchasing health services. The way the health insurance system is organized can have a profound impact on the equity, efficiency, and organization of the health care delivery system.

Purchasing arrangements can be broadly classified into two groups. In single-payer systems, one organization—typically the government—collects and pools revenues and purchases health services for the entire population. All citizens are included within a single risk pool. Single-payer systems have monopsony power in purchasing health services. In multiple-payer systems, by contrast, several different organizations perform all four functions for specific segments of the population. Those insured by multipayer systems potentially have different health risks, and members can choose their own purchaser. Multiple-payer systems have to compete for demand from patients and providers for market share in purchasing health services. Under such systems, competitive forces are, therefore, in play both among purchasers and providers. In the past, a belief—which can be traced to insurance market failure—that competition in health financing is bad led many developing countries to favor single-payer systems. The underlying premise was that in a single-payer system a monopsony purchaser, owing to its power, could provide all the market advantages available while avoiding all the known problems of insurance market failure.

But single-payer systems have not performed as well as expected. First, it has become clear that these systems are vulnerable to the same abuse of power and inefficiencies as monopolies: bureaucratic capture, rent-seeking behavior, unresponsiveness to consumers, and a breakdown in information flows and transparency. Second, analysts have observed that there are limits to the benefits of competition among providers unless there are also some competitive pressures on purchasers. Third, many low- and middle-income countries already have multipayer systems in the form of a Ministry of Health, social health insurance, voluntary health insurance (community and private health insurance), special free-standing vertical programs financed by the international donor community, and direct purchasing of health care by households. In many low-income countries, the latter comprises as much as 80 percent of total health care expenditure. In these countries, policy makers are not asking, "Should we introduce a multipayer system?" They are asking, "Why should we introduce a single-payer system?" These issues are explored in greater detail in chapters 18–20.

In chapter 18, "Single-Payer Health Insurance Systems: What Are the Advantages?" Gerard F. Anderson and Peter Sotir Hussey briefly compare single-payer and multiple-payer systems before concentrating on the organization and operation of single-payer systems.

The authors show how single-payer systems can be classified into four generic models: regional-private, regional-public, central-private, and central-public. These models differ in the extent of centralization of financing and administration (regional or central) and in the ownership of health care providers (mainly public or mainly private). The locus of financing and administration affects the way revenues are generated, benefits are determined, and the system is regulated. The ownership of health care providers affects the purchasing relationship between insurers and providers. The authors first examine several dimensions of each of the four models: revenue collection, risk pooling, purchasing, and social solidarity. They then compare these same dimensions under single-payer and multi-payer models.

Anderson and Hussey conclude that there is no universal paradigm for the design of health care purchasers. Countries vary greatly in their priorities, populations, development, and systems of government. Each of the two major types of health insurance system—single-payer and multiple-payer—has strengths and weaknesses. Countries deciding on the reform or development of health care purchasing should evaluate these strengths and weaknesses against their own priorities and needs, political and economic constraints, and administrative capabilities.

In chapter 19, "Multiple Payers in Health Care: A Framework for Assessment," Peter Zweifel examines the flip side of this debate by focusing on the strengths and weaknesses of multipurchasers. Both consumers of health care and governments suspect they are not getting their money's worth. Governments point to a high and often rising share of health care expenditure in the GDP. However, it is not clear that simply reducing this share would be in the interest of consumers and voters, who in their daily lives seek to obtain "value for their money" at least as much if not more than a reduction in their spending.

One way to improve the ratio of benefits to cost in the health sector is to choose payment systems that give providers of health services incentives to behave efficiently and meet other policy objectives such as equity. In principle, this could be achieved through either a single- or a multiple-payer system. Economic theory, however, indicates that the optimal choice of a payment system depends heavily on the amount of information available to the prospective patient. Three scenarios are considered: full information, asymmetric information with regard to provider effort only, and asymmetric information with regard to both effort and type of provider. In each case, the optimal payment function is stated and discussed. The author concludes that patients, without complementary agents to help in the purchasing process, are unlikely to find the optimal health care provider because they do not know some of the crucial parameters.

Zweifel concludes that the choice of a complementary agent and the concomitant payment system should be made in view of objectives and priorities that policy makers have set for the health care system. Governments acting as complementary agents have a comparative advantage in managing challenges that originate domestically, such as aging and the increasing number of one-person households. But they are also more likely to abuse their power as monopsony purchasers seeking to reduce health care expenditure beyond the preference of the society they represent. By contrast, competitive health insurers as complementary agents are better at adjusting to challenges posed by globalization and changing medical technology. Thus, multiple-payer systems hold the promise of keeping the incentives of service providers aligned with the changing world around them, something that governments as single payers often neglect. This is particularly true in low- and middle-income countries.

In chapter 20, "Influencing the Demand Side of Purchasing," Tim Ensor and Stephanie Cooper look at the role of demand-side barriers in impeding access to the use of health services. Demand-side barriers are defined as determinants of use of health care that are not dependent on service delivery or price, or on the direct price of those services. They include distance, education, opportunity cost, and cultural and social barriers. There is some evidence that these barriers are at least as important in determining access to services as the quality, volume, and price of services delivered by health care providers.

The authors recall that although much of public health spending is supposed to target and help the poor and vulnerable, according to a growing body of evidence it often benefits the better-off instead. Statistics point to persistent differences in access to health services and health care between rich and poor groups, and substantial barriers to access for the poorest. An example is provided of an average British citizen who falls ill and goes to a general practitioner or a nearby hospital emergency department where referral is a normal part of treatment. An average citizen in Bangladesh who ends up in a similar situation has a myriad of confusing choices to make. A rural resident may have to decide whether to go to a local subdistrict or union health center, a facility run by a nongovernmental organization, a minimally trained village doctor, or a local drugstore (where the owners, qualified pharmacists or not, offer advice). Reaching the nearest district hospital can mean hiring a rickshaw and then paying for a bus ticket. Tight household finances can force choices about which household members receive treatment. Thousands of sick people every day have to navigate through these complex decisions in low-income countries, where the supply of supply of services is only one of the many factors in decisions taken by patients.

Ensor and Cooper conclude that despite the importance of demand-side barriers, those who make resource allocation and purchasing decisions direct policies mainly toward improving the supply-side constraints. Most government planning models are supply driven, with staff size and capacity of facilities being key determinants of funding flows. The authors recommend that to address known demand-side constraints, policy makers involved in resource allocation and purchasers shift more attention to population determinants of health care needs, poverty dimensions, and demand-side policy objectives. Few of the studies reported have an explicit poverty focus, although many of the interventions are conducted in poor areas. There is a clear need for further work to examine the most cost-effective ways of reducing barriers to accessing services and in particular to investigate what methods are most effective in expanding access to essential care among the poor.

PART VI: LEGAL AND REGULATORY ISSUES

Part 6 examines some of the institutional dimensions of resource allocation and purchasing of priority health services for the poor. Unlike the significant attention that has been paid to regulation of health insurance and quality of care, regulation of resource allocation and purchasing is at a much earlier and more primitive stage of development.

Health systems that have social or private health insurance underpinnings also have a variety of laws governing revenue collection and risk pooling, which may overlap or complement those related to resource allocation and purchasing behavior. These rules are particularly important when the statutory structure of collective financing of health care does not explicitly incorporate all of the population into a single-risk pool or scheme. For example, recent reforms in the regulation of South African health insurance schemes explicitly address abuses that can arise when only a portion of the population is included under formal insurance schemes and government-provided health services.

Furthermore, many laws governing the provision of health services—notably provider licensing and liability for professional negligence—influence but were not designed to address issues in resource allocation and purchasing; nor do they address the role of purchasers acting as an "agent" on behalf of patients. Some aspects of these laws may enhance service delivery but unwittingly act as constraints on strategic purchasing.

In chapter 21, "Law and Regulation," Frank G. Feeley examines the effect that existing and proposed laws and regulations can have on the feasibility and effectiveness of arrangements for RAP in developing and transitional economies.

The authors review categories of law and regulation, including provider licensing, monopoly and competition legislation, liability for professional negligence, mandated benefits and permitted exclusions, antidiscrimination laws, appeals procedures and other methods of asserting patient entitlement, rate setting and prohibitions on unauthorized provider charges, capacity controls and purchaser discretion in selecting providers, and patient confidentiality and collection of payment-related data. Specific reference is made to recent experience in the Russian Federation, South Africa, Chile, and the Philippines, as well as possible precedents from more developed countries.

Feeley concludes that moving from passive budgeting and resource allocation to strategic purchasing of priority health services will require policy makers to revisit the underlying regulatory framework for buying health services for the poor and other high-priority target population groups. In many instances, new laws may be needed to ensure that the poor benefit, that the benefit package includes priority services, and that services are purchased from the public and private providers most likely to offer the best services at affordable prices and using payment incentives that respond to the desired policy objectives.

In "Quality-Based Purchasing in the United States: Applications in Developing Countries?" the 22nd and final chapter of the book, Peggy McNamara observes that policy makers increasingly recognize the potential power of the purchasing function—whether led by national and regional governments, social insurance funds, community-based insurance organizations, employers, health plans, or consumers—to achieve not only efficiency and equity but also quality goals.

Evidence provided by the author suggests that, when presented with credible information about their performance relative to their peers, providers *do* make improvements in the quality of services they offer—particularly when this information is made available to the public at large. Perhaps previously—in the absence of comparative data to the contrary—providers presumed that their performance was state of the art. Or perhaps they instituted quality improvement initiatives out of fear of losing patients. Regardless, purchasers that collect and disseminate comparative performance data on hospitals and physicians seem to contribute to quality improvement.

McNamara concludes the chapter by emphasizing that no matter what it is called—quality-based purchasing, value-based purchasing, performance-based purchasing, responsible purchasing, or strategic contracting—the concept of leveraging payer clout to promote high-quality care and improve health outcomes has a compelling logic and broad appeal. When combined with a pro-poor focus, such approaches ensure that health services not only allocate resources to the poor but also address their health problems effectively.

PART I

The Conceptual Framework

CHAPTER 1

Managing Scarcity through Strategic Purchasing of Health Care

Alexander S. Preker

Throughout the 20th century great progress was made in securing better access and financial protection against the cost of illness through collective financing of health care. Although governments and households spend substantial resources on health care, they fail to secure access to quality health services or respond, through publicly funded programs, to the needs of many ordinary people who are sick. They fail to prevent known diseases or promote good health. And they fail to prevent people from falling into poverty when seeking health care. Yet these are the very problems that collective financing arrangements were supposed to address. What went wrong?

Promoting health and confronting disease challenges requires action across a range of activities in the health system. This includes improvements in the policymaking and stewardship role of governments; better access to human resources, drugs, medical equipment, and consumables; and a greater engagement of both public and private providers of services. But ultimately it is resource allocation and purchasing (RAP) mechanisms that are instrumental in setting new directions and introducing the needed incentives for a change to occur. Managing scarcity and making RAP arrangements work better for poor and ordinary people is an important part of this story.

This book reviews ways to make public spending on health care more efficient and equitable in developing countries, with a special focus on strategic purchasing and contracting of services from nongovernmental providers. The use of purchasing as a tool to enhance public sector performance is well documented in the literature on institutional economics and industrial organizations. The extension to the health sector has recently been the focus of increased attention among policymakers. Lessons learned from this experience are now being successfully applied to developing countries). The first section examines the evolution of collective financing arrangements, provides arguments for strategic purchasing rather than passive resource allocation, and proposes a framework for analyzing existing RAP arrangements.

THE EVOLUTION OF HEALTH SYSTEMS AND COLLECTIVE FINANCING OF HEALTH CARE

Why do individuals need help in purchasing health services from providers? Is the "middle man" really necessary? Can individuals not just buy health services in the same way they would go to the local market to buy bread, milk, or fruit?

Throughout most of history, that is what most people did. When sick, they contacted local healers directly. Public policy was limited largely to protecting the sick against charlatans and enforced through ethical codes such as the Hippocratic oath. There was no expensive technology, and most serious conditions led to death. Loss of employment and burial costs were the most expensive parts of illness.

With industrialization and the scientific revolution, all of this changed. As understanding about the causes, prevention, and treatment of illness expanded, interventions become more complex and expensive. Health care was no longer the exclusive domain of traditional healers. Other actors became involved. This included policymakers, specialized institutions involved in regulation and financing, complex organizations specialized in delivery of services (for example, hospitals, clinics, diagnostics), and a range of specialized providers (for example, doctors, nurses, pharmacists, dentists, allied health workers). Through this process, the health system slowly became differentiated beyond the simple patient-healer relationship (figure 1.1).

Though often merged in a single organization or agency under a government department, health care financing can be broken down into several activities, each with its own set of objectives, priorities, and constraints. This includes activities related to the collection of revenues, the pooling of funds, and their subsequent use within the service delivery system. There are important interactions among these specialized subactivities. This book deals mainly with the transfer of funds from RAP arrangements to providers. Other than the short overview provided in the next section, this book does not deal with issues related to the collection of revenues, spreading of risk through the pooling subactivities, or internal use of funds by providers.

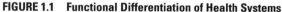

FIGURE 1.1   Functional Differentiation of Health Systems

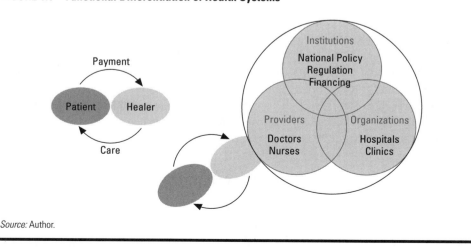

Source: Author.

Differentiation of Financing Subactivities

The revenue collection side of the health care financing story is now well understood, having received much attention in both industrial and developing countries in recent years. Money for collective financing of health care may come from a variety of public and private sources (taxes, public charges, mandates, grants, loans, charity, private insurance). In addition, providers often collect some revenues themselves directly in the form of out-of-pocket payments at the time of treatment. The implications of the efficiency-equity tradeoff associated with such direct payments for the poor in low-income countries are now better understood.

The revenue pooling and risk sharing side of health care financing is also well understood in both industrial and developing countries. Some people are much sicker than others. Sharing risks across population groups is a fundamental aspect of financial protection in the health sector. Furthermore, people use health care most during childhood, the childbearing years, and old age—when they are the least productive economically. Income smoothing across the life cycle can, therefore, also contribute to financial protection in the health sector. Finally, the rich are better able to contribute than the poor, yet the poor shoulder a larger share of the disease burden. Pooling allows the financial burden of illness to be shared between the rich and poor, between the healthy and sick, and between the gainfully employed and economically inactive years of the life cycle. Such pooling also provides insurance against the expenditure variance related to uncertainty in the severity and cost of illness, a mechanism that is equally needed at low income levels.

Revenues that are collected and pooled in this manner are then transferred to a variety of different agencies involved in the resource allocation process or purchasing of health services from providers. Four organizational modalities predominate: (a) a government department in the Ministry of Health, Ministry of Finance, or Ministry of Social Security, for example; (b) a social health insurance agency; (c) private health insurance funds; and (d) individual medical savings accounts. In the case of private health insurance and medical savings accounts, there is a direct link between the individuals who contributed to the program and the entitlement to benefits. In the case of the resources available to social health insurance agencies, usually entitlement is loosely established, based on contribution status of the covered population. In the case of resources available to government departments, there is usually no link at all. Coverage is usually conferred by category of population (the poor, civil servants, or the whole population in the case of universal entitlement).

The differentiation of collective financing into these subactivities offers several advantage over direct out-of-pocket spending in the health sector. Collecting money to pay for health care before the individual becomes ill provides a more predictable source of income to pay for health care and permits the application of a progressive contribution scale, where the size of the payment is proportional to the ability to pay. Pooling the money allows cross-subsidies from the gainfully employed to inactive participants, from the rich to poor, and across the lifecycle. The resulting funds can be channeled through specialized financing arrangements or agencies that have greater purchasing power, provide a more predictable income stream for providers, and allow better strategic decisions to be made about priorities and spending patterns than would be possible in the case of direct patient-healer financial transactions.

Over time, collective financing arrangements have replaced direct out-of-pocket payments for health care in most industrial countries. By the early 20th century, employment-based friendly societies and sickness funds began offering income support and access to doctors and hospitals at the time of illness. With the exception of Mexico, Turkey, and the United States, today all countries in the Organisation for Economic Co-operation and Development (OECD) offer their populations universal protection against the cost of illness. Many lower- and middle-income countries have tried to follow the same path, with varying success.

Some authors have tried to characterize health care systems on the basis of the type of financing arrangement and organization or ownership of providers. Four dominant patterns emerge: (a) the U.K.- or Beveridge-styled national health system (general revenue taxes with allocation to an integrated network of public providers through a government department); (b) the German- or Bismark-styled social insurance system (payroll taxes with allocation or purchasing of services from both public and private providers through autonomous health insurance funds); (c) U.S.- or free market-styled private health insurance system (insurance premiums with purchasing of services largely from private providers through health plans); and (d) 19th-century laissez-faire system (user fees with direct spot transaction between patients and providers).

In reality, however, all countries rely on several sources of financing and often have more than one RAP agency involved in resource allocation and purchasing. For example, private health insurance exists in the United Kingdom, and the United States has very large Medicare and Medicaid programs that are based on social insurance principles. All developing countries have some government or social insurance programs to finance health care. Furthermore, economic units (centralized or decentralized) of a national health service are just like social insurance funds. The discussion of RAP arrangements that follows is therefore equally relevant to all, not just to countries that have a past history of German- or Bismark-styled social insurance funds.

Unique Problems in Health Financing at Low Income Levels

The resources available to low- and middle-income countries are much less in both absolute and relative terms than at higher income levels.

At the global level, although 84 percent of the world's poor shoulder 93 percent of the global burden of disease, only 11 percent (US$280 billion) of total global spending on health care (US$2.5 trillion) reaches low- and middle-income countries. Recent work has shown that developing counties have an annual expenditure shortfall of between US$30 billion and US$60 billion in meeting the financing requirements of the Millennium Development Goals (MDGs). The slow anticipated economic growth over the next few years means that domestic growth alone is not likely to fill the expenditure gap in countries that need additional resources the most.

Furthermore, like pre-19th-century Europe, households in many developing countries still rely largely on direct out-of-pocket, spot market purchase of health services from public and private providers rather than collective financing mechanisms. There are several reasons for this trend in collective financing in developing countries.

First, low-income countries often have large rural and informal sector populations, limiting the taxation capacity of their governments. Despite these constraints, there are good examples from many low- and middle-income countries that more spending could be made available to collective RAP arrangements if fiscal objectives are respected and watched carefully.

A related set of problems is faced during the pooling of financial resources at low income levels. Pooling requires some transfer of resources from rich to poor, healthy to sick, and gainfully employed to inactive. Tax evasion by the rich and middle class is widespread in low-income countries, allowing higher income groups to avoid contributing their share to the overall revenue pool. Household expenditure often accounts for as much as 80 percent of total health expenditures owing to high user charges (official or unofficial) in both public and private facilities.

Finally, for a variety of reasons that will be described in greater detail in the following section, the rich often benefit more than the poor from public expenditure and subsidies on health care. And scarce public resources that are available to the poor are often squandered on ineffective care.

Government Failure in Delivering Efficient and Equitable Services for the Poor

Governments in many countries are unfortunately failing to address these problems in public spending on health care. In principle public financing should lead to an efficient and equitable spending on health care. In practice the incidence of spending on public services is often prorich, and outcomes for the poor are much worse (figures 1.2 and 1.3).

Until recently, financing of public services in most low- and middle-income countries was done through inflation-adjusted historical budgets and transfers of funds from one government department to another with little strategic thinking behind the allocation decisions. Often there were no internal markets or purchasing of services from nongovernmental providers. Everything was public, ranging from financing to service delivery to management. Although there are exceptions, the resulting services were fraught with a range of production failures of now well-documented and understood origins.

Similar problems have been observed in the health sector of countries such as Australia and Canada, and in Scandinavia, Eastern Europe, Costa Rica, Sri Lanka,

FIGURE 1.2   Incidence of Spending on Public Services

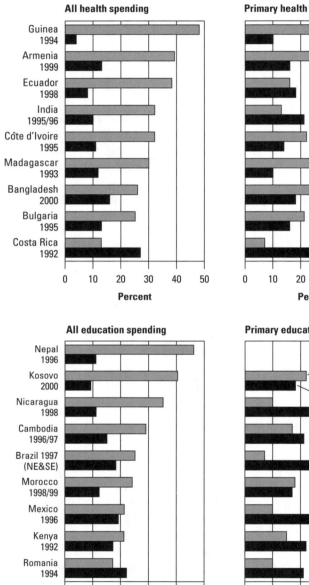
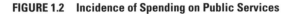

All health spending

Primary health

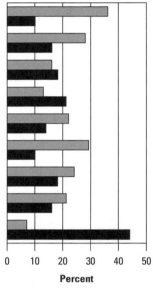
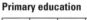

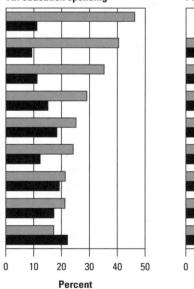

All education spending

Primary education

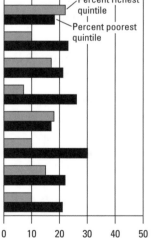
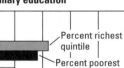

FIGURE 1.3   Outcomes Are Worse for Poor People

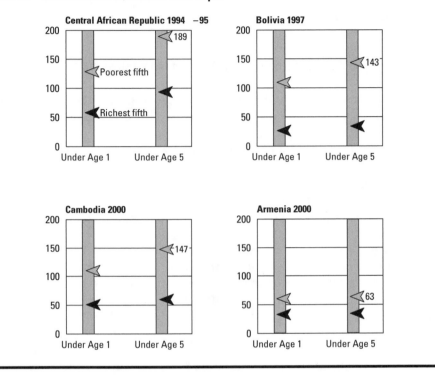

and Cuba, which were once regarded as having model health care systems. The resulting services are often beset by low productivity, inefficient use of scarce resources, poor consumer quality, lack of responsiveness to consumer expectations, public sector accountability problems, and lack of innovation. Figures 1.2 and 1.3 provide an illustration of the widespread problems of inequitable health outcomes and prorich spending patterns in many government-run health services today.

REFORM TRENDS IN PUBLIC SPENDING ON HEALTH CARE

It is in this context that there is a call for reform in public spending on health care through the world today. It is high on the political agenda of many western countries such Australia, Canada, France, Sweden, the United Kingdom, and the United States. And it is a central part of government reform agendas in low- and middle-income countries such as China, Colombia, Ghana, Hungary, Islamic Republic of Iran, India, Kenya, Lebanon, Malaysia, Nepal, Rond_nia (Brazil), and the Russian Federation.

A central theme of these reforms is the urgent need for change, a redefined role of governments as policymakers and oversight organizations, and more direct involvement by the private sector in producing and financing health services. They usually involve complementary financing reforms, including a separation of purchasing from direct provision of health services.

CONTINUED NEED FOR STRONG PUBLIC POLICY IN MANAGING SCARCE RESOURCES

If public production and spending on health care is so bad, why not let individuals buy health services in an open marketplace as they would buy most consumer goods?

Although approaches to reform vary, with some countries pursuing strategies that are more market oriented than others, even in countries with active private participation in the health sector good public policies are still needed for managing scarce public resources. No country has the luxury of making an unlimited public budget available to the health sector—not even rich countries. In low-income countries, where the disease burden is overwhelming, the need is even greater for strong public policies to set realistic priorities and ration scarce health care resources. As a result, cost containment and getting better value for money has become a major preoccupation for many developing as well as most Western countries.

In such settings, there are significant advantages to collective financing of health care over direct transactions between patients and providers. The advantages include a need to secure an equitable source of financing and steady income stream for providers; a need for some redistribution of resources from rich to poor, from healthy to sick, and from gainfully employed to economically inactive; and a need to set priorities and manage scarcity at the systems level. Markets do not perform well in meeting such distributive objectives when services are bought through direct transactions between patients and providers.

Redefining the Appropriate Role of the State and New Public Sector Management

During the 1980s and early 1990s, attempts were made to reform public services under the rubric of "New Public Sector Management." These reforms tried to emulate market conditions. This included better training of staff, improved management techniques, and market-based incentive structures. Many countries set up semiautonomous agencies that were subjected to private corporate law and antitrust regulations in the hope of exposing them to marketlike incentives.

Similar approaches were tried in the health sector, leading to heavy investments in training of clinical staff and managers. Human resources police introduced performance-based payment systems and the most advanced management practices from some of the world's leading business schools. The list of production techniques tried is extensive, including business-process reengineering, patient-focused care, and quality-improvement techniques. Reforms included activities such as establishing clinical directorates, introducing improved information systems to facilitate effective decisionmaking, and performance benchmarking.

Although the application of New Public Sector Management techniques in the public sector resulted in some early successes, old habits are hard to break, and services often deteriorated again after the heightened attention waned. During economic crisis and for political reasons, governments often weaken the high-powered economic incentives that should have been built into the reforms (risk of bankruptcy). Accountability arrangements remained weak (box 1.1).

BOX 1.1   IMPERFECT PUBLIC ACCOUNTABILITY ARRANGEMENTS

In an ideal setting (left-hand diagram in the figure), good public accountability is secured through a large overlap *(authorizing environment)* between fairly homogeneous social values, the existing political agenda, and vested bureaucratic interests. In democratic societies, patients can exert their influence on this process through voting, representation on hospital boards or other governing bodies, and consumer interest groups. The greater the resulting intersection, the more likely it will be that patients' interests will be reflected through national health policies, available health services, and the behavior of doctors, nurses, and other personnel.

Unfortunately, individual preferences are often not translated into public policies in this way. People's values are almost never homogeneous. The more diverse the society, the less chance there is for a large overlap among the political agenda that drives the institutional environment for purchasing (policymaking, regulations, financing), the bureaucratic interest of the managers who run health care organizations such as hospitals or clinics, and the social values of the health care providers who treat patients (right-hand diagram in the figure). The interest of individual patients is often left out.

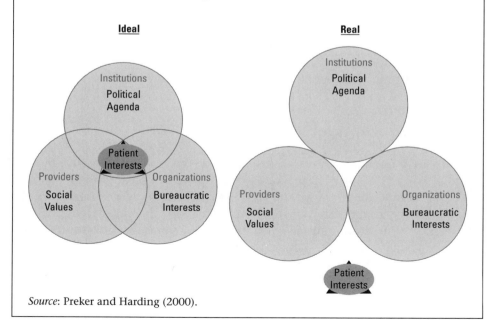

Source: Preker and Harding (2000).

Over time, this approach to reforming public service delivery became marred by spectacular failures in many developing counties. The experience in the health sector is similar.

Why has the public sector been so impervious to such reforms? There are several explanations, all with clear parallels in the market failure. Simply stated, when already overextended governments also try to do even more with too few resources and too little capability, they usually end up with a bloated and inefficient public sector that produces low-quality services that are unresponsive to the people that use them. In this context, management reforms alone are not enough.

Difficulties with public accountability and information asymmetry often lead to monopoly power of public providers due to (box 1.1): (a) legal restrictions on competition; (b) access to subsidized capital and revenues, creating an uneven playing field; (c) below-cost distribution of goods and services to achieve equity goals; or (d) production of public goods or goods where markets are not viable. Such public monopolies allow public providers to extract *rents* in the form of informal user charges and engage in other aspects of public sector corruption.

The resulting public monopoly suppliers have strong incentives to lower expenditures through decreased output when staff members benefit from the financial residuals. Time-keeping is often not enforced rigorously (doctors often work short hours in public institutions). And public assets are often used to pursue personal agendas (discretionary spending on special projects, research or private practice in public facilities).

Similar stories abound in the health sector. Services delivered by public providers remain notably unresponsive and unaccountable to users despite valiant efforts to improve them through better management techniques. Countless stories recount poor staff treatment of patients in government health facilities. Quality is often low—both clinical and consumer quality. Equipment is frequently broken or poorly functioning. Key problem areas include weak public accountability, information asymmetry, abuse of monopoly power in the public sector, failure to provide public goods, and most notably loss in strategic policy formulation.

Complementary Financing Reforms

Three types of financing reforms usually precede the move from passive budgeting to active purchasing of health care by the public : (a) separation of financing from provision (purchaser-provider splits); (b) separation of governance of the funding agency from the stewardship function of governments (decentralization and agency formation); and (c) reintroduction of some form of direct out-of-pocket copayments (user fees) to deal with moral hazard and policies to address adverse selection. Following these reforms, information disclosure, contracts, and regulations are used to secure service delivery objectives rather than hierarchical controls over staff (figure 1.4).

FIGURE 1.4   Recent Reforms

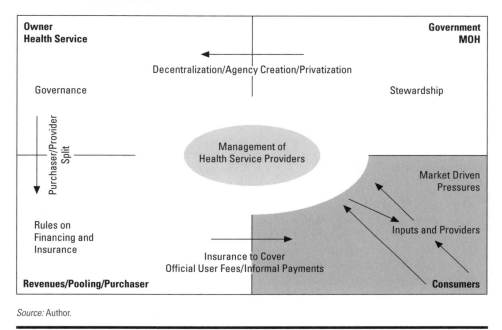

Source: Author.

THE PURCHASER-PROVIDER SPLIT

How can the spending of public money be made more effective and efficient ? Experience has shown that, by itself, collective financing of health care is not a guarantee that money will be spent wisely or benefit the individuals in greatest need. Without strategic policies and focused spending mechanisms, the poor and other ordinary people are likely to get left out.

The shift from hiring staff to produce services in house to purchasing services—moving from "a" to "b"—has been at the center of a lively debate on collective financing of health care during recent years and efforts to make health care systems more effective and efficient in performing their function. It is a central part of reforms that attempt to improve responsibility, accountability, and performance in health care through a separation in the responsibilities of purchasers and providers. (See box 1.2 for definitions of contracting, purchasing, and commissioning.)

Make or Buy Decisions

Are there different ways to spend money wisely on health care? How can you ensure that scarce resources benefit the very poor? What are the alternatives?

In settings of intractable public sector production failure, buying services from nongovernmental providers is often a real alternative to public production.

BOX 1.2   CONTRACTING, PURCHASING, AND COMMISSIONING OF HEALTH CARE: FLIP SIDES, SAME COIN?

"The time has come," the Walrus said, "to speak of many things,
Of buy, and sell, and contracts hard, and soft commissionings [sic].
To settle once and evermore the terms in wide profusion,
And bring to bear our insights proud, and add to the confusion."

Robert Taylor interpreting Lewis Carroll (2003)

"It is hard to see what the fuss is all about, and hard to understand why the land that gave us Alice in Wonderland should make so much ado about what these words are used to mean . . ."

Loraine Hawkins (2003)

Contracting, purchasing, and commissioning are relatively new terms that apply experiences from commercial settings to the payment of health services. All are part of health reforms that have tried to introduce market incentives. The terms are often used interchangeably and have strong emotional overtones. No precise definition can be found in a dictionary of economic terms. Yet in common usage, each of the three terms has a distinct meaning that has mutated over time. All emphasize a trend in paying for health services that moves from passive and input-based funding (line item or historical global budgets) to more active and output/outcome-based funding (facilities, population, or other specified level of coverage).

Contracting conveys the notion of "buying" health services rather than simply allocating a budget to pay for health care. There is a buyer and a seller. The sale may be a one-off "spot market" transaction or it may lead to the beginning of a longer-term relationship between the buyer and seller. Contracting almost always refers to services acquired from the private sector (for profit or not for profit). Strictly speaking—in most countries—internal contracts are not even legally binding or governed by contract law even if the term is used in this context. The term soon fell into disrepute among critics for being reductionist— focused too narrowly on the relationship between payers and providers, on "widget counting," on cost, and on volumes. "Where, in all of this, was the patient?" they would ask.

Purchasing tried to address these shortcomings by including elements of "strategic direction" and "intelligence" in the contractual arrangement. Buyers are supposed to ask critical questions about who benefits from the purchase (the poor, sick, children?), what services are acquired (primary care, hospitals, cost-effective interventions?), who can provide the services (public, private, nongovernmental organizations?), the mechanism used to pay for the services (global budgets, capitation, or fee for service?), and the price (market prices, reference prices, subsidies?). Purchasing can and often does refer to relationships with both public and private providers. Many social health insurance funds "purchase" services from networks of public providers run by ministries of health and local governments as well as the private sector. But "purchasing"

soon met much the same fate. It connoted an even more aggressive and con-
flictual relationship between the payer/provider.

Commissioning was a new, softer, fluffier, cuddlier term favored for a short
period by the British Left, only to be replaced recently by "planning and delivery." It connotes a multifaceted approach to relations between purchasers and
providers, intended to cover everything from health needs assessment and service planning through to monitoring and evaluation. At the time this lingo
was coined, there was increased attention on fostering a more open and
"mature" relationship between purchasers and providers. Competition is
muted and longer term, and less contestable relationships are favored.

Whichever term is preferred—purchasing, contracting, or commissioning—
all convey a sense of strategic direction in paying for health services. Historical
budget allocations, even when adjusted for health needs, income, future demographic trends, geographic location, and other factors, still convey the image
of a passive ATM that is unintelligent and nonstrategic.

Source: Author.

In addition to securing needed services that the public sector has difficulties in
producing, it also allows governments to focus their attention on critical areas of
known market failure such as: (a) public goods (policymaking and information);
(b) goods with large externalities (disease prevention); and (c) goods with
intractable market failure (insurance). Most goods and services in the health sector do not belong to these three categories, suggesting that they could be competently produced and bought from others.

But is it really worth the effort? Why purchase services rather than hire staff
to produce the needed services in house? Why should one level of government
purchase services from other levels of government, from parastatal agencies, or
from private providers? Is it not easier to just set aside a budget to produce services that are needed and let providers get on with their business? Would this
not avoid the added hassle of letting and managing contracts, monitoring outcomes, and settling disputes when disagreements arise during this process? Is
public production not the only solution when capacity to contract and regulate
is low?

These were precisely the questions that policymakers began asking during the
1980s and 1990s. There was a growing consensus that the path to greater state
effectiveness and rapid development depends on matching the role of governments to their capabilities and changing the incentive structure in the public
sector.

After two decades of success in many other areas of the economy, notably
public enterprise reform, infrastructure, telecommunications, and water and
sanitation, the use of quasi markets and the private sector to reform public services delivery has now also been successfully extended to the social sectors,

including health. Many low-income countries are now using quasi markets, purchasing, outsourcing, and a variety of other market techniques to improve efficiency, productivity, quality, and consumer satisfaction in the health sector.

There is now an overwhelming body of evidence that most goods and services in the health sector can be produced at good quality and low price by nongovernmental producers and that the state can achieve both efficiency and equity objectives through an active process of contracting, purchasing, and commissioning such services from those providers rather than passive subsidies.

In most low- and middle-income countries the private sector is already very active. Use of such services often comprises a large share of health care expenditure. If such private providers already exist, why not use them rather than engage in public production of services that are often of low consumer and clinical quality, unresponsive to patient expectation, and costly in terms of associated informal payments that patients have to make to providers?

Countries that finance their health services through social security systems—France, Germany, Singapore, South Africa, Switzerland, Ronz_nia (Brazil)—have been doing this successfully for years. The issue is therefore not "can it work" but "how to get from here to there" in countries that have a long history of service production through the public sector and restrictive private sector policies.

For governments to purchase services from such private providers means doing business in a different way. It means focusing on outputs and outcomes rather than inputs. It means learning new skills. It takes time and must be accompanied by capacity building in areas such as competitive bidding, contracting, regulation, and the coordination of nongovernmental providers. And it means challenging vested stakeholders whose power and influence often come from being one of the largest employers in the economy.

A three-step process can be used to move gradually from one balance to another in the public-private mix in service delivery —making better use of the existing private sector, expanding areas that are already successful, and converting public to private ownership and management in areas where the latter has a demonstrated superior performance.

If a large, contestable private sector is already producing goods and services whose output is easily measurable, the public sector can benefit from its existence by slowly increasing the use of these resources through coordination, contracting, and establishing a constructive regulatory environment for this sector to grow. Once experience has been gained in coordinating and contracting with providers, the lessons learned can be transferred to other priority areas where there may be scope for expansion in the activities of nongovernmental providers. Finally, where the public sector is clearly engaged in inefficient activities, as is the case with the production of many inputs and basic services, they can be converted to private ownership and subsequently bought as needed from the new nongovernmental providers.

Such involvement by the private sector through contracting, purchasing, or commissioning of services from nongovernmental providers does not mean a disengagement of the state in the health sector. On the contrary, it means a greater engagement by securing sustainable financing (through public mandates and subsidies for the poor), stimulating the generation of context-specific knowledge, and fostering an appropriate labor market for the health sector.

From Policy Design to Implementation

Private and nongovernmental organizations have been contracting in, contracting out, and using collective purchasing services for decades. Countries that use social health insurance to finance health care have also been purchasing services through parastatal agencies for years. Individuals have been purchasing health care directly from providers for centuries. Purchasing is, therefore, not new in the health sector. The question is not "Does it work?" The question is "How does the public sector get from where it is today to becoming an active purchaser of health services and what can it do to ensure that, in doing so, it buys health gains, preserves equity objectives, and is responsive to the needs and expectations of the patients it is supposed to serve?"

Three types of purchaser-provider splits predominate : (a) total split (the purchaser does not own or manage any services or employ any staff who provide such services); (b) partial split (the purchaser retains some ownership and continues to employ some staff but is allowed to outsource and purchase some services); and (c) noncompetitive split.

In the 1990s, the formerly unified British National Health Service (NHS) was split into purchasers and providers, with the NHS District Health Authorities becoming purchasers and the NHS hospitals becoming providers. During the same time period, the U.S. health care system, driven by market forces rather than government fiat, moved toward greater functional integration of financing and service delivery under health maintenance organizations (HMOs). Many countries have followed the U.K. trend toward purchaser-provider splits in Europe and developing countries.

Although much has been written about the added transaction cost of such, at least some of the criticism has been tactical and ideological rather than based on real evaluation of their successes and failures. In many cases, such as in Italy, the reforms were focused more on decentralization and regionalization with a continuation of former cost-reimbursement than a purchaser-provider split with competitive tendering for contracts. Reforms in New Zealand failed at least in part because of a lack of sustainable political commitment and follow through. When done properly, potential cost saving due to a switch from budget-based allocation to output-based purchasing of services can be significant. Such savings have been estimated to be almost 10 percent in Sweden.

A review of such experiences highlights both advantages and disadvantages to reforms that introduce purchaser-provider splits. A few of the advantages include a shift in the balance of power away from providers toward purchasers; a greater focus by purchasers on policy objectives than on managing services; the need to make running costs and investments more explicit; and a possibility of increased patient choice if a large number of providers are allowed to contract with the purchaser. A few of the disadvantages include some loss of control over providers; planning and coordination may become more difficult; increased transaction costs; a need to learn new skills in letting contracts and managing and monitoring contracts; and a possibility of decreased patient choice if the range of providers who can contract with the purchaser is restricted to only a few.

GETTING VALUE FOR PUBLIC MONEY SPENT ON HEALTH CARE

Typically, the flow of funds from collective financing arrangements to providers takes one of three forms : (a) passive allocation of funds from one branch or one level of government to another with an integration of funding and service delivery; (b) prospective contracting or commissioning of services by one branch of government from another or from nongovernmental providers (for profit and not for profit) with payment linked to an explicit agreement on volume and quality of services to be provided; or (c) retrospective reimbursement for services delivered.

Replacing the Passive Cashiers with an Intelligent Purchasing Agent

Many funding departments or agencies still behave like passive cashiers (like ATM machines). They focus on paying what they are supposed to pay. Someone else decides who benefits, what services should be included, which providers are eligible for reimbursement, what prices are to be paid, and which payment mechanism should be used. By contrast, "strategic purchasing involves a continuous search for the best ways to maximize health system performance by deciding which interventions should be purchased, how, and from whom".

Countries that retain hierarchical structures continue to spend money on health care on the basis of decisions made elsewhere (for example, the centralized national health services of many developing countries). Countries that have semiautonomous health insurance funds (for example, the Health Insurance Commission in Australia) usually confer some decision rights on these bodies. Finally, countries that use fully autonomous agencies or private health insurance (for example, the Czech Republic, Germany, or the United States) transfer almost all of the "intelligent" policymaking function to the funding arrangements, while their governments retain only a high-level policy oversight.

Shift in Focus from Inputs to Outcomes and Well-Defined Client Groups

The key to managing scarcity more effectively lies in shifting the emphasis of collective financing from its traditional focus on inputs to a new focus on better outcomes. Improved health is only one of several potential desirable outcomes from strategic purchasing.

Others desirable outcomes include protection against the impoverishing effects of illness or coverage of specific target populations. The latter may include (a) vulnerable groups such as mothers and their children; (b) patients suffering from specific diseases such as tuberculosis, malaria, or human immunodeficiency virus/acquired immunodeficiency syndrome (HIV/AIDS); or (c) high-risk social groups such as the poor.

Such a multidimensional approach to health outcomes is not new. And it is consistent with the MDGs relating to achievement of better health and protection against impoverishment by the year 2015.

FORTHCOMING BOOKS ON RESOURCE ALLOCATION AND PURCHASING IN THE HEALTH SECTOR

These above-mentioned topics will be explored in the remainder of this book, *Spending Wisely: Buying Health Services for the Poor*. The underlying economics for purchasing of health services will be published in a forthcoming companion volume, *The Economics of Resource Allocation and Purchasing of Health Care*. A third volume will provide a collection of regional and country case studies that were used to inform volume one and underpin the economic theory of volume two. Finally, the Bank is working with various other partners to produce a series of applied manuals on provider payments.

REFERENCES

Aaron, H. J. 1994. "Health Spending Analysis: Thinking Straight about Medical Costs." *Health Affairs (Millwood)* 13(5): 7–13.

Akin, J., N. Birdsall, and others. 1987. "Financing Health Services in Developing countries: An Agenda for Reform." World Bank, Washington, D.C.

Allen, R. 1999. "New Public Management: Pitfalls for Central and Eastern Europe." *Public Management Forum* 1(4).

Arrow, K. W. 1963. "Uncertainty and the Welfare Economics of Medical Care." *American Economic Review* 53: 940–73.

Bartlett, W. and J. Le Grand. 1993. *Quasi-markets and Social Policy*. Basingstoke: Macmillan.

———. 1980. *Arrow's Theorem: The Paradox of Social Choice*. New Haven, Conn.: Yale University Press.

Beauchamp, T. L., and J. F. Childress. 1983. *Principles of Biomedical Ethics*. Oxford: Oxford University Press.

Belli, P. 2002. "The Impact of Resource Allocation and Purchasing Reforms on Equity." HNP Discussion Paper, World Bank, Washington, D.C.

Bennett, S., B. McPake, and others, eds. 1997. Private Health Providers in Developing Countries. London: ZED Publishers.

Bitran, R., and U. Giedion. 2002. "Waivers and Exemptions for Health Services in Developing Countries." HNP Discussion Paper, World Bank, Washington, D.C.

Bitran, R., J. Munoz, and others 2000. "Equity in the Financing of Social Security for Health in Chile." *Health Policy* 50(3): 171–96.

Broomberg J., A. Masobe and A. Mills. 1997. "To Purchase or to Provide? The Relative Efficiency of Contracting Out Versus Direct Public Provision of Hospital Services in South Africa." *Private Health Providers in Developing Countries: Serving the Public Interest?* ed. S. Bennett, B. McPake, and A. Mills. London: Zed Books.

Carrin G., M. Jancloes and J. Perrot. 1998. "Towards New Partnerships for Health Development in Developing Countries: The Contractual Approach as a Policy Tool." *Tropical Medicine and International Health* 6: 512–14.

Carrin, G., R. Zeramdini, and others. 2001. "The Impact of the Degree of Risk-Sharing in Health Financing on Health System Attainment." HNP Discussion Paper, World Bank, Washington, D.C.

Chalkley, M., and J. M. Malcomson. 2000. "Government Purchasing of Health Services." In *Handbook of Health Economics*, ed. A. J. Culyer and J. P. Newhouse, 848–90. Amsterdam: Elsevier.

Chernichovsky D. 1995. "Health System Reforms in Industrialized Democracies: An Emerging Paradigm." *Milbank Quarterly* 73(3): 339–72.

———. 2002. "Pluralism, Public Choice, and the State in the Emerging Paradigm in Health Systems." *Milbank Quarterly* 80(1): 5–39.

Claeson, M., C. C. Griffin, and others. 2001. *Health, Nutrition, and Population Sourcebook for the Poverty Reduction Strategy Paper*. Washington, D.C.: World Bank.

Coulter, A. and C. Ham, eds. 2000. *The Global Challenge of Health Care Rationing. State of Health*. Buckingham: Open University Press.

Creese, A. L. 1991. "User Charges for Health Care: A Review of Recent Experience." *Health Policy and Planning* 6(4): 309–19.

Demone H. and M. Gibeleman, eds. 1989. *Services for Sale: Purchasing of Helath and Human Services*. New Brunswick, NJ: Rutgers University Press.

Devarajan, S., M. J. Miller, and others. 2002. "Goals for Development: History, Prospects and Costs." World Bank Discussion Paper, World Bank, Washington, D.C.

Diderichsen, F. 2002. "Resource Allocation for Health Equity: Issues and Methods." HNP Discussion Paper, World Bank, Washington, D.C.

Dionne, G. 2000. *Handbook of Insurance*. Boston, Mass.: Kluwer.

Domberger S. 1999. *The Contracting Organization: A Strategic Guide to Out-sourcing*. New York: Oxford University Press.

Dror, D., and A. S. Preker, eds. 2002. *Social Re-Insurance: A New Approach to Sustainable Community Health Financing*. Washington, D.C.: World Bank/International Labour Organisation.

Dunleavy, P., and C. Hood. 1994. "From Old Public Administration to New Public Management." *Public Money and Management* 14(3): 9–16.

Eisenhardt, K. M. 1988. "Control: Organization and Economic Approaches." *Management Science* 31: 134–49.

Ellis R. and M. Chawla. 1993. *Public and Private Interaction in the Health Sector in Developing Countries*. Boston, Mass.: Management Sciences for Health.

England R. 1997. *Contracting in the Health Sector: A Guide to the Use of Contracting in Developing Countries*. Washington, D.C.: World Bank, WBI.

Epp J. 1999. *A Guide for Bank Operations on "Contracting-Out" for Reproductive Health Services*. Washington, D.C.: World Bank.

Evans, R. G. 1983. "The Welfare Economics Public Health Insurance: Theory and Canadian Practice." In *Social Insurance*, ed. L. Soderstrom, 71–104. Amsterdam: North-Holland.

Figueras, J., R. Robinson, and others, eds. 2005. *Effective Purchasing of Health Gain*. Buckingham: Open University Press. Flanagan, H., and P. Spurgeon. 1996. *Public Sector Managerial Effectiveness: Theory and Practice in the National Health Service*. Buckingham: Open University Press.

Fougere G. 2001. "Transforming Health Sectors: New Logics of Organizing in the New Zealand Health System." *Social Science and Medicine* 52(8): 1233–42.

Gerdtham U.G., M. Lothgren, M. Tambour and C. Rehnberg. 1999. "Internal Markets and Health Care Efficiency: A Multiple-Output Stochastic Frontier Analysis." *Journal of Health Economics* 8(2): 151–64.

Gertler, P. J., and J. Hammer. 1997. "Strategies for Pricing Publicly Provided Health Services." In *Innovations in Health Financing*, ed.G. Schieber, 127–154. Washington, D.C.: World Bank.

Gilson, L. 1997. "The Lessons User Fee Experience in Africa." *Health Policy and Planning* 12(4): 273–85.

Gottret, P. 2004. "Financing Accelerated Progress Toward Achieving the Millennium Development Goals." HNP Discussion Paper, World Bank, Washington, D.C.

Griffin C.C. 1989. "Strengthening Health Services in Developing Coungtries through the Private Sector." Discussion Paper Number 4, International Finance Corporation, Washington, D.C.

Gupta, S. 2001. "Fiscal Requirements." HNP Discussion Paper, World Bank, Washington, D.C.

Gwatkin, D. 2000. "Health Inequalities and the Health of the Poor: What Do We Know? What Can We Do?" *Bulletin of the World Health Organization* 78(1): 3–17.

———. 2001. "Poverty and Inequalities in Health Within Developing Countries: Filling the Information Gap." In *Poverty, Inequality, and Health: An International Perspective*, eds. D. Leon and G. Walt, 217–246. Oxford: Oxford University Press.

———. 2002a. "Free Government Health Services: Are They the Best Way to Serve the Poor?" HNP Discussion Paper, World Bank, Washington, D.C.

———. 2002b. "Who Would Gain Most from Efforts to Reach the Millennium Development Goals: An Inquiry into the Possibility of Progress that Fails to Reach the Poor." HNP Discussion Paper, World Bank, Washington, D.C.

Hanson K. and P. Berman. 1998. "Private Health Care Provision in Developing Countries: A Preliminary Analysis of Levels and Composition." *Health Policy and Planning* 13(3): 195–211.

Harding, A., and A. S. Preker, eds. 2003. *Private Participation in Health Services*. Health, Nutrition, and Population Series. Washington, D.C.: World Bank.

Hauck, K., P. C. Smith, and others. 2002. "The Economics of Priority Setting for Health Care: A Literature Review." HNP Discussion Paper, World Bank, Washington, D.C.

Heffler, S., S. Smith, and others. 2002. "Health Spending Projections for 2001–2011: The Latest Outlook. Faster Health Spending Growth and a Slowing Economy Drive the Health Spending Projection for 2001 Up Sharply." *Health Affairs (Millwood)* 21(2):207–18.

Hermans H. and J. Nooren. 1998. "Contracting and the Purchaser-Provider Split in Western Europe: A Legal-Organizational Analysis." *Medicine and Law* 17(2): 167–88.

Hillman D. and J. Christianson. 1984. "Competitive Bidding as a Cost-containment Strategy for Indigent Medical Care: The Implementation Experience in Arizona." *Journal of Health Policy, Politics and Law* 9(3): 427–51.

Hutchison J., P. Hardee and C. Barns. 1997. "Bureaucracy of Purchaser-Provider Split Delays Treatment." *British Medical Journal* 314(7089): 1275.

Jakab, M., A. S. Preker, and others. 2002. "The Introduction of Market Forces in the Public Hospital Sector: From New Public Sector Management to Organizational Reform." HNP Discussion Paper, World Bank, Washington, D.C.

Jenkinson T. and C. Mayer. 1996. "The Assessment: Contracts and Competitive Bidding to Health Care." *Oxford Review of Economic Policy* 12(4): 9.

Jommi C., E. Cantu and E. Anessi-Pessina. 2001. "New Funding Arrangements in the Italian National Health Service." *International Journal of Health Planning and Management* 16(4): 347–68.

Jost T. S., D. Hughes, J. Mchale and L. Griffiths. 1995. "The British Health Care Reforms, the American Health Care Revolution, and Purchaser/Provider Contracts." *Journal of Health Politics, Policy and Law* 20(4): 885–908.

Kaufmann, D., and R. Ryterman. 1998. *Global Corruption Survey*. Washington, D.C.: World Bank.

Klein, R., P. Day, and others. 1996. *Managing Scarcity: Priority Setting and Rationing in the National Health Service*. Buckingham: Open University Press.

Kumaranayake, L., C. Kurowski, and others. 2001. *Costs of Scaling-up Priority Health Interventions in Low and Selected Middle Income Countries: Methodology and Estimates*. Geneva: World Health Organization.

Kutzin, J. 2000. "Towards Universal Health Coverage: A Goal Oriented Framework for Policy Analysis, Washington." HNP Discussion Paper, World Bank, Washington, D.C.

Lewis M. 1988. *The Private Sector and Health Care Delivery in Developing Countries: Definition, Experience, and Potential*. Washington, D.C.: USAID, Resources for Child Health Project (REACH).

Liu, X., and W. C. Hsiao. 1995. "The Cost Escalation of Social Health Insurance Plans in China: Its Implication for Public Policy." *Social Science and Medicine* 41(8):1095–101.

Lyons, A. S., and R. J. Petrucelli. 1978. *Medicine: An Illustrated History*. New York: Harry N. Abrams.

McCombs J.S. and J.B. Christianson. 1987. "Applying Competitive Bidding to Health Care." *Journal of Health Politics, Policy and Law* 12(4): 703–22.

McPake B. and E. Ngalande Bande. 1994. "Contracting Out of Health Services in Developing Countries." *Health Policy and Planning* 9(1): 25–30.

Milgrom, P. and J. Robers. 1992. *Economics of Organization and Management.* Englewood Cliffs, N.J.: Prentice-Hall.

Mills A. 1996. "Government Capacity to Contract with the Private Sector: Health Sector Experience and Lessons." *HEFP.*

Mills A. and J. Broomberg. 1998. "Experiences of Contracting: An Overview of the Literature. Macroeconomics, Health and Development Series." Technical Paper 33, WHO/CO/MESD.33. World Health Organization, Geneva.

Moore, M. 1995. *Creating Public Value.* Boston, Mass.: Harvard University Press.

Mossalios, E., J. Figueras, and others, eds. 2002. *Funding Health Care: Options for Europe.* Buckingham: Open University Press/World Health Organization.

Mossialos, E., and J. LeGrand, eds. 1999. *Health Care and Cost Containment in the European Union.* Ashgate: Aldershot.

Musgrove, P. 1996. *Public and Private Roles in Health: Theory and Financing Patterns.* Washington, D.C.: World Bank.

Musgrove, P., R. Zeramdini, and others. 2002. "Basic Patterns in National Health Expenditure." *Bulletin of the World Health Organization* 80(2): 134–42.

Newbrander, W., D. Collins, and others. 2001. *Ensuring Equal Access to Health Services: User Fee Systems and the Poor.* Boston, Mass.: Management Sciences for Health.

Nitayarumphong, S., and A. Mills. 1998. *Achieving Universal Coverage of Health Care.* Bangkok: Ministry of Public Health.

OECD (Organization for Economic Co-operation and Development). 1992. *The Reform of Health Care: A Comparative Analysis of Seven OECD Countries.* Paris: OECD.

Oevretveit, J. 1995. *Purchasing for Health.* Buckingham: Open University Press.

Osborne, D., and T. Gaebler. 1993. *Reinventing Government.* New York: Plume.

Outreville, J. F. 1998. *Theory and Practice of Insurance.* Boston, Mass.: Kluwer.

Oxley, H. 1995. *New Directions in Health Care Policy.* Paris: Organisation for Economic Co-operation and Development.

Paton C. 1995. "Present Dangers and Future Threats: Some Perverse Incentives in the NHS Reforms." *British Medical Journal* 310(6989): 1245–8.

Pauly, M. 1971. *Medical Care at Public Expense: A Study in Applied Welfare Economics.* New York: Praeger Publishers.

———. 2000. "Insurance Reimbursement." In A. J. Culyer and J. P. Newhouse, eds., *Handbook of Health Economics.* Amsterdam: Elsevier.

Peacock, A. 1980. "On the Anatomy of Collective Failure, Public Finance." *Public Finance* 35(1): 33–43.

Peters, D. H., A. S. Yazbeck, and others, eds. 2002. *Better Health Systems for India's Poor: Finding, Analysis, and Options.* HNP Publication Series. Washington, D.C.: World Bank.

Polidano, C. 1999. *The New Public Management in Developing Countries.* Manchester: University of Manchester, Institute for Development Policy and Management.

Polidano, C., M. Minogue, and others, eds. 1998. *Beyond the New Public Management: Changing Ideas and Practices in Governance*. Cheltenham, United Kingdom: Edward Elgar.

Preker, A. S. 1989. *The Introduction of Universality in Health Care*. London: IIHS, Organisation for Economic Co-operation and Development.

———. 2001. "Global Development Challenges and Health Care Reform." *World Hospitals and Health Services Journal* 37(3): 2–8, 40, 42.

Preker, A. S., and G. Carrin, eds. 2004. *Health Financing for Poor People: Resource Mobilization and Risk Sharing*. Health, Nutrition and Population Series. Washington, D.C.: World Bank/International Labour Organisation.

Preker, A. S., G. Carrrin, and others. 2001. "Role of Communities in Resource Mobilization and Risk Sharing: A Synthesis Report." HNP Discussion Paper, World Bank, Washington, D.C.

Preker, A. S., and R. G. A. Feachem. 1996. "Market Mechanisms and the Health Sector in Central and Eastern Europe. Technical Paper Series No. 293, World Bank, Washington, D.C.

Preker, A. S., and A. Harding. 2000. "The Economics of Public and Private Roles in Health Care: Insights from Institutional Economics and Organizational Theory." HNP Discussion Paper, World Bank, Washington, D.C.

Preker, A. S., and A. Harding, eds. 2003. *Innovations in Health Service Delivery: The Corporatization of Public Hospitals*. Health, Nutrition, and Population Series. Washington, D.C.: World Bank.

Preker, A. S., M. Jakab, and others. 2002. "Health Financing Reform in Central and Easter Europe and the Former Soviet Union." In *Funding Health Care: Options for Europe*, eds. E. Mossalios, J. Figueras, and A. Dixon, 80–108. Buckingham: Open University Press/World Health Organization.

Preker, A. S., and J. Langenbrunner, eds. 2004. *Spending Wisely: Buying Health Services for the Poor*. Health, Nutrition and Population Series. Washington, D.C.: World Bank.

Preker, A. S., E. Suzuki, and others. 2003. "Costing Accelerated Progress Toward Achieving the Millennium Development Goals." HNP Discussion Paper, World Bank, Washington, D.C.

Rice J.A. 1995. *New Contracting for Health Gain: A Discussion Paper for Developing Health Insurance and Health Services Purchasing*. Washington, D.C.: USAID, Zdrav Reform Project.

Robinson J. 1999. *The Corporate Practice of Medicine: Competition and Innovation in Health Care*. Berkeley, CA: University of California Press.

Rosen J.E. 2000. "Contracting for Reproductive Health Care: A Guide." HNP Discussion Paper, World Bank, Washington, D.C.

Saltman R. and O. Ferroussier-Davis. 1995. "Applying Planned Market Logic to Developing Countries' Health Systems: An Initial Exploration." Discussion Paper No.4., World Health Organization, Geneva.

Savoie, D. 1995. "What Is Wrong with the New Public Management?" *Canadian Public Administration* 1(1): 112–21.

Schick, A. 1998. "Why Most Developing Countries Should Not Try New Zealand's Reforms." *World Bank Research Observer* 13(1): 23–31.

Schieber, G., ed. 1996. *Innovations in Health Financing*. Washington, D.C.: World Bank.

———. 1997. *Innovations in Health Financing*. Washington, D.C.: World Bank.

Shaw P. 2002. "New Public Sector Management in Health." HNP Discussion Paper, World Bank, Washington, D.C.

Slater S. and C. Saade. 1996. *Mobilizing the Commercial Sector for Public Health Objectives: A Practical Guide*. Washington, D.C.: UNAIDS with BASICS and UNICEF.

Torres G. and S. Mathur. 1996. *The Third Wave of Privatization: Privatization of Social Sectors in Developing Countries*. Washington, D.C.: World Bank, Private Sector Development.

United Nations. 2000. *A Better World for All: Progress Towards the International Development Goals*. New York: United Nations.

———. 2001. *Road Map Towards the Implementation of the United Nations Millennium Declaration*. New York: United Nations.

Vining, A. R., and D. L. Weimer. 1990. "Government Supply and Government Production Failure: A Framework Based on Contestability." *Journal of Public Policy* 10(1): 1–22.

Wagstaff, A. 2002a. "Health Spending and Aid as Escape Routes from the Vicious Circle of Poverty and Health." HNP Discussion Paper, World Bank, Washington, D.C.

———. 2002b. "Intersectoral Synergies and the Health MDGs: Preliminary Cross-Country Findings, Collaboration and Policy Simulations." World Bank, Washington, D.C.

Wagstaff, A., and E. van Doorslaer. 2001. "What Makes the Personal Income Tax Progressive? A Comparative Analysis of Fifteen OECD Countries." *International Tax and Public Finance* 8(3): 299–315.

Wagstaff, A., E. van Doorslaer, and others. 1992. "Equity in the Finance of Health Care: Some International Comparisons." *Journal of Health Economics* 11(4): 361–88.

Wagstaff, A., N. Watanabe, and others. 2001. "Impoverishment, Insurance, and Health Care Payments." World Bank, Washington, D.C. Walsh, K. 1995. *Public Services and Market Mechanisms: Competition, Contracting and the New Public Management*. Basingstoke, United Kingdom: Macmillan.

Waters H., L. Hatt and H. Axelsson 2002. "Working with the Private Sector for Child Health." HNP Discussion Paper, World Bank, Washington, D.C.

Weimer, D. L., and A. R. Vining. 1989. *Policy Analysis: Concept and Practice*. Englewood Cliffs, N.J.: Prentice Hall.

WHO (World Health Organization). 2000. *Health Systems: Measuring Performance*. Geneva: WHO.

———. 2001. *Macroeconomics and Health: Investing in Health for Economic Development*. Geneva: WHO.

———. 2002a. *Development Assistance and Health*. Geneva: WHO.

———. 2002b. *Improving Health Outcomes of the Poor*. Geneva: WHO.

———. 2002c. *Mobilisation of Domestic Resources for Health*. Geneva: WHO.

Williamson, O. 1985. *The Economic Institutions of Capitalism: Firms, Markets and Relational Contracting*. New York: Free Press.

Wilson, C. 1977. "A Model of Insurance Markets with Imperfect Information." *Journal of Economic Theory* 16(2): 167–207.

Wilson, J. Q. 1989. *Bureaucracy*. New York: Basic Books.

Wolf, C. J. 1979. "A Theory of Non-Market Failure." *Journal of Law and Economics* 22(1): 107–39.

World Bank. 1993. *World Development Report 1993: Investing in Health*. New York and Oxford: Oxford University Press.

———. 1995. *Bureaucrats in Business: The Economics and Politics of Government Ownership*. Washington, D.C.: World Bank.

———. 1996. *World Development Report 1996: From Plan to Market*. Oxford: Oxford University Press.

———. 1997a. *Sector Strategy for HNP*. Washington, D.C.: World Bank.

———. 1997b. *World Development Report 1997: The State in a Changing World*. Oxford: Oxford University Press.

———. 2000. *Reforming Public Institutions and Strengthening Governance: A World Bank Strategy*. Washington, D.C.: World Bank.

———. 2002a. *Global Economic Prospects and the Developing Countries 2003*. Washington, D.C.: World Bank.

———. 2002b. *World Development Report 2002: Building Institutions for Markets*. Oxford: Oxford University Press.

———. 2003. *World Development Report 2003: Making Services Work for the Poor*. Oxford: Oxford University Press.

Zeckhauser, R. 1970. "Medical Insurance: A Study of the Trade-Off between Risk Sharing and Appropriate Incentives." *Journal of Economic Theory* 2(1): 10–26.

CHAPTER 2

For Whom to Buy? Are Free Government Health Services the Best Way to Reach the Poor?

Davidson R. Gwatkin

Equity is a frequently stated justification for government involvement in the health care market. This is often taken to mean directly providing all segments of the population with a wide range of government-operated health services at no cost: free universal care.

Yet a look at the record suggests that this goal all too often remains elusive, especially in poor countries; that governments in fact serve only some of the population; and that the people served are disproportionately concentrated among the better-off. When this happens, government health services, far from promoting equity, work against it.

What is to be done? One option is to persist: to increase the resources devoted to existing government-operated service programs, in order to expand coverage beyond the high-income areas, where they usually concentrate, out toward the poorer periphery. With enough time and resources, this strategy should eventually lead to inclusion of increasing numbers of poor people and a diminution or elimination of inequalities in government coverage.

To many observers, this would be the ideal situation, but the ideal can be a formidable enemy of the good. For example, it is difficult to envisage the availability of adequate government funds to permit significant progress toward a universal coverage goal in most, if not all, developing and transition economies. Where resources are scarce, a continued concentration on the expansion of government services as they currently exist would be much more likely to produce frustration than progress, and a limited, if any, increase in affordable services for the neediest.

Such constraints need not be fatal, however, because the continued pursuit of universal coverage by widening the range of free government services is not the only, or necessarily the best, approach to benefit the poor. Even when equity-oriented governments do not wish to abandon altogether their universal free coverage aspirations, they have the option of limiting universal coverage efforts to a few interventions of particular epidemiological effectiveness, and of finding alternative ways to achieve equity for other services.

Many alternative ways are available. For example, often the pattern of government expenditures can be modified to increase the proportion that benefits the disadvantaged. Or, to cite another possibility, one might try encouraging upper-income people to cover a larger share of their health care costs, thereby freeing up government health service resources to serve previously excluded groups.

The purpose of this chapter is to make and illustrate the basic point made above: there are many ways for governments to pursue the goal of ensuring that the poor receive adequate, affordable services through alternative approaches to resource allocation and purchasing. This assertion is explored in the three sections that follow. The first section summarizes the information known about the distribution of benefits from government health services across social groups, to document the regressive pattern that now frequently exists and the need for significant changes in approach if the poor are to benefit. The second and third sections illustrate the kinds of changes that might be considered, discussing in further detail the two examples noted briefly above.

THE BENEFICIARIES OF GOVERNMENT HEALTH SERVICE EXPENDITURES

There are two principal sources of information about who benefits from government health service expenditures. One is a series of reports, using different variants of a methodology known as *benefit incidence,* which present information about overall government health service expenditures. The second is a set of 45 comparable country studies on socioeconomic inequalities in health status and service use, showing who uses a set of specific maternal and child health services.

Both sources, while varied in nature, show that overall government health service programs usually—though not always—benefit the better-off more than the disadvantaged. This is true especially for secondary and tertiary care, which usually accounts for most government health care expenditures, less so for primary care and preventive services.

The First Source: Benefit-Incidence Reports

The many ins and outs of benefit-incidence methodology, used in some 25 to 30 country studies thus far, have been explained elsewhere (Castro-Leal and others 2000; Demery 2002; Gwatkin 2000). Briefly put, this methodology is the equity analogue to the better known cost-effectiveness analysis. That is, where cost-effectiveness analysis examines the amount of output produced per unit of resources invested in a health service program, benefit-incidence analysis is concerned with how that output is distributed across socioeconomic groups. It typically draws on two types of data: household surveys with information about socioeconomic status and utilization of health services, to estimate the use of different types of government services by each of several socioeconomic groups; and government statistics and financial records, which permit construction of an estimate for the unit cost of each type of government service covered. The volume of each service used by each socioeconomic group is multiplied by the unit cost of that service, adjusted to account for any user fees paid by group members, and then the results are summed for each socioeconomic group. The

TABLE 2.1   How Much Do the Poor Gain from Government Health Service Expenditures in Africa? (percent)

	Primary care		Total care	
	Percentage of benefit of gained by:		Percentage of benefit of gained by:	
Country	Poorest population quintile	Richest population quintile	Poorest population quintile	Richest population quintile
Côte d'Ivoire (1995)	14	22	11	32
Ghana (1992)	10	31	12	33
Guinea (1994)	10	36	4	48
Kenya (rural, 1992)	22	14	14	24
Madagascar (1993)	10	29	12	30
Tanzania (1992–93)	18	21	17	29
South Africa (1994)	18	10	16	17
Unweighted average	15	23	12	30

Note: The percentages refer to the total financial benefits from government health care expenditures accruing to the poorest and richest population quintiles.

Source: Castro-Leal and others 2000.

result is an estimate of the total amount of government health service resources used by the different groups.

Perhaps the best known set of cost-benefit estimates is a set of seven country studies for Africa, whose findings are summarized in table 2.1. As can be seen, 30 percent of total government health care expenditures went to benefit the top 20 percent of the population—more than two-and-a-half times the 12 percent that benefited the poorest 20 percent. The record was better with respect to primary care; but even there, the top 20 percent of the population received on average one-and-a-half times as much gain as did the bottom 20 percent (23 percent of total financial benefit for the top quintile versus 15 percent of total financial benefit for the bottom quintile).

Table 2.2 presents summary figures from a collection of 22 benefit-incidence studies (including the 7 included in table 2.1), from four developing and transitional regions. The figures need to be interpreted with considerable caution because of possible interstudy methodological differences but are nonetheless of interest in showing that higher gains for the better-off are the norm in all regions, with the exception of Latin America (about which more later). All in all, the top quintile received more than the bottom quintile in 13 of the 22 countries—in 12 of the 14 countries outside of Latin America. This is similar to the findings from a more recent compilation showing a regressive pattern of overall expenditures in 17 of 25 developing societies covered and in 15 of the 17 societies outside of Latin America (Wagstaff 2002).

TABLE 2.2   Financial Subsidy from Government Health Services Accruing to Poorest and Richest 20 Percent of the Population (regional averages in percentage)

| Region | Primary care | | Hospital care | | | | | | Total health care | |
| | | | Outpatient | | Inpatient | | Total | | | |
	Poorest quintile	Richest quintile	Poorest quintile	Richest quintile	Poorest quintile	Richest quintile	Poorest quintile	Richest quintile	Poorest quintile	Richest quintile
Africa	15 (7)	23 (7)	12 (2)	36 (2)	16 (2)	34 (2)	10 (5)	33 (5)	12 (7)	30 (7)
Asia	21 (2)	16 (2)	7 (1)	41 (1)	5 (1)	41 (1)	13 (1)	22 (1)	19 (5)	21 (5)
Eastern Europe	16 (2)	22 (2)	—	—	—	—	12 (2)	29 (2)	13 (2)	27 (2)
Latin America	—	—	—	—	—	—	—	—	29 (8)	14 (8)

— Not available.

Note: Each figure in parentheses indicates the number of countries included in the average that appears immediately to the left of the parentheses.

Source: Gwatkin 2001.

The Second Source: Comparable Country Studies of Socioeconomic Inequalities in Health Service Use

The 45 country studies (Gwatkin and others 2000) constituting the second source of information are based on the household data from the intercountry Demographic and Health Study (DHS) program. These data are from comparable large-scale household surveys that focus on maternal, child, and reproductive health. The data sets also include information about household assets or attributes (for example, type of roof and flooring; availability of electricity; possession of bicycle, radio, watch; source of drinking water). This information was combined to form a single wealth index. The index was used to divide the study population into wealth quintiles, and the values were tabulated for about 30 health status and service use indicators (for example, infant mortality, total fertility, immunization, use of modern contraception).[1]

Three of the indicators available for most, but not all, of the studies referred to use of public facilities: for treatment of childrens' diarrhea and acute respiratory infections among children and for obstetrical deliveries. The results are summarized in table 2.3.

TABLE 2.3   Distribution of Benefits of Three Government Maternal and Child Health Programs across Socioeconomic Classes

A. Treatment rates by socioeconomic population quintile

Intervention	Percentage of cases receiving treatment in a government facility (unweighted country averages)					Number of countries
	Bottom population quintile	Second population quintile	Middle population quintile	Fourth population quintile	Top population quintile	
Medical treatment, diarrhea	20.3	21.2	22.4	23.1	23.3	37
Medical treatment, acute respiratory infections	24.5	28.5	30.9	31.7	31.8	34
Obstetric deliveries	25.6	34.1	41.7	52.1	60.2	45

B. Intercountry differences in treatment inequality rates

Intervention (1)	Number of countries (2)	Number of countries with higher treatment rate in top than in bottom quintile (3)	Percentage of countries with higher treatment rate in top than in bottom quintile[a] (4)
Medical treatment, diarrhea	37	24	64.9
Medical treatment, acute respiratory infections	34	26	76.4
Obstetric deliveries	45	43	95.6

a. Col.3/col.2 × 100.

Source: Gwatkin and others 2000.

As can be seen in section A of that table, coverage rates increase steadily across quintiles for each of the three interventions, with the coverage in each quintile being higher than that in the quintiles below it. The rate of increase is modest for relatively simple interventions such as medical treatment of diarrhea or acute respiratory infection. As shown in section B, in a substantial minority of countries, the coverage rate is somewhat higher in the bottom quintile than in the top quintile. For more complex treatments such as attended deliveries, the picture is starker: the upper-income groups are much more likely to receive care in public services in almost all countries. The coverage rate in the top quintile is on average nearly three times greater than in the lowest quintile.

In brief, even the simplest interventions offered through government facilities usually reach the better-off at least somewhat more frequently than they do the neediest, for whom they are especially intended. For more complicated and expensive interventions to which most government health service resources are dedicated, coverage inequalities favoring the better-off are much larger.

FOCUSING GOVERNMENT SERVICES ON THE POOR

For observers who believe that lessening disparities between the better-off and the disadvantaged is an important role of government health service provision, the figures presented in tables 2.1 through 2.3 are not encouraging. The picture, while by no means totally black, is certainly a much darker shade of gray than is often realized.

What, then, if anything, can be done to reorient government services more toward the disadvantaged groups who must be reached to achieve the equity objective? Although no definitive answer is available, strong suggestions emerge from a long tradition of experience in the health and other social sectors in trying to reach the poor.

Types of Targeting

The measures used for this purpose, generally known by the infelicitous term "targeting," are of several types. Different authors employ different taxonomies and terminology in describing these types, but almost all differentiate between what might be called "individual," "categorical," and "self"-targeting.[2]

Individual or "direct targeting" applies to programs that, through some sort of means testing, seek to direct their benefits toward particular individuals who are poor. The means testing can be direct, through a careful, objective assessment of an individual's income, wealth, or both. Or it can be indirect, using "proxy means testing," under which individuals are selected on the basis of a few selected characteristics (for example, type of roof on house, level of education) shown to be closely associated with poverty through careful statistical analysis of large household data sets.

Categorical targeting also goes under a variety of other names—such as "indirect," "broad," "characteristic," or "indicator" targeting—each with a somewhat different connotation. The methods referred to by these different names share an emphasis on particular categories or groups of people or types of programs, rather than on individuals. Such emphasis is adopted in full recognition that it cannot produce the degree of precision theoretically available through an individual approach; but in the belief that the greater administrative feasibility and political benefits of indirect targeting will outweigh its theoretical shortcomings. Examples of indirect targeting include targeting particular population groups (say, landless agricultural workers) in which the prevalence of poverty is especially high; targeting geographic areas in which most people are poor; giving priority to services that are primarily relevant for the poor (such as clean water supplies in settings where most of the better-off already have access to clean water); and targeting through initiatives to deal with problems concentrated among the poor (for example, communicable diseases).

Self-targeting, or "self-selection," relies on programs that are made universally available but are thought likely to be attractive only to the poor. It is used especially in public works programs. There, low-paying temporary manual labor jobs are made available to anyone who comes for them, but the low remuneration and short duration make them attract only people in severe need. A health example would be offering free hospitalization in large wards for anybody who wishes it, in anticipation that all but the poor will prefer to pay for a private room.

These different types of targeting are by no means mutually exclusive. Programs that apply two or three simultaneously are common.

The Effectiveness of Targeting

There is no known instance of a targeting program's approaching perfection—that is, of reaching all poor people within a society, while excluding all those who are not poor. There are many cases where targeting appears to make no difference. Upon occasion, it even ends up subsidizing the better-off more than the disadvantaged. But, in many other instances, targeted programs have resulted in a significantly larger portion of benefits going to the poor than under the typical government service programs described in the preceding section.

Many of these instances are from outside the health sector. The most comprehensive recent review, covering 67 programs from a wide range of sectors, found that the poor got more benefits in 70 to 75 percent of cases than they would have had the benefits been evenly distributed across the population (which would in itself be an improvement over the present situation with respect to government health service expenditure programs). On average, the poor got a bit over one-third more. None of the numerous targeting methods used by the various programs seemed clearly superior to the others (Coady, Grosh, and Hoddinott 2002).

A similar result emerged from another widely cited review that compared 18 carefully targeted Latin American government programs in a wide range of fields (including health) with 30 less-well-targeted programs. The principal findings were:

- In eight untargeted programs offering general food subsidies to entire populations, an average of 33 percent of the total benefit went to the poorest 40 percent of households.

- In 22 government primary care and education programs that were "loosely targeted"—that is, provided benefits not specifically targeted but considerably more relevant for the poor because the services provided were already readily accessible to the better-off—58 percent of the total benefit accrued to the poorest 40 percent.

- In the 18 more carefully targeted programs, the poorest 40 percent of the households got 72 percent of the total program benefits—over twice as high a percentage as the 33 percent that went to this poor group under the untargeted programs just mentioned (Grosh 1994).[3]

Within the health sector, by far the greatest amount of attention has gone to one particular type of individual targeting: that is, the identification of poor individuals qualified to receive exemptions from the user fees frequently introduced as a component of health sector reforms. Here, the record has been widely varied.

At one end of the spectrum are the many countries, especially in Africa, whose governments simply issued decrees that the poor should be exempted and then largely forgot about them. Several reviews have shown that these have had little impact (Gilson, Russell, and Buse 1995; Nolan and Turbat 1995; Russell and Gilson 1997; Waters 1994).

In other places sustained effort and resources have been applied, and there the record is much different. Examples include some of the Latin American initiatives included in the general review described above and a set of nine successful efforts identified in another overall review of the exemption experience (Willis 1993).

Perhaps the largest and best known of the more promising experience has been Thailand, which has been offering free medical care to low-income groups since 1975 through an initiative known as the Low-Income Support Program.[4] The program was modified numerous times as the government gained experience with it, and by the late 1990s was open to the some 25 percent of Thai families living below the country's nationally determined poverty line. Local officials of the Ministry of Home Affairs determined which families were qualified to participate and issued identification cards to the families that qualified. The cardholders presenting their cards at government health facilities were exempted from the usual fees. The cost was covered by a special allocation to the service-providing facilities from the Ministry of Public Health, which used about 8 percent of its budget for this purpose. By the late 1990s, some 11 million people—20 percent of

Thailand's population—were participating in the initiative. Independent surveys suggest that about 80 percent of these people were indeed poor and that about 65 percent of Thailand's poor were covered.

While some observers would argue that a certain amount of "leakage"— coverage of nonpoor—should be tolerated to win support from politically important groups,[5] many Thais were seriously disturbed about the 20 percent of nonpoor who were inappropriately receiving benefits. Thus in 2001 the initiative was merged with a policy of universal care introduced by a new government. Though by no means perfect in its targeting accuracy, and thus controversial within Thailand, the Thai program's record nonetheless stands in stark contrast to the usual pattern of health service beneficiaries outlined in the preceding section and serves to indicate that exemption programs can be developed in which most benefits do flow to the poor.

This and the other instances covered by the reviews also point to several guidelines for developing such programs. One is to have clear and easily verifiable eligibility criteria and arranging for people other than clinical personnel to determine who is and is not eligible (for example, by having responsible people thoroughly familiar with local financial conditions issue identification cards to the poor for presentation at health facilities). Another is to provide for financial support from an outside source to reimburse service providers for the revenue they forgo in providing free or subsidized services. Yet another is to be willing to experiment continually over the extended period of time that may be needed to get an exemption to work correctly.

In brief, effectively focusing government services on the poor is by no means easy. Effective targeting programs cannot be painlessly achieved simply by waving a wand or issuing a decree or two. Rather, they require determination, time, and money. But where these factors are present, they can make enough of a difference in the benefits across social classes to deserve serious consideration.

ENCOURAGING THE BETTER-OFF TO PAY FOR THEIR OWN SERVICES

Another option is to encourage the better-off to pick up a greater part of their own health bills. This can be done in many ways. One is to charge more for the government health services used by high-income people. Another is to use governmental authority to establish alternative, self-financed mechanisms through which the better-off can obtain services at their own expense.

Payment for Government Services

As long as government health services are free to and used by everyone, any service use by members of an upper-income group represents a government subsidy to that group. However, the introduction of user fees presents an opportunity to employ differential financing that could alter the amount of subsidy going to different segments of the population. One way that differential financing can be used to promote equity is to reduce the amount that the poor must pay through the fee exemptions for the disadvantaged that have just been discussed. Another way of achieving the same objective is to get upper-income groups to pay more.

For example, the highest price possible could be charged for higher-level medical care, which typically accounts for most government health care expenditures and which, as noted earlier, is almost always used disproportionately by the better-off. Given this pattern of use, any cost-recovery measures would be borne primarily by the upper-income groups. Concerns about protecting the small minority of service users who are poor could be addressed through a fee waiver system.

An approach of this sort would probably be considerably more feasible politically—and more justifiable on substantive grounds, as well—if accompanied by a health insurance program covering specified upper-income groups. One obvious possibility is gradually introduced mandatory catastrophe insurance for all workers in the formal sector, financed through some combination of employee and employer contributions. This would protect the few but extremely unfortunate upper-income households faced with medical bills that lie far beyond even their means.

Establishment of Alternative Mechanisms

A more radical approach would be to get the better-off out of government facilities altogether—that is, by getting the government out of the business of providing or financing services for the better-off. This might be done by, say, using government regulatory powers to foster the establishment of a fully self-financing private commercial health sector serving the better-off.

Although few if any countries are known to have tried such an approach in the "pure" form just described, a rough approximation of it exists in the social security programs for formal sector workers in many places, especially in Latin America. Latin American countries have a long tradition of government social security programs that include health insurance for formally employed workers financed through payroll taxes and employee contributions. The programs often operate their own health facilities open only to enrolled workers, reimburse workers for services they obtain through the private sector, or both.

As of the mid-1990s, such programs existed in 17 countries in Latin America and the Caribbean. The programs were generally large: in 9 of the 17 countries, the funds flowing through them represented one-half or more of government health expenditures; in 5 of the 17, the programs covered more than half the population. In the 2 leading countries, Chile and Costa Rica, the social security health programs covered about 90 percent of the population and accounted for a comparable percentage of government health expenditures (Suárez-Berenguela 1998).

In most of these programs, the middle- and upper-income groups that constitute the majority of participants were directly covering most of the programs' costs, although some degree of government contribution to the programs was often involved. As of 1977 (the latest year with readily available comparative data), systems in four of the nine countries that provide figures were entirely self-financing, with no government subsidies; in the others, the amount of subsidy from government revenues ranged from 4 to 15 percent (World Bank 1987).

Beyond this, evidence from one national initiative, in Chile, suggests that social security health programs can be used as a mechanism for channeling government subsidies to the poor. The Chilean program, Fondo Nacional de Salud (FONASA), delivers no services itself, instead covering the costs of services provided by others, both government facilities and private practitioners. FONASA reaches about 70 percent of the country's population; some 40 percent of its beneficiaries are legally indigent and pay no premiums. Of the government subsidy that FONASA receives, more than 90 percent goes to services that reach these legally indigent. This suggests that governments of countries with effective social security health programs can think of grants to or contracts with those social security programs as a means of providing health services to the poor, as an alternative to direct service provision through government clinics, in much the same manner that nongovernmental and community organizations are used elsewhere (Bitran 1998).

The social security programs as just described, however, are far from ideal. Leaving aside the questions often raised about their efficiency, there are equity issues as well. The most frequently mentioned one concerns the two-tier health system in most countries with social security programs—well-equipped and staffed facilities for the better-off, who constitute the majority of social security program participants, and much less adequate health ministry services for the neediest, who are largely excluded from social security systems. In addition, it is not possible to be sure that the volume of government health resources available for the poor is greater than would otherwise have been the case. While data inadequacies prevent any clear judgment, the possibility cannot be ruled out that without the political pressure created by upper-income groups concerned about health services for themselves, government health service budgets are lower for each person served than they would have been had they been required to serve all income groups rather than just the needy.

All in all, as is often the case, the record is far from entirely clear or unambiguous. But at least part of it is striking: namely, just how much better government health care expenditures are oriented toward the poor in Latin America than in other regions. Particularly stark is the contrast with Africa, where there is rarely any significant alternative to government health services for upper-income groups. In Africa, as shown earlier, the top 20 percent of the population gets two-and-a-half times as much benefit from government health expenditures as does the bottom 20 percent. In Latin America, the figures from eight countries reproduced in table 2.2 show a situation that is almost exactly opposite: on average, the poorest 20 percent of the population gets more than twice as much benefit as the richest 20 percent (29 percent versus 14 percent of total benefit). Although this difference is no doubt attributable to many factors, it is difficult to resist the strong sense that Latin America's reliance on social security programs for the better-off has played a significant role.

CONCLUSIONS

Perhaps the best way to conclude is by returning to the question posed at the outset: Does the pursuit of universal coverage by a wide range of free government services constitute the most promising approach to meeting the needs of disadvantaged population groups? The response to that question presented in the preceding sections is "probably not." The record to date points clearly to the danger that the benefits of subsidized government health services will flow primarily to the better-off, rather than to the poor for whom the services are intended. Although there is no perfect approach to dealing with this issue, the record also points to several approaches that can significantly ameliorate the situation. Two of them, discussed here, are the adoption of targeting measures to increase the proportion of benefits from government expenditures that flow to the poor and the development of alternative, self-sustaining service financing and delivery mechanisms to serve the better-off. Successful implementation of approaches such as these would allow governments to focus their efforts to achieve universal free coverage on a limited number of interventions that are particularly important for poor groups.

NOTES

The author acknowledges with appreciation the helpful advice and suggestions received from Cristian Baeza and Pablo Gottret. But neither should be held responsible for whatever errors may remain despite their efforts.

1. The service indicator data available do not indicate the amounts paid for public services. This introduces the possibility of distortion that would occur if, say, the better-off were to pay fully for their services, while the poor receive theirs for free. Although this consideration deserves to be borne in mind while assessing the statistics, such anecdotal evidence as exists provides little basis for believing that it introduces a major distortion.

2. For a fuller, recent discussion of targeting types, on which this section draws heavily, see Coady, Grosh, and Hoddinott (2002).

3. The figures cited refer to medians rather than means and pertain to the poorest 40 percent of households rather than individuals. Because of higher fertility among the poor, the 40 percent of poorest households can be expected to contain more than 40 percent of individuals in the population. A report on benefits based on the poorest 40 percent of individuals would thus be likely to show at least somewhat lower figures for all three types of program described; but because each of the three types would be affected in a similar manner, their relative effectiveness in reaching the poor would not necessarily be changed.

4. The information in this section is drawn primarily from Khoman (1997). For an earlier report on the Thai experience, see Mills (1991).

5. See, for example, Gelbach and Pritchett (1997a, 1997b).

REFERENCES

Bitran, R. 1998. "Equity in the Financing of Social Security for Health in Latin America." Major Applied Research Paper. Abt Associates Inc., Partnerships for Health Reform, Bethesda, Md.

Castro-Leal, F., J. Dayton, L. Demery, and K. Mehtra. 2000. "Public Spending on Health Care in Africa: Do The Poor Benefit?" *Bulletin of the World Health Organization* 78(1): 66–74.

Coady, D., M. Grosh, and J. Hoddinott. 2002. "The Targeting of Transfers in Developing Countries: Review of Experience and Lessons." Draft paper for Safety Nets Primer Series. World Bank, Social Protection Anchor Unit, Washington, D.C.

Demery, L. 2002. "Benefit Incidence Analysis." In *Tool Kit: Techniques for Evaluating the Poverty Impact of Economic Policies*. Washington, D.C.: World Bank. http://poverty.worldbank.org/files/12995_TKWeb_Toolkit_all.pdf

Gelbach, J. B., and L. H. Pritchett. 1997a. "More for the Poor Is Less for the Poor: The Politics of Targeting." World Bank Policy Research Working Paper 1799. World Bank, Washington, D.C.

———. 1997b. "Indicator Targeting in a Political Economy: Leakier Can Be Better." Unpublished manuscript. World Bank, Washington, D.C.

Gilson, L. S. Russell, and K. Buse. 1995. "The Political Economy of User Fees with Targeting: Developing Health Financing Policy." *Journal of International Development* 7(3): 369–401.

Grosh, M. 1994. *Administering Targeted Social Programs in Latin America: From Platitudes to Practice*. Washington, D.C.: World Bank.

Gwatkin, D. R. 2000. "The Current State of Knowledge about Targeting Health Programs to Reach the Poor." World Bank, Washington, D.C. http://www.worldbank.org/poverty/health/library/targeting.pdf

———. 2001. "Poverty and Inequalities in Health within Developing Countries: Filling the Information Gap." In D. Leon and G. Walt, eds., *Poverty and Inequality in Health: An International Perspective*. London: Oxford University Press.

Gwatkin, D. R., S. Rutstein, K. Johnson, R. P. Pande, and A. Wagstaff. 2000. *Socioeconomic Differences in Health, Nutrition, and Population*. Washington, D.C.: World Bank, Health, Nutrition, and Population Department.

Khoman, S. 1997. "Rural Health Care Financing in Thailand." In G. J. Schieber, ed., *Innovations in Health Care Financing: Proceedings of a World Bank Conference, March 10–11, 1997*. Washington, D.C.: World Bank.

Mills, A. 1991. "Exempting the Poor: The Experience of Thailand." *Social Science and Medicine* 33(11): 1241–52.

Nolan, B., and V. Turbat. 1995. *Cost Recovery in Public Health Services in Sub-Saharan Africa*. Washington, D.C.: World Bank, Economic Development Institute.

Russell, S., and L. Gilson. 1997. "User Fee Policy to Promote Health Service Access for the Poor: A Wolf in Sheep's Clothing?" *International Journal of Health Services* 27(2): 359–79.

Suárez-Berenguela, R. 1998. "El Gasto Nacional en Salud en las Américas, 1995." Consultancy Report ACS-0298-ASC9. Pan American Health Organization, Washington, D.C.

Waters, H. 1994. "Literature Review: Equity in the Health Sector in Developing Countries, with Lessons Learned for Sub-Saharan Africa." BASICS Project Document PN-ABW-162. BASICS Project, AFR/SD, HHRAA Project, Washington, D.C.

Wagstaff, A. 2002. "Inequalities in Health in Developing Countries: Swimming against the Tide?" Policy Research Working Paper 2795. World Bank, Washington, D.C.

Willis, C. Y. 1993. "Means Testing in Cost Recovery of Health Services in Developing Countries, Phase I: Review of Concepts and Literature and Preliminary Field Work Design." Major Applied Research Paper 7. Abt Associates Inc., Health Financing and Sustainability Project, Bethesda, Md.

World Bank. 1987. *Financing Health Services in Developing Countries: An Agenda for Reform.* Washington, D.C.: World Bank.

CHAPTER 3

What to Buy? Revisiting Priority Setting in Health Care

Katharina Hauck, Peter C. Smith, and Maria Goddard

Most countries face high demands on their health care systems and a limited budget to meet them. Policymakers therefore try to get the best value for their money. Priority setting is a systematic approach toward distributing the available health care resources optimally among competing demands subject to constraints. In practice, priority setting often takes place implicitly, but recognition is growing that a transparent process is needed.

Some Approaches to Priority Setting

The best approach toward priority setting depends on local circumstances. Applying simple "rules" fails to take into account the many case-specific factors and constraints that may influence the priority-setting process. In addition, different societies have different objectives and therefore different ideas of what is "optimal." However, two key objectives for using the available resources have received worldwide attention:

- *Maximization of health:* to achieve the best possible health status for the entire population

- *Reduction of inequities in health:* to minimize differences in health status between individuals or societal groups.

The simplest form of priority setting can be formulated as a linear program. The goal is to maximize benefits from health care interventions within the budget. Equity considerations can be incorporated by assigning different weights to benefits realized by different individuals or groups. Ranking programs according to their (equity-weighted) cost-effectiveness ratios is a logical consequence of this approach.

The apparent simplicity of this approach, however, masks problems that arise when attempting to make it operational. Some of these problems relate to weaknesses in the cost-effectiveness methodology. The incorporation of equity considerations into this approach is also far from straightforward when seeking to make the simple academic concepts operational. A third set of problems arises from the political, institutional, and environmental context in which priorities are set and implemented. In reality, decisionmakers pay attention to a wide variety of objectives and face many practical constraints that often render the use of unadulterated cost-effectiveness rules inappropriate.

This chapter summarizes the results of a review of the literature on priority setting in health care (Hauck, Smith, and Goddard 2003). We take an economic perspective and offer a critical look at economic models to see whether they are useful for priority setting, in theory and in practice. Throughout we focus on priority setting from a national policymaker's viewpoint. Decisionmakers at higher levels (such as donor agencies) and lower levels (local governments, individual clinicians) may also profoundly influence resource allocation, and these issues are alluded to in relevant sections of the report.

ECONOMIC EVALUATION

Economic evaluation, predominantly in the form of cost-effectiveness analysis, has powerfully influenced the theory of priority setting. In practice, however, decisionmakers do not widely use the results of economic evaluation (Anell and Svarvar 2000; Drummond, Cooke, and Walley 1997; Grizzle and others 2000; Hoffman and Graf von der Schulenburg 2000; Hoffmann and others 2002; Sloan, Whetten-Goldstein, and Wilson 1997). This is to some extent due to the existence of methodological and practical barriers. We consider these below.

Methodological barriers affect the applicability, generalizability, and reliability of studies. As a result, programs may be cost-effective in one setting but not in another. We identify six classes of reason for inconsistencies between cost-effectiveness studies.

First, studies can be undertaken from a variety of *perspectives* (for example, society, a health care institution, or third-party payers), and rankings of interventions may differ depending on the perspective adopted (Torrance, Siegel, and Luce 1996).

Second, studies might not be *generalizable* to other settings (other countries), because health care systems, disease incidence, or relative prices and costs are different. Drummond, Cooke, and Walley (1997), Phelps (1997), and Phillips (1993) discuss factors likely to affect cost-effectiveness estimates of programs in different countries.

Third, choice of the *target population*—the population for whom a program is intended—can affect the cost-effectiveness of interventions (Mandelblatt and others 1996; Torrance, Siegel, and Luce 1996).

Fourth, *uncertainty* surrounds the parameters used in evaluations, and different methods of dealing with it can produce different estimates of cost-effectiveness (Briggs 2001; Manning, Fryback, and Weinstein 1996).

Fifth, *timing* is an issue. Economic evaluation studies must be conducted before medical technologies are in widespread use, and established behaviors are difficult to change.

Sixth, costs and effectiveness of different programs may exhibit important interactions, and the incremental costs of establishing a new program depend on the existing infrastructure (O'Brien and Sculpher 2000). Therefore, economic evaluation studies should ideally consider *portfolios of programs*.

A powerful criticism of conventional cost-effectiveness analysis is that it fails to model the general economic environment in which health care takes place. Ideally, a general equilibrium approach should be used in order to analyze the full impact of choices made in the health care sector on overall social welfare. In practice, this is difficult, but awareness of the limitations of operating within a partial equilibrium framework can help us understand why governments may make priority-setting decisions for economic reasons other than apparent relative cost-effectiveness of programs. Jack (2000) uses positive externalities as an example. Examples include immunization against disease and completion of curative therapy, both reducing the likelihood that others will contract the illness. If the consumer of such a good does not take into account the benefit to others, she will consume too little. In this situation, a government can improve overall welfare by inducing the individual to consume more, typically by subsidizing the price of the good.

Moreover, health system activities may generate important outputs in addition to their impact on the level and distribution of health. The *World Health Report 2000* (World Health Organization [WHO] 2000; Darby and others 2000) recognized some of these by examining the health system's "responsiveness" to users. This is defined as "how the system performs relative to nonhealth aspects" and embraces respect for the person (dignity, confidentiality, autonomy) and client orientation (prompt attention, quality of amenities, access to social support, and freedom of provider choice). There is much debate about the exact nature and importance of responsiveness but little doubt about the important influence the health system can have on individual welfare, independent of its impact on health. Most politicians are sensitive to responsiveness issues such as patient satisfaction and waiting times and, if those have become important political issues, may want to take them into account in priority setting.

The ramifications of health system performance extend beyond individual welfare, to affect national productivity and other macroeconomic factors. The WHO (2001) report on macroeconomics and health argued that, besides saving lives, investment in health can "reduce poverty, spur economic development, and promote global security." The lower life expectancy in poor countries means lower lifetime earnings. For example, average undiscounted lifetime incomes in Botswana are one-tenth of those in the United States. However, poor health influences not only absolute incomes. According to WHO estimates, each 10 percent improvement in life expectancy at birth is associated with a rise in economic growth of at least 0.3 to 0.4 percent per year, holding other growth factors constant. High prevalence of diseases such as malaria and human immunodeficiency virus/acquired immunodeficiency syndrome (HIV/AIDS) is associated with persistently low economic growth rates.

The effect of better health on macroeconomic factors can work through numerous mechanisms such as promoting increased worker productivity, improving educational status, and reducing personal uncertainty associated with health.

Some health system interventions have wider implications for the economy than others, although outputs may appear identical when measured purely in terms of health outcomes. The existence of various types of externalities may explain, in economic terms, priority-setting decisions that appear to run contrary to an approach based on simple cost-effectiveness ratios alone.

Finally, practical barriers to the use of economic evaluation studies arise from the different perspectives of decisionmakers operating in the political and clinical environment and researchers who produce cost-effectiveness data. Others have considered these issues (Anell and Svarvar 2000; Burns and others 2000; Cox, Motheral, and Griffis 2000; Drummond and Weatherly 2000; Duthie and others 1999; Ginsberg, Kravitz, and Sandberg 2000; Grizzle and others 2000; Hoffmann and Graf von der Schulenburg 2000). We nevertheless conclude that cost-effectiveness analysis is a powerful tool for priority setting. The shortcomings we identify do not imply it should be abandoned, but that improvements in methodology and coverage may enhance the practical usefulness of cost-effectiveness analysis.

EQUITY ISSUES

Cost-effectiveness analysis, in its simplest form, addresses only the efficiency concern of maximizing health subject to a budget constraint. In practice, policymakers usually want to set priorities that also address equity concerns to produce a "fair" allocation of resources.

We can identify seven concepts of equity: *egalitarianism,* which implies that everybody should have identical health status (Culyer and Wagstaff 1993; Le Grand 1982; Roemer 1998); *allocation according to need,* which relies on an adequate definition of "need" (Culyer and Wagstaff 1993; Hurley 2000; Nord 1996; Nord and others 1999; Williams 1978); the concept of *rule of rescue,* which posits an ethical duty to do everything possible to help people in immediate life-threatening situations (Hadorn 1991); *equality of access,* which is often used to operationalize the concept of equity but itself requires a definition of "access" as well as need (Culyer and Wagstaff 1993; Hurley 2000); the notion of providing a *decent minimum,* which involves definition of an essential package of health services (New 1997; New and Le Grand 1996); Rawls' *maximin principle,* which demands that social policy should seek to maximize the position of the worst-off (Bommier and Stecklov 2002; Olsen 1997; Rawls 1977); and *libertarianism,* which favors a distribution of resources according to entitlement.

It is important to recognize that any notion of fairness is ultimately a personal construct and that no concept is in any sense more legitimate than another. It is the politician's job to formulate a societal notion of the preferred concept of equity in the light of these individual viewpoints. However, many discussions of equity concepts are theoretical and remote from practical implementation issues, and therefore offer limited help to politicians. Most equity considerations can be captured under two broad headings: equity related to some *concept of need* (or "deservingness"), and equity related to *access to services*. In principle, these equity concerns can readily be incorporated into an economic approach to priority setting but require adjustments in the benefits and the costs of each intervention considered.

Regarding the first equity category, deservingness, among the possible criteria for allocating resources are:

- Capacity to benefit from health care (the only equity criterion consistent with the health maximization criterion)

- Expected future health (skewing resources toward individuals with lower potential for health)

- Previous health experience (skewing resources toward historically less healthy individuals)

- Rule of rescue (skewing resources toward individuals with immediate needs)

- Some other concept of need.

Each of these criteria except the first implies the existence of some dimension of social condition, or "need," against which otherwise identical health gains should be weighted differently. Suppose θ indicates an individual's need status (say life expectancy) and $f(\theta)$ indicates the population's probability density function. Consider an intervention i with expected benefit for any individual in need of b_i. Then, if the relative incidence of intervention i is given by $g_i(\theta)$, the total benefits B_i are given by

$$B_i \int b_i g_i(\theta) f(\theta) d(\theta)$$

A concern with equity implies a need to weight the benefits differently for each population group under consideration. That is, assuming a higher level of θ indicates a higher level of priority, there exists a function $w_B(\theta)$ such that

$$\int w_B(\theta) f(\theta) d\theta = 1$$

where $w_B(\theta_1) \geq w_B(\theta_2)$ if and only if $\theta_1 \geq \theta_2$. Weighted benefits are now written as

$$B_i^w = \int b_i g_i(\theta) w_B(\theta) f(\theta) d(\theta).$$

In some circumstances, the effectiveness of the intervention b_i also varies with the degree of need θ. This is readily incorporated into this formulation of aggregate benefits.

In other words, the health gains arising from an intervention will be valued differentially, depending on the beneficiary population group. This equity-weighted formulation of benefits will increase measured benefits for interventions used disproportionately by disadvantaged populations, at the expense of interventions used more by less needy populations. Williams' (1988) notion of an equity adjusted QALY (quality adjusted life year) is an example of such a construct. In a priority-setting context, therefore, such needs weighting should effect a shift toward programs favoring disadvantaged populations.

The second equity category, equity of access, implies an interest in increasing utilization among disadvantaged populations and recognition of their current unmet needs. Any strategy to improve access is likely to affect both the benefits and the costs of the intervention. Benefits will increase to the extent that more citizens receive the intervention. This means that we must change the incidence distribution from $g_i^1(\theta)$ (incidence without the access strategy) to $g_i^2(\theta)$ (incidence with the access strategy), where $g_i^2(\theta) \geq g_i^1(\theta)$. The increase in benefits is therefore

$$\Delta B_i = \int b_i g_i^2(\theta) f(\theta) d\theta - \int b_i g_i^1(\theta) f(\theta) d\theta$$

However, the strategy will also require additional resources to secure access to the intervention for disadvantaged groups, for example, in the form of a subsidy to encourage use. By definition, the expected costs of securing use of the intervention are greater for disadvantaged groups than for others. So we must now define a function $x_i^2(\theta)$ to reflect the differential unit costs of securing benefits b_i depending on social condition θ, where $x_i^2(\theta) \geq x_i$, the original unit costs of providing the intervention. Then the increased costs are recalculated as

$$\Delta X_i = \int x_i^2(\theta) g_i^2(\theta) f(\theta) d\theta - \int x_i g_i^1(\theta) f(\theta) d\theta$$

where it will usually be the case that $x_i^2(\theta_1) \geq x_i^2(\theta_2)$ if and only if $\theta_1 \geq \theta_2$.

In a priority-setting context, this second category of equity consideration may discriminate against conditions with a high incidence among disadvantaged groups or against programs with high relative costs of securing equity of access among disadvantaged groups. The desire to effect equity of access may disproportionately increase the costs of such interventions, making them less attractive for a priority setter.

Thus, introducing both outcome and access equity concepts is not inconsistent with the cost-effectiveness criterion. However, their introduction will change the cost-effectiveness rankings of individual interventions and therefore their priority ranking. Also, within a fixed budget, the incorporation of equity criteria will usually result in a reduction of the health gains secured by the chosen package, as some efficiency is sacrificed.

The nature and importance of the equity concept to be employed in priority setting is ultimately a political judgment. But the decisionmaker may wish to seek public views on what constitutes a "fair" distribution of health and health care. Attempts to elicit equity concepts from the general public have been made, applying ideas of fairness to operational priority-setting principles. For example, many people in the United Kingdom are keen to redirect considerable resources toward disadvantaged people, at the expense of other aspects of health care (Dolan and others 2000; Shaw and others 2001). The median respondent deems an intervention offering six months' improvement in life expectancy to the lowest social class equivalent to an intervention offering two years' improvement to the highest social class.

We have outlined the main equity concepts addressed in the literature. However, even if the theoretical issues set out above are addressed satisfactorily, the problem of how to use equity concepts in a practical way in the priority-setting process would still remain. For example, decisionmakers at different levels of the health care system may pursue different equity concepts. There is no guarantee that equity concepts framed at the national level are respected by regional or local administrators or by clinicians in their dealings with patients. Therefore, it may be necessary to change incentive structures, set up guidelines, or introduce audit procedures to implement successfully a chosen equity concept.

We nevertheless believe that—if clearly formulated—theoretical principles of equity can be made consistent with cost-effectiveness notions. However, to date they have contributed little to solving practical problems in setting priorities. The most promising areas—which are still fraught with difficulties—include the development of equity-weighted measures of health benefits, estimates of the additional costs of ensuring equity of access to health care services, attempts to define a decent minimum, and progress in eliciting the public's views about what constitutes a "fair" distribution of health and health care.

PRACTICAL CONSTRAINTS

Practical considerations often force decisionmakers to deviate from the decisions they would make if faced only with the simple efficiency–equity maximization problem. These can be considered under three headings: the political economy of priority setting, institutional constraints, and the links between health care financing and priority setting.

The Political Economy of Priority Setting

A spectrum of government utility functions can be envisaged with respect to health care. At one extreme, the government might be concerned solely with the long-run efficiency and equity concerns discussed above. At the other end of the spectrum, a government might set health priorities solely to offer the best prospect of its remaining in power, which may imply major departures from such long run-criteria. The most realistic scenario is likely to lie between these two extremes. The political economy models are therefore useful as an additional explanation for priority-setting decisions in practice. We briefly consider models of *majority voting, interest groups, bureaucratic decisionmaking,* and *rent-seeking* behavior.

MAJORITY VOTING MODELS

A government depends for its survival on the support of key interest groups. In principle, in democratic societies, the ultimate arbiter will be the electorate. A rich *theory of voting behavior* has been developed (Anderson 1999; Mueller 1989), but there is little evidence of its direct application in the health domain, despite the important role played by health in local and national elections. Prominent among the theories of majority rule voting is the notion of the median voter (Hotelling 1929). It focuses on the politician as a maximizer of votes, who seeks to develop policies that capture the vote of the median voter. Empirical results suggest that this model is often better—or as good—in explaining government spending decisions than competing models, at least in the United States (Ahmed and Greene 2000; Congleton and Bennett 1995; Congleton and Shugart 1990).

Models of voting behavior may explain why governments find it difficult to direct resources toward certain patient groups, even where justified on efficiency or equity grounds. For example, all citizens believe that they (or their relatives) may need emergency health care or maternity services, so expenditure on these services is likely to be widely supported. However, services directed at certain chronic conditions (for example,, certain mental illnesses) may receive less popular support because the median voter cannot perceive any personal need for them. Even if interventions for those chronic conditions are more cost-effective, the government may find it difficult to assign them high priority.

In many low-income countries, a small minority of wealthy citizens suffer mainly from noncommunicable and chronic conditions, whereas a large majority of the poor suffer mainly from communicable diseases and diseases associated with poor living conditions. Because there are more poor than wealthy individuals in the overall electorate, the median voter is likely to belong to the poor group. The median voter model predicts that most health care expenditure would be devoted to illnesses of the poor to win the median voter's support.

However, this is often not the case. The proportion of health care expenditure devoted to illnesses of the wealthy is often much higher than would be justified by the prevalence of these illnesses in the general population (World Bank 1993). An amended model can explain this by incorporating information about health care financing. Small groups of wealthy citizens pay a large proportion of taxes in low-income countries. To retain this tax base, the government may provide health care services to treat illnesses of the wealthy. This anomaly implies the need for a "tax-weighted" median voter model, which would shift the median voter into the wealthy rather than the poor group.

KEY INTEREST-GROUP MODELS

An alternative way of examining priority setting is to focus on key *interest groups* that influence the government's decisions. If, for example, a government relies for its survival on urban support, it may favor programs in such urban areas, even if they are less cost-effective than programs that benefit rural areas. A substantial body of literature has analyzed the interest group model of government and has shed light on why political institutions may fail to allocate resources efficiently (Holcombe 1985; McCormick and Tollison 1981; Weingast, Shepsle, and Johnsen 1981).

The interest-group model assumes that coalitions of individuals that have the lowest costs of organizing themselves (for example, becoming informed, lobbying, and securing group cohesion) have a comparative advantage in skewing resources in their interests (Olson 1971). For an overview of interest group models in low-income countries see Shugart (1999).

Many countries devolve stewardship of the health system to local governments, which may have broad autonomy over the choice of priorities and level of funding. Devolution can therefore lead to wide divergences between local and national priorities. Such variations may be both efficient and legitimate. For example, the urban services pattern would likely be inefficient or (in most people's view) inequitable if applied in remote rural areas.

Variations between local governments may, however, reflect inefficiencies or rigidities that inhibit pursuit of national priorities. National governments may wish to encourage local governments to change policies. Mechanisms for doing this, examined in the fiscal federalism literature (King 1984), are based mainly on grants-in-aid paid by national governments to localities. Grants can be used to deter undesirable activities or to encourage activity that would not otherwise take place.

This principle can also be applied to individual physicians or households whose behavior can influence the implementation of priorities. For example, poor compliance may compromise a national vaccination program that, in theory, is highly cost-effective. Because there is no guarantee that national policies will be reflected in local actions, a government may have to offer incentives for compliance and include their costs in any cost-effectiveness analysis.

Donor agencies often make their finance and support conditional on national actions, and their preoccupations may therefore be an important influence on national priority setting. For example, the Millennium Development Goals (MDGs) include several health-related topics and are therefore likely to materially influence national policies (IMF, OECD, U.N., World Bank Group 2000).

BUREAUCRATIC MODELS

Another locus of potential self-interest is represented by the *bureaucratic models* developed by commentators such as Tullock (1965) and Niskanen (1971). These focus on bureaucrats' interest in maximizing their influence and the effects of their behavior on the level and nature of government output. At the center of bureaucratic models is the implication that bureaucrats receive power and remuneration in proportion to the size of their "empires."

Such models for priority setting in health imply that government agencies will promote policies that enlarge their own enterprises and undermine proposals for activities outside their direct control. The key issue is that bureaucrats have informational advantages over their political counterparts. Ministers are therefore at a comparative disadvantage in setting policies in line with their own objectives (Niskanen 1975).

RENT-SEEKING MODELS

More generally, health systems result from a complex mixture of institutions, regulations, conventions, and historical accidents. These arrangements give great scope for what Tullock (1967) and Krueger (1974) refer to as *rent-seeking,* where various parties compete to appropriate the producer surpluses created by imperfectly competitive market structures. When the government undertakes projects, the possibility of transfers is created, triggering rent-seeking activity that dissipates society's potential gains from the project. Therefore, rent-seeking is another reason priority setting may fail to maximize societal welfare. Pedersen (1997) uses this approach to explain why, in low-income countries, urban social groups have gained more income than most of the population, who live in rural areas or urban shantytowns.

We have discussed various ways government failure influences the priority-setting process. Economic models of public choice represent the "dismal science" at its most dismal. Many of the models discussed are relevant to only a minority of countries, and the effects described may be counterbalanced by other mechanisms. We nevertheless believe it is vital to have a clear understanding of the potential for self-serving behavior in any political process and to develop a priority-setting policy that can either challenge or accommodate political realities and imperatives.

Institutional Constraints

An important consideration for any priority-setting endeavor is the managerial burden it imposes on the government. The informational requirements for priority setting are enormous, and judgments must often be made in the absence of relevant information. Limited managerial capacity and information resources may give rise to disagreement and instability in the priority-setting process. In its purest form, the rational cost-effectiveness model assumes that information capture is costless and that the required analytic capacity exists. However Simon (1957, 1959) characterizes the policymaking process as one of "satisficing" rather than optimizing. Instead of maximizing the benefit from a portfolio of health care programs, the politician's goal is to attain a satisfactory level of benefit.

INCREMENTAL DECISIONMAKING

The model of satisficing is linked to the long tradition of viewing government activity as an incremental process, in which problems are tackled on the basis of perceived urgency and importance. Lindblom (1959) characterizes the process as one of "muddling through." This incremental view conflicts with the "rational comprehensive" model assumed by cost-effectiveness models, and assumes that in practice a government should progressively remove ineffective programs and replace them with more effective actions. The incremental model implies that priorities are set on the basis of criteria that are ignored in conventional cost-effectiveness models, such as the magnitude of the program involved or practical considerations such as the feasibility and costs of change.

PROGRAM BUDGETING AND MARGINAL ANALYSIS

Program budgeting and marginal analysis, developed as a practical approach to priority setting, attempts to rationalize the incremental budgeting approach. Mitton and Donaldson (2002) have analyzed how key Canadian decisionmakers in regional health authorities set priorities. The decisionmakers reported that a clear process of setting priorities does not exist, and that resources are generally allocated on the basis of historical trends. Program budgeting and marginal analysis may be useful in such a context.

ROBUSTNESS ANALYSIS

Robustness analysis, originating from operational research, can be used as a means of incorporating uncertainty and transition costs into decisionmaking. Decisionmakers often exhibit considerable risk aversion, and reversing a decision that proves wrong may be extremely costly, either politically or in terms of real resources. Thus, it may be optimal for decisionmakers to adopt "robust" rather than optimal decisions (Gupta and Rosenhead 1968). For an overview of this theory, see Rosenhead (1980, 1989). The concept of robustness can take two forms: the decision is "good" (if not optimal) under a wide range of future scenarios, or the decision is readily reversed or altered if later information indicates a change in strategy is required.

OPTION PRICING THEORY

Option pricing theory offers a more formal approach to modeling the robustness of a decision to adopt a health care technology (Palmer and Smith 2000). The options approach is useful whenever a program's future costs and benefits are uncertain, subsequent abandonment would be costly, and a decision can be postponed. Option pricing adjusts the calculated cost-effectiveness ratio according to the degree of uncertainty and the costs of change, and explains why politicians are reluctant to make radical changes in existing priority-setting schemes. It explains why decisionmakers often appear conservative in retaining existing technologies and requiring a high rate of return from new technologies.

Links with the Financing System

The traditional priority-setting model considers choice of technologies independently of the health care finance system, although, in practice, the health system and the financing system may interact in important ways. Some financial mechanisms may have implications for provider or patient behavior (for example, stimulating or suppressing demand or changing insurance arrangements). These responses may influence who gains access to health care and how they do so, which in turn may affect health outcomes and equity. They may also affect the size of the revenue base available for funding collective health care.

The priority-setting literature generally presumes that a form of collective insurance is in place, with funding contributions independent of utilization. However, in practice all health systems use a mixture of funding mechanisms, and lower-income countries often rely heavily on direct user charges. We consider the additional methods of funding health care under three headings: private health insurance, complementary insurance, and direct user charges or informal payments.

PRIVATE HEALTH INSURANCE

Citizens can replace collective health care coverage with *private insurance.* Individuals who opt out may receive a rebate on the collective payment, which effectively subsidizes private insurance premiums. People will choose private coverage if the expected utility from the private package is greater than the expected utility from the proposed collective package, after taking account of the (possibly subsidized) private premium. Private insurance will be attractive to individuals with relatively high incomes, good health, and expected health care needs not covered by the collective benefit package.

Widespread reliance on private insurance has implications for activity and costs in the collective priority-setting process. Where the private premium is subsidized, the subsidy also effectively results in a loss of revenue for the collective system. Widespread opting out may reduce revenue-raising capacity, possibly leading to a downward spiral of increasing restrictions in the collective package and expanding private coverage. In short, the budget available for the collective package may be endogenous to the choice of package. In designing priorities under these arrangements, therefore, policymakers must consider the attractiveness of the collective package for anyone who is in a position to choose private insurance instead.

COMPLEMENTARY INSURANCE

Complementary insurance offers the opportunity to purchase coverage beyond the priorities encompassed in the basic package. Assuming no citizens can opt out of the basic package, this arrangement can allow some divergence from pure cost-effectiveness criteria in setting priorities. For example, the collective package could be targeted at interventions needed by the poor or at interventions needed to avoid widespread catastrophic payments.

FORMAL OR INFORMAL USER CHARGES

We now consider a system of *formal or informal user charges* operating alongside a collective health system. In the extreme case, user charges might be set at market clearing prices, and there would be little role for priority setting or collective provision. User charges are therefore generally lower than market prices for high-priority interventions. They then fulfill a dual role of moderating demand and partially financing the health system. However, they also leave room for catastrophic payments, substantial barriers to access, and therefore serious inequity.

When user charges are in place, a patient must decide whether the expected utility of an intervention exceeds the expected utility of forgoing the intervention, after taking into account the user charge. Where user charges cause impoverishment or inability to access care, their reduction or removal for the poor has to be considered. This will increase expenditures under the collective system (through increased demand) and reduce its income (through the subsidy). It may also alter political support for the collective system, depending on which individuals qualify for the subsidy. The implications of a user charge system can be examined mathematically, and this analysis reinforces the view that—when resources are limited—free access should be targeted at low-probability, high-cost conditions that would otherwise lead to catastrophic payments for the poor.

CONCLUSIONS

Priority setting in health care is a complex task. This brief survey illustrates the many theoretical, political, and practical obstacles confronting decisionmakers. It would be easy—but too pessimistic—to conclude that the priority-setting task is unmanageable, rather than merely difficult.

We believe that an economic approach to priority setting offers many advantages, not least that it forces decisionmakers to define the objectives of the priority-setting process. The process will often involve conflicts, but they will be made explicit. An economic perspective provides a framework for exploring conflicts and making tradeoffs clear.

However, the economic approach is just one element of the priority-setting process, and cannot be used to the exclusion of the many other factors that influence decisionmakers, some hard to incorporate into economists' models. Optimal approaches to the priority-setting process will depend on local circumstances and constraints. We nevertheless believe that the traditional economic approach can be expanded to incorporate both equity concerns and a wealth of practical constraints that influence decisions. Making these principles operational offers a rich and challenging agenda for researchers and policymakers.

REFERENCES

Ahmed, S., and K. V. Greene. 2000. "Is the Median Voter a Clear-Cut Winner? Comparing the Median Voter Theory and Competing Theories in Explaining Local Government Spending." *Public Choice* 105: 207–30.

Anderson, G. M. 1999. "Electoral Limits." In D. P. Racheter and R. E. Wagner, eds., *Limiting Leviathan*. Cheltenham, U.K. and Northampton, Mass.: Edward Elgar.

Anell, A., and P. Svarvar. 2000. "Pharmacoeconomics and Clinical Practice Guidelines: A Survey of Attitudes in Swedish Formulary Committees." *PharmacoEconomics* 17(2): 175–85.

Bommier, A., and G. Stecklov. 2002. "Defining Health Inequality: Why Rawls Succeeds Where Social Welfare Theory Fails." *Journal of Health Economics* 21(3): 497–513.

Briggs, A. 2001. "Handling Uncertainty in Economic Evaluation and Presenting the Results." In M. F. Drummond and A. McGuire, eds., *Economic Evaluation in Health Care: Merging Theory with Practice*. Oxford: Oxford University Press.

Burns, A., P. Charlwood, P. Darling, D. M. Fox, and L. Greenfield. 2000. *Better Information, Better Outcomes: The Use of Health Technology Assessment and Clinical Effectiveness Data in Health Care Purchasing Decisions in the United Kingdom and the United States*. Washington D.C.: Millbank Memorial Fund.

Congleton, R. D., and R. W. Bennett. 1995. "On the Political Economy of State Highway Expenditures: Some Evidence of the Relative Performance of Alternative Public Choice Models." *Public Choice* 84: 1–24.

Congleton, R. D., and W. F. Shugart. 1990. "The Growth of Social Security: Electoral Push or Political Pull." *Economic Inquiry* 28: 109–32.

Cox, E. R., B. R. Motheral, and D. Griffis. 2000. "Relevance of Pharmacoeconomics and Health Outcomes Information to Health Care Decisionmakers in the United States." *Value in Health* 3(2): 162 (abstract).

Culyer, A. J., and A. Wagstaff. 1993. "Equity and Equality in Health and Health Care." *Journal of Health Economics* 12(4): 431–57.

Darby, C., N. Valentine, A. DeSilva, and C. J. L. Murray. 2000. *World Health Organization (WHO): Strategy on Measuring Responsiveness*. Geneva: World Health Organization.

Dolan, P., R. Shaw, P. C. Smith, A. Tsuchiya, and A. Williams. 2000. *To Maximize Health or to Reduce Inequalities in Health? Toward a Social Welfare Function Based on Stated Preference Data*. York, U.K.: University of York, Centre for Health Economics.

Drummond, M. F., J. Cooke, and T. Walley. 1997. "Economic Evaluation under Managed Competition." *Social Science and Medicine* 45(4):583–95.

Drummond, M. F., and H. Weatherly. 2000. "Implementing the Findings of Health Technology Assessments: If the CAT Got Out of the Bag, Can the TAIL Wag the Dog?" *International Journal of Technology Assessment in Health Care* 16(1): 1–12.

Duthie, T., P. Trueman, J. Chancellor, and L. Diez. 1999. "Research into the Use of Health Economics in Decisionmaking in the United Kingdom." *Health Policy* 46: 143–57.

Ginsberg, M. E., R. L. Kravitz, and W. A. Sandberg. 2000. "A Survey of Physician Attitudes and Practices Concerning Cost-Effectiveness in Patient Care." *Western Journal of Medicine* 173: 390–93.

Grizzle, A. J., B. M. Olsen, B. R. Motheral, E. P. Armstrong, J. Abarca, and E. R. Cox. 2000. "Therapeutic Value: Who Decides?" *Pharmaceutical Executive* November: 84–90.

Gupta, S. K., and J. Rosenhead. 1968. "Robustness in Sequential Investment Decisions." *Management Science* 15: 18–29.

Hadorn, D.C. 1991. "Setting Health Priorities in Oregon: Cost-Effectiveness Meets the Rule of Rescue." *Journal of the American Medical Association* 265: 2218–25.

Hauck, K., P. Smith, and M. Goddard. 2003. *The Economics of Priority Setting for Health: A Literature Review*. Washington, D.C.: World Bank.

Hoffmann, C., and J. M. Graf von der Schulenburg. 2000. "The Influence of Economic Evaluation Studies on Decisionmaking. A European Survey." *Health Policy* 52: 179–92.

Hoffmann, C., B. A. Stoykova, J. Nixon, J. M. Glanville, K. Misso, and M. F. Drummond. 2002. "Do Health-Care Decisionmakers Find Economic Evaluations Useful? The Findings of Focus Group Research in U.K. Health Authorities." *Value in Health* 5(2): 71–78.

Holcombe, R. G. 1985. *An Economic Analysis of Democracy*. Carbondale: Southern Illinois University Press.

Hotelling, H. 1929. "Stability in Competition." *Economic Journal* 39: 41–57.

Hurley, J. 2000. "An Overview of the Normative Economics of the Health Sector." In A. J. Culyer and J. P. Newhouse, eds., *North-Holland Handbook of Health Economics*. Amsterdam: Elsevier.

IMF, OECD, U.N., World Bank Group (International Monetary Fund, Organisation for Economic Co-operation and Development, United Nations, and World Bank Group). 2000. *A Better World for All: Progress toward the International Development Goals*. Washington, D.C., and London: Communications Development and Grundy and Northedge.

Jack, W. 2000. "Public Spending on Health Care: How Are Different Criteria Related? A Second Opinion." *Health Policy* 53: 61–67.

King, D.N. 1984. *Fiscal Tiers: The Economics of Multilevel Government*. London: Allen and Unwin.

Krueger, A. O. 1974. "The Political Economy of the Rent-Seeking Society." *American Economic Review* 64:291–303.

Le Grand, J. 1982. *The Strategy of Equality*. London: Allen and Unwin.

Lindblom, C. E. 1959. "The 'Science' of Muddling Through." *Public Administration* 19: 79–88.

Mandelblatt, J. S., D. G. Fryback, M. C. Weinstein, L. B. Russell, M. R. Gold, and D. C. Hadorn. 1996. "Assessing the Effectiveness of Health Interventions." In M. R. Gold, J. E. Siegel, L. B. Russell, and M. C. Weinstein, eds., *Cost-Effectiveness in Health and Medicine*, New York: Oxford University Press.

Manning, W. G., D. G. Fryback, and M. C. Weinstein. 1996. "Reflecting Uncertainty in Cost-Effectiveness Analysis." In M. R. Gold, J. E. Siegel, L. B. Russell, and M. C. Weinstein, eds., *Cost-Effectiveness in Health and Medicine*. New York: Oxford University Press.

McCormick, R. E., and R. D. Tollison. 1981. *Politicians, Legislation, and the Economy: An Inquiry into the Interest-Group Theory of Government*. Boston: Martinus Nijhoff.

Mitton, C., and C. Donaldson. 2002. "Setting Priorities in Canadian Regional Health Authorities: A Survey of Key Decisionmakers." *Health Policy* 60: 39–58.

Mueller, D. C. 1989. *Public Choice II*. Cambridge: Cambridge University Press.

New, B. 1997. "Defining a Package of Health Care Services the NHS Is Responsible For: The Case For." In B. New, ed., *Rationing: Talk and Action in Health Care*. London: King's Fund and BMJ.

New, B., and J. Le Grand. 1996. *Rationing in the NHS: Principles and Pragmatism.* London: King's Fund.

Niskanen, W. A. 1971. *Bureaucracy and Representative Government.* Chicago: Aldine-Atherton.

———. 1975. "Bureaucrats and Politicians." *Journal of Law and Economics* 18: 617–644.

Nord, E. 1996. "Health Status Index Models for Use in Resource Allocation Decisions. A Critical Review in the Light of Observed Preferences for Social Choice." *International Journal of Technology Assessment in Health Care* 12: 31–44.

Nord, E., J. L. Pinto, J. Richardson, P. Menzel, and P. Ubel. 1999. "Incorporating Societal Concerns for Fairness in Numerical Valuations of Health Programs." *Health Economics* 8: 25–39.

O'Brien, B. J., and M. J. Sculpher. 2000. "Building Uncertainty into Cost-Effectiveness Rankings: Portfolio Risk-Return Tradeoffs and Implications for Decision Rules." *Medical Care* 38(5): 460–68.

Olsen, E. O. 1997. "Theories of Justice and Their Implications for Priority Setting in Health Care." *Journal of Health Economics* 16: 625–39.

Olson, M. 1971. *The Logic of Collective Action: Public Goods and the Theory of Groups.* Cambridge, Mass.: Harvard University Press.

Palmer, S., and P. C. Smith. 2000. "Incorporating Option Values into the Economic Evaluation of Health Care Technologies." *Journal of Health Economics* 19: 755–66.

Pedersen, K. R. 1997. "The Political Economy of Distribution in Developing Countries: A Rent-Seeking Approach." *Public Choice* 91: 351–73.

Phelps, C. E. 1997. "Good Technologies Gone Bad. How and Why the Cost-Effectiveness of Medical Intervention Changes for Different Populations." *Medical Decisionmaking* 17: 107–17.

Phillips, M. 1993. "Setting Global Priorities for Strategies to Control Diarrhoeal Disease: The Contribution of Cost-Effectiveness Analysis." In A. Mills and K. Lee, eds., *Health Economics Research in Developing Countries.* Oxford: Oxford University Press.

Rawls, J. 1977. *A Theory of Justice.* Cambridge, Mass.: Harvard University Press.

Roemer, J. 1998. *Equality of Opportunity.* Cambridge, Mass.: Harvard University Press.

Rosenhead, J. 1980. "Planning under Uncertainty 2: A Methodology for Robustness Analysis." *Journal of Operational Research Society* 31: 331–41.

Rosenhead, J. 1989. "Robustness Analysis: Keeping Your Options Open." In J. Rosenhead, ed., *Rational Analysis for a Problematic World: Problem Structuring Methods for Complexity, Uncertainty and Conflict.* Chichester: John Wiley and Sons Ltd.

Shaw, R., P. Dolan, A. Tsuchiya, A. Williams, P. C. Smith, and R. Burrows. 2001. *Development of a Questionnaire to Elicit People's Preferences Regarding Health Inequalities.* York, U.K.: University of York, Centre for Health Economics.

Shugart, W. F. 1999. "The Interest-Group Theory of Government in Developing Economy Perspective." In M. S. Kimenyi and J. M. Mbaku, eds., *Institutions and Collective Choice in Developing Countries.* Aldershot: Ashgate Publishing Ltd.

Simon, H. A. 1957. *Models of Man.* New York: John Wiley and Sons.

————. 1959. "Theories of Decisionmaking in Economics and Behavioral Science." *American Economic Review* 49: 253–83.

Sloan, F. A., K. Whetten-Goldstein, and A. Wilson. 1997. "Hospital Pharmacy Decisions, Cost-Containment, and the Use of Cost-Effectiveness Analysis." *Social Science and Medicine* 45(4): 523–33.

Torrance, G. W., J. E. Siegel, and B. R. Luce. 1996. "Framing and Designing the Cost-Effectiveness Analysis." In M. R. Gold, J. E. Siegel, L. B. Russell, and M. C. Weinstein, eds., *Cost-Effectiveness in Health and Medicine.* New York: Oxford University Press.

Tullock, G. 1965. *The Politics of Bureaucracy.* Washington, D.C.: Public Affairs Press.

————. 1967. "The Welfare Costs of Tariffs, Monopolies and Theft." *Western Economic Journal* 5: 224–32.

Weingast, B. R., K. A. Shepsle, and C. Johnsen. 1981. "The Political Economy of Benefits and Costs: A Neoclassical Approach to Distributive Politics." *Journal of Political Economy* 89: 642–46.

Williams, A. 1978. "Need: An Economic Exegesis." In A. J. Culyer and K. G. Wright, eds., *Economic Aspects of Health Services.* London: Martin Robertson.

————. 1988. "Ethics and Efficiency in the Provision of Health Care." In J. M. Bell and S. Mendus, eds., *Philosophy and Medical Welfare.* Cambridge: Cambridge University Press.

World Bank. 1993. *World Development Report 1993: Investing in Health.* New York, Oxford University Press for the World Bank.

WHO (World Health Organization). 2000. *The World Health Report 2000. Health Systems: Improving Performance.* Geneva.

————. 2001. *Macroeconomics and Health: Investing in Health for Economic Development. Report of the Commission on Macroeconomics and Health.* Chaired by J. D. Sachs. Geneva.

CHAPTER 4

From Whom to Buy? Selecting Providers

Fernando Montenegro Torres and Cristian Baeza

From whom should medical services be purchased? In answering this important question, we argue that, for a strategic purchaser, the central objective is to achieve the necessary correspondence between the interventions the purchaser wants and the provider that can deliver the intervention within an appropriate time frame, with the best quality standards, and at the lowest price possible. We call this correspondence the *intervention-provider matching*. Strategic purchasing in this context means that purchasers can and do act selectively in choosing their suppliers. Although this might seem all too obvious, in reality the necessary correspondence between intervention and provider is at the core of the problem of purchasing selectivity.

For a purchaser to "match" the intervention with the appropriate provider, some basic conditions must be met. First, the purchaser must be entitled institutionally, legally, and administratively to be selective and therefore to take part in the decisions regarding the selection of providers. Second, there must be multiple providers to choose from, a variety of providers offering comparable products. Finally, the purchaser and the providers must be able to establish a purchasing-providing relationship within the regulatory and legal environment in which the purchaser carries out its decisions.

We focus on three principal criteria for selecting a provider and establishing a successful relationship with the purchaser. They can be summarized as follows:

- Can the purchaser identify the intervention that has to be purchased and appropriately match the intervention to an eligible provider?

- Has the purchaser the necessary institutional and technical capabilities to be selective in the purchasing process?

- Is the purchaser entitled to be selective, and is there more than one type of provider to choose from?

DEFINING AND IDENTIFYING ELIGIBLE PROVIDERS AND MATCHING THE INTERVENTION

Irrespective of the type or complexity of the intervention, the purchaser should carefully define the intervention before beginning the negotiation and contracting process with providers. The success or failure of this task of definition can greatly influence the contracting process, the purchaser–provider relationship, and the final results.

In a *fee-for-service payment system,* the purchasing process is highly fragmented and unintegrated. The provider ultimately decides which health care goods and services to buy and in what volumes. The relationship between provider and purchaser is essentially a mere reimbursement transaction not comprehensively influenced by health outcomes. At the other side of the spectrum, in developing countries where traditional historical budgets often provide operating funds for public providers, the decisions regarding the services to be financed are made de facto at the provider level. These decisions are the result of a combination of provider limitations and the population's actual demand for services.

In both fee for service in private health insurance in the United States and historic budgets of public health ministries in Latin America (just to mention two radically different examples); the emphasis is placed on health care services and not on outcomes. In reviewing the budgeting process, ministries of health seldom attempt to measure the health status of a population using proxy variables (mortality of children under five years of age, maternal mortality). Typically, within the framework it is assumed that the financial risk is borne by the purchaser (fee-for-service model) or by the objective constraints imposed by the lack of resources in public facilities (historical budgets of ministries of health).

However, when a split between purchaser and provider occurs and an explicit separation emerges between the purchasing and the provision functions, more precise definitions of the health interventions to be purchased are needed. With a focus on outcomes and not on services provided, and a more precise definition of what to purchase, the purchaser can now strategize between health interventions. These interventions can be measured, monitored, and linked to outcomes in reimbursing providers, thus establishing new sets of incentives for better outcomes.

A strategic purchaser should establish a clear correspondence between the desired intervention and the selection of the best provider. The criteria and information a purchaser uses to buy individual services are different from those used by a purchaser to buy more comprehensive health outcomes. Therefore the matching between the provider and the product or outcomes can occur within a broad spectrum of types of health care services. The purchaser may want to buy very precise interventions or services or may need to purchase more comprehensive outcomes such as health care services for individuals with specific diseases or for population groups (for example, patients with acquired immunodeficiency syndrome, mental health care services, mothers and children from lower income groups) or integrated health care services to promote and take care of the health of a whole population living within a specific geographical area.

For well-defined services limited in scope, such as weight and height control of children under five years of age (under-5), the strategic purchaser should seek a provider that can offer those specific services most effectively and at the lowest possible cost. In this case, contracting with medical specialists (here, pediatricians) may not be necessary to get what the purchaser wants. Other health care professionals such as a nurse, skilled nurses' aide, or even a trained community member might provide the service more effectively and efficiently and most probably as a stand-alone provider.

However, if permitted by the regulatory environment and the purchaser can develop more strategic purchasing options, outcomes that are more comprehensive might be preferred over isolated services. If the purchaser wants to buy a complex set of interventions and focuses on outcomes such as maternal-and-child health indicators, a variety of providers representing many specialties and types of professional skills (for example, pediatricians, obstetrician-gynecologists, and nurses) is probably a more suitable alternative.

For the provision of complex health outcomes, the network of participating providers needed is not merely an expansion or agglomeration of different types of primary health care physicians, specialists and ancillary services, and administrative professionals. Rather, it is a complex system that commands more than just medical knowledge and management capacity. Moreover, the purchaser has to bear in mind that, both for the purchaser and for the provider, important opportunity costs are associated with providing a continuum of services via the integration of providers and services. The delivery of health care services to an entire population or subgroups of a population necessitates complex organizations having the capacity for integrating different functions and structures that are not always available in developing countries but that can emerge as a result of a new regulatory environment and the emergence of strategic purchasers focusing on broader outcomes.

What Are the Special Challenges of Aiming to Purchase Outcomes Related to the Health of Populations?

The best way to use outcomes as a tool for strategic purchasing is to aim for the most comprehensive outcome interventions whenever these outcomes can be measured and monitored. In an ideal world, a healthy population would be the ultimate outcome. However, owing to the multidimensionality of the health of a population, the contributions of health care services to this complex outcome are difficult to measure.

Nevertheless, some operational tools have been suggested for linking reimbursement of comprehensive services to combined measures of health within the environment of integrated delivery of health care services (Studnicki and others 2002). Shortell (1992), for instance, describes the health promotion accountability region (HPAR), a type of integrated delivery system at a regional level, as a geographical unit for reimbursement mechanisms that would be partially tied to improvements in population health status. These improvements could be measured by a combined index of morbidity and disability. Kindig (1997, 1998) suggests a financial mechanism that rewards integrated delivery systems for improvements in an index combining life expectancy, morbidity, and disability in what he labels as HALE, health-adjusted life expectancy. In any case, it seems more feasible to develop payment mechanisms for reimbursing integrated delivery systems than individual providers when considering broad outcomes such as those mentioned above.

In a few, well-defined situations, however, a strategic purchaser may not wish to buy a comprehensive product from an integrated network of providers. For instance, when the probability of requiring an intervention is low, but the intervention is costly and complex, purchasers and providers may be better off excluding it from the comprehensive outcome-focused contract. In that case, the purchaser may be better off managing direct access to services for that special health condition or contracting with a provider specializing in it, so that the provider has the minimum number of cases to maintain the technical skills and the economies of scale required for such complex interventions. Providers are better off because they do not have to bear the risk of providing such interventions, and the risk is pooled at the highest level possible by the purchaser itself.

The definition of the product or service that the purchaser wants to buy is related to the degree of the separation of functions. Some public institutions may purchase only services not offered by public providers, which represents a limited form of purchasing. Other public organizations may have already started a process of separating functions and may have begun to contract out with private providers with the goal of eventually purchasing all services from private and public providers. Strategic purchasing and the definitions of the desired product must be carefully analyzed within the context of the institutional and organization changes of the institutions and organizations in which the purchaser exists, but must also be developed as a capacity-building tool within the context of longer-term objectives. In this sense, strategic purchasing can be a useful tool in the health care reform process.

Do the Providers Have the Organizational and Institutional Capacity to Deliver the Intervention?

As the intervention that the purchaser wants to buy increases in complexity and gets closer to broader outcomes, so too does the range of the providers' professional and technical profiles, the intricacy of the related administrative functions, and the institutional and organizational capabilities needed to work as an integrated network of health care services.

THE HANDS-OFF APPROACH

The necessary network of health care service providers is not merely an expansion or agglomeration of different types of primary health care physicians, specialists and ancillary services, and administrative professionals. It is a complex system that requires more than just medical knowledge or management capacity. It requires a provider capable of integrating different functions and structures, bonded by the "glue" of the goal of achieving a variety of health outcomes within the limits of specific organizational and institutional incentives. If the provider has the required "integrating tissue" for delivering a continuum of care, the purchaser can have a more "hands-off" approach. The purchaser does not need to focus on the problem of integrating services and can concentrate on monitoring outcomes, thus avoiding micromanagement of the health care services to obtain the desired outcomes.

At the same time, when the purchaser buys isolated, limited interventions, the entire burden of integration needed to achieve the best outcomes falls upon the purchaser. If the purchaser cannot become the integrating tissue in the absence of capacity or willingness of providers to do so, the purchasing process will become fragmented and focused on isolated interventions.

THE HANDS-ON APPROACH

In developing countries without such providers, organizational capacity typically does not exist. An environment in which many individual providers can offer only fragmented services poses a challenge to the purchaser to work with independent providers and simultaneously support them with organizational capacity that gives patients access to a seamless continuum of services. Alternatively, the purchaser can encourage the development of such organizational capacity during the contracting and purchasing process. Fragmented providers can eventually develop the required integrating tissue as a result of several actions by the purchaser and the establishment of changing financial incentives that promote the integration of delivery organizations. This is what we call a hands-on approach on the part of the purchaser.

In most low-income countries, however, providers' low organizational and weak institutional capacity undermines effective coordination among providers, and frequently this applies to public purchasers as well. Before implementing broader separation of the functions of purchasing and providing services and aiming to work with independent providers, an investment in building up institutional capacity in the public and private sectors must be ensured.

CAN THE PURCHASER BUY THE DESIRED INTERVENTION FROM THE ELIGIBLE PROVIDERS?

In middle- and low-income countries, physicians, nurses, and nurses' aides make up a vast group of independent providers, but in most cases their practice is largely unregulated, and out-of-pocket expenditures pay for their services.

Identifying Eligible Providers and the Public and Private Institutional and Organizational Capabilities

In some middle-income countries, groups of physicians have started to merge into new forms of association, sometimes integrated with inpatient services. This type of integration offers some opportunities for public purchasers; however, it is important that contracts with these types of providers be carried out in the appropriate regulatory environment. In most low- and middle-income countries, most physicians who work for publicly funded organizations also have their own practices. Contracting with this type of provider has to take into account the risks of contracting with private providers who are allowed to work for both public and private organizations. In such an unregulated environment, purchasing can promote perverse incentives. Additionally, identifying an eligible provider is directly related to the particularities of the geographical area and the population for whom the purchaser buys services. For instance, if the purchaser wants to identify primary health care physicians and specialists in areas with a high concentration of accredited physicians, human resources might not be a problem. However, the situation is different in remote rural areas where the population is scattered over large geographical areas or in hard-to-reach places.

In developing countries, public institutions (social security and ministries of health) and policymakers are quite familiar with vertically integrated systems, because they are the classical model for health services delivery under historical budgets. Rigid vertical integration models are not, however, the only type of integrated delivery that can meet the demands of strategic purchasers. *Virtual integration,* for instance, can occur in developing countries when public purchasers work with a network of private providers with different capacities to provide integrated health care services.

To provide health care services for a defined population, the purchaser can also aim to contract with a fully integrated network of private providers, also known as *integrated delivery organizations*. However, effective integrated systems require not only health care services management but also tools for collecting and analyzing data collection and financial and risk-management capabilities. In the context of developing countries, these prerequisites imply real limitations for integrated delivery organizations that have only rudimentary information, financial, and risk-management capabilities.

If the purchaser has enough purchasing power and buys health care services directly from independent providers and providers with some integrated services, the purchaser can determine the rules that will govern the delivery of health care services and the management of information. However, if the providers lack the resources to develop and manage health information systems, the purchaser may have to take over these functions.

When acquiring services from both public providers and private integrated delivery systems, a purchaser has to ask some important questions. How should consumers be allocated to the different parts of the mixed system? Should they be permitted to choose between seeing a "public" provider and signing with an integrated delivery organization? To what extent does geographical location limit the availability of eligible providers? The choice of options can vary according to socioeconomic considerations (for example, household income) as in Colombia where the better-off must join the equivalent of a health maintenance organization, but the poor can also choose a public provider, or according to geographical location, as in Chile, where only public providers practice in rural areas.

Another important issue to be resolved is related to human resources. Should health care professionals be permitted to work both for an integrated delivery organization (that has a public contract) and as an independent provider with whom a public purchaser can establish a contract? This question is important for most developing countries where physicians can both work in the public sector and simultaneously run independent practices and where lack of regulation gives physicians the wrong incentives to move patients back and forth between public and private environments.

These issues are closely related to inequities in the quality of health care services, especially when policies target demographic subgroups.

Are There Eligible Providers and Is the Purchaser Allowed to Be Selective?

At first, it seems evident that a purchaser should be entitled to select the best providers available to serve its clients' needs. Such a selective approach toward providers, however, is not always feasible for two main reasons: first, purchasers may not have a mandate to contract selectively and may be required to have funding agreements with all public providers regardless of their performance; second, even if purchasers have the legal mandate to contract with eligible providers, the provider market may not be competitive.

Lack of supply and natural monopolies in the provision of health care services can occur in the case of complex health interventions. Multiple providers are most likely when there are no or small barriers to market entry. Providers of highly complex interventions face significant barriers to entry and are not usually subject to contestability. In contrast, low-complexity interventions tend to behave like commodities, and providers face few barriers to entry, which makes for a highly contestable market.

Monopolies in provision can also occur because of limitations in selectivity by the regulatory and legal framework. The purchaser may not be entitled to be selective because of its legal and regulatory operating environment or because of its governance structure and accountability (table 4.1).

TABLE 4.1   Modalities between Purchaser and Provider Market Structures

Purchaser provider	Single	Multiple
Single	Bilateral monopoly (rural Hungary)	Competitive purchasing with monopolistic provision (rural Chile)
Multiple	Monopolistic purchasing with competitive provision (urban Hungary, Brazil, Kyrgyzstan)	Competitive purchasing and provision (urban Chile, Lebanon)

Source: Authors.

If natural monopolies and legal and regulatory restrictions to selectivity occur and selectivity is impossible or will take a long time to happen, imposing performance targets on providers is an alternative. These performance targets—imitating performance pressures from fully free selection purchasing—can be applied in contexts where, in the short run, the purchaser action is constrained to only periodic changes in the conditions and targets specified in the contracts.

Even when selectivity is not possible, correct incentives have to be created for the purchaser to set targets for providers through such noncompeting initiatives as management contestability and yardstick competition.

Management contestability implies competition not for market share at any specific time but competition over time. The management of a monopoly hospital may be open to public bid. The winner will not have any competitive pressures for market share for the duration of the contract because the hospital has a monopoly and no competitors can enter that market. However, the management company is still under competitive pressure because the contract and funding will expire and will be advertised again. The management company's performance during the contract period will influence its chances of winning the next contract.

Benchmark or *yardstick competition* refers to the use of comparative provider performance indicators to put pressure on providers to improve performance, or as a basis for determining service prices. The introduction of *quasi contracts* (performance agreements) has been used extensively in public sector reform to achieve this goal. This mechanism relies on the monopolistic purchasing power of single-payer purchasers that allows them to attach performance conditions to funding.

Trends in separating purchasing and provision in public sector reforms are oriented to these noncompetitive settings. It is frequently argued that the change in the incentive environment of providers (both public and private monopolies), even without selectivity, through management contestability, yardstick competition, or similar approaches, would be enough to create the right incentives for providers to significantly increase efficiency, quality, and responsiveness. But does it really work? The evidence suggests that such an approach is insufficient and that true competition and selectivity are required to set correct incentives for providers to improve efficiency (Baeza and others 2001).

When the purchaser's regulatory and legal environment limits selectivity and provider monopolies exist, the purchaser's main goal should be to achieve selectivity as soon as possible. During the transition, management contestability and yardstick competition can be solutions but only when designed as temporary alternatives. Several problems have to be solved to achieve selectivity.

In actuality, many public purchasers are forced to buy from specific public providers to avoid creating operational deficits as a result of restrictive and rigid management rules for production inputs, as is frequently the case with manpower (some examples and good case studies are the national health services of Chile, New Zealand, and the United Kingdom).

REFERENCES

Baeza, C., A. Harding, M. Nuñez, and A. S. Preker. 2001. "From Whom to Purchase? Selecting Providers." Paper prepared for the Conference on Resource Allocation and Purchasing, May 14, 2001, World Bank, Washington, D.C.

Baeza, C., M. Jakab, J. Langenbrunner, and A. S. Preker. 2000. "Resource Allocation and Purchasing (RAP) Arrangements that Benefit the Poor and Excluded Groups: Concept Note." World Bank/ILO/WHO RAP Project, Washington, D.C.

Kindig, D. 1997. *Purchasing Population Health: Paying for Results*. Ann Arbor: University of Michigan Press.

———. 1998. "Purchasing Population Health: Aligning Financial Incentives to Improve Health Outcomes." *Health Services Research* 33(2): 223–42.

Shortell, S. 1992. "A Model for State Health Reform." *Health Affairs* 11(1): 108–27.

Studnicki, J., F. Murphy, D. Malvey, R. Costello, S. Luther, and D. Werner. 2002. "Toward a Population Health Delivery System: First Steps in Performance Measurement." *Health Care Management Review* 27(1): 76–95.

CHAPTER 5

How to Pay? Understanding and Using Payment Incentives

John C. Langenbrunner and Xingzhu Liu

Many countries have experimented with alternative ways of paying providers of health care services. This chapter illustrates different methods, suggests some of the theoretical advantages and limitations of each, and provides a framework for evaluating alternatives.

Under resource allocation and purchasing (RAP) arrangements, payments to health care providers can be approached in three ways:

- Direct payment to providers by the patient

- Direct payment to providers by the patient, but with later full or partial reimbursement

- Direct payment to the provider by the RAP mechanism, with only a limited copayment or informal charge paid by the patient.

Direct payment by the patient sends the consumer a clear signal about the price of the service. However, poor patients or patients receiving expensive care for major illnesses may not have the disposable income. Even full or partial reimbursement later may not be able to bridge the period between paying for the service and receiving a full or partial reimbursement.

When providers are reimbursed primarily through RAP arrangements rather than patients, the payment incentives and mechanism used, rather than prices and demand, create the behavioral environment for suppliers of services.

Owing to information asymmetry, neither consumers nor producers have full information about preferences, prices, or the market in which they operate. The level, mix, and quality of care for patients can be ascertained only after the fact, and good health depends on other factors besides the health services consumed. Physicians act as agents for their patients (Arrow 1963), but often not even they know the full impact of the interventions that they are recommending. Both consumer and provider behavior is therefore important. Pricing and payment mechanisms provide an opportunity to shape the behavior of both through incentives.

PAYMENT SYSTEM TYPES AND A CONCEPTUAL FRAMEWORK FOR INCENTIVES

Oxley (1995) characterizes the financial relationship between funders (purchasers) and providers of health services in three categories:

- The *reimbursement approach* in which providers are funded *retrospectively* for services delivered. Under this open-ended "fee-for-service" model, the agents determine the nature and quality of health service (that is, the patients and the physicians) and face little in the way of financial consequences.

- The *contract approach* involving some kind of *prospective* agreement between purchaser and provider regarding the terms and conditions of payment. The contract approach allows specification of the intensity and quality of care.

- An *integrated approach* to health systems design, combining the roles of purchaser and provider under a single institutional umbrella (often a local or central government).

This characterization of payment mechanisms can be applied to funding of both hospital and individual providers (for example, physicians). Impacts of these alternative payment mechanisms should be assessed in the context of objectives such as quality of care, cost, and targeting to the poor. But often the objectives are multiple and competing, and conflicts or tensions arise across the multiple behaviors of purchasers, providers, and patients. Several parties' objectives may be equally desirable but mutually irreconcilable in the sense that payment systems' capacity to achieve each objective are not the same, and multiple objectives may compete or conflict with each other. Among the tensions illustrated by the literature on provider payments are:

- Quality-enhancement and cost containment (Ellis and McGuire 1990)

- Provider risk and production efficiency (Jack forthcoming)

- Risk-selection and production efficiency (Newhouse 1998)

- "Fairness" in levels of payment and optimal levels of service (Jencks and others 1984).

Provider response to payment incentives has been analyzed through both principal-agent models and monopolistic competitive models. Principal-agent theory recognizes and explicitly models the potential conflicts of interest between different actors, emphasizing asymmetry of information as the critical problem in disciplining providers. Going principal-agent models one better, monopolistic competitive models explicitly consider the effects of competition among a plurality of health providers.

Using these models from the perspective of the tensions outlined above, the literature suggests that retrospective payment systems address issues of access, acceptable levels of provider risk, adequate revenues, patient selection, and quality enhancement. Prospective payments do better on optimal levels of services, efficiency, and cost containment. With integrated models, cost containment is often an outcome, but the overall impact depends upon how internal managers allocate resources within these integrated environments.

WHICH PAYMENT SYSTEM SHOULD BE CHOSEN?

Payment systems should respond to an explicit hierarchy of policy priorities as well as practical considerations.

Purchasers first have to decide on policy objectives—increased revenues, efficiency, cost containment, access, quality, administrative simplicity, or some combination. The payment system chosen and the incentives used have to address one or more health sector policy objectives at that particular time. Incentives must be chosen in tandem with other factors such as improved knowledge about clinical outcomes, cultural factors, and providers' professional ethics.

On the practical side, owing to asymmetry of information, payments are often linked to outputs, which are more easily observable and verified (by both parties) than the attainment of health outcomes or policy objectives such as improved efficiency or equity. In addition, when purchasers begin to consider new incentives, decisions are typically based on readily available information, technical capacity, and time available to design, implement, and then monitor payment systems.

Purchasers have to grapple with the basic mechanics of developing a payment system for providers. Purchasers view payment mechanisms along two axes (figure 5.1): the unit of payment and the level of payment.

FIGURE 5.1   Dimensions of Developing a Payment System

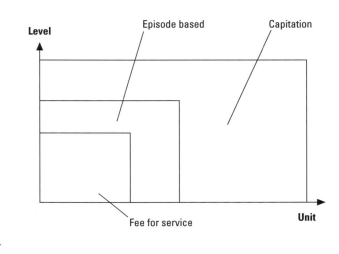

Source: Authors.

The unit of payment can be discrete, say, a visit or a test, but even these units can be further subdivided. At the other extreme, the unit of payment can be much more aggregate—an episode of care or even some bundle of needed services for a defined period of time such as one year.

The rate or level of payment will be based on

- Standard and perceived cost of the services

- Number of providers

- Competition among providers

- Health product volume

- Availability of good information

- Ability of patients to copay.

Other factors, such as provider influence and governance issues, are also important (see chapter 6, this volume, by Waters and Hussey regarding price setting).

Often when purchasers have to develop a payment system, they have too little time and technical resources to design a good one. The purchasers' lack of technical capacity and sound baseline information on cost and volume of needed care may force them initially to merge these two dimensions, allocating resources on a historical basis or on the basis of gross categories of inputs. This is closest aligned with the Oxley notion of an integrated approach; specific examples of such mechanisms are discussed below.

Line-Item Budgets

This lack of information often results in use of the line-item budgeting approach. The provider is paid an amount per given period (usually per year) for a defined responsibility of service provision. The total amount is broken down into, for instance, salaries, drugs, equipment, maintenance, and the like. Managers cannot switch funds across the line items without approval by the funding agency such as the ministry of finance. Line-item budgets are typically provided by governments directly for publicly run facilities, where there is no purchaser–provider split. This approach was common in Eastern bloc and former Soviet Union republics, as well as in many Soviet-influenced systems in the Arab Republic of Egypt, some African countries, and Vietnam. It is also still found in many government-run systems in all regions of the world, regardless of income (for example, Bahrain, Bangladesh, Mozambique).

Line-item budgeting does offer strong administrative controls, often valued by government-run providers. At a theoretical level, technical and allocative efficiency of health interventions can be optimized by manipulating the government budget lines over time to increase delivery of cost-effective health interventions and decrease delivery of less-cost-effective interventions. This assumes governments can track and understand the right combination to achieve these outputs, but in reality, they cannot for lack of good monitoring information. That is why line-item budgeting is being abandoned across the world. Too frequently, line-item budgets have been based on poor or inappropriate information (table 5.1) and they have provided incentives for inefficient use of resources, with fast spend-outs by the end of the budget year. The line budget is rigid in use of resources and discourages use of the best and the least costly combination of inputs for providers to produce services (Ensor and Langenbrunner 2002).

Salary

Closely related to line-item budgeting, and often used in conjunction with it, is use of salary as a payment method for doctors on the basis of the time worked. A part-time or full-time salary can be paid depending on the pattern of employment. Salary payment to doctors is quite common. For example, all hospital-based doctors in China and the United Kingdom are salaried. Doctors who provide care in outpatient health centers are often salaried in Finland, the former U.S.S.R., Greece, India, Indonesia, Israel, Portugal, Spain, Sweden, Turkey, and many Latin American countries (Ron, Abel-Smith, and Tamburi 1990).

Salary facilitates planning and execution of public or insurance budgets and is neutral with regard to economic incentive for either over- or underproviding services (Culyer, Donaldson, and Gerard 1988). The salary system encourages doctors to conduct group consultations and referrals necessary for appropriate treatment and costs less to administer than performance-based approaches.

At the same time, fixed salary provides no incentives for doctors to work productively—or at all, if salaries are very low, as in many low-income countries in Africa and Asia. Salaried physicians may require illegal payments from the patients and gain under-the-table money from kickbacks provided by pharmaceutical industries and high-tech equipment owners. Salary payment provides no direct incentive for doctors to recommend the most cost-effective health interventions, decrease costs, and improve health outcomes.

**TABLE 5.1   Basis for Allocating Resources by Line Items
in Former Soviet Union Republics**

Budget line item	Basis of funding level
1 and 2. Salaries and social security	Number and grade of staff in post
3. Operating expenditures	Last year's budget
9. Meals	Bed days
10. Medicines	Bed days
12. Equipment	Number of beds
14. Furniture and fixtures	Number of beds
16. Maintenance	Number of beds

Source: Ensor and Langenbrunner (2002).

Gosden, Pedersen, and Torgerson (1999) reviewed 23 papers and found that payment by salary was associated with the lowest use of tests and referrals, fewer procedures per patient, lower throughput of patients per doctor, longer consultation, and more preventive care. However, the review did not look at the links between utilization and case mix (patient needs) and outcomes.

LINKING PAYMENTS WITH PERFORMANCE

Many countries have moved away from line-item budgets. Initially, simple units of retrospective payment were introduced (for example, per service). This payment mechanism is typically referred to as fee for service (FFS) for outpatient care and per diem (per day) for inpatient care (for example, in India, Malaysia, parts of Russia, and Sri Lanka). Initially, some are relatively easy to introduce, and the change can encourage provider participation and improvements in productivity (as measured by volume) and performance. Several are discussed below, starting with retrospective mechanisms and moving to more sophisticated prospective mechanisms.

Fee for service. FFS is a payment method whereby providers are reimbursed based on specific items provided (for example, doctor consultations, specific x-ray tests, specific surgical operations). FFS also includes itemized charges for medical products and drugs, because material products are often furnished with medical labor services.

FFS payment can be further divided into three subgroups:

• Open-ended fees

• Negotiated fee schedule

• Regulated fee schedule (Ron, Abel-Smith, and Tamburi 1990).

The traditional type of FFS is an open-ended fee charged by the doctor according to the market. This was the most common type of payment in the medical market during the time medical care was less organized, regulated, and planned than it is today. Although the share of this type of FFS payment has been shrinking since the early 20th century, it is still popular in such countries as Canada, China, the Republic of Korea, and the United States (under its indemnity plans). The experience in industrial countries, and increasingly in other parts of the world, is that FFS correlates with a pronounced increase in volume and overall health expenditure (the Czech Republic and Taiwan). One short-term response to expenditure growth under FFS has been to cap overall spending on the supply side (Croatia), and to encourage some patient cost sharing to minimize moral hazard (parts of Canada, the Philippines).

The negotiated fee schedule came into existence with the establishment of health insurance schemes. To reduce the cost of services, purchasers (often social health insurance schemes or private health insurance companies) negotiate with providers or provider associations a set of standards of charges for the items of services. This system exists in countries such as Belgium, France, and Germany

(Normand and Weber 1994). The United States and Canada are increasingly using the negotiated fee schedule for their social health insurance programs and managed care organizations for both preventive and curative services in combination with capitation payment. Some governments regulate this schedule, as in Japan and China.

The FFS model does have advantages. First, it can be easily developed and implemented, with little capacity. Community financing schemes in Asia and Africa have utilized it at start-up (Diop 2002). A second important advantage is that FFS payment more accurately reflects the work actually done and the efforts expended (Ron, Abel-Smith, and Tamburi 1990). Thus, this method of payment encourages providers to work longer hours or provide more services. In general, this is thought to improve access and utilization for underserved areas (rural areas as in the Philippines), for underserved populations (the poor), or for high-priority services (the Czech Republic, Denmark, Haiti, United Kingdom); (Eicher, Auxilia, and Pollock 2001).[1] Third, if costs are understood, scheduled fees can be set to encourage the provision of cost-effective services.

If prices and marginal costs do not correlate, either there is overuse (if the price is set too high) or underuse (if the price is set too low). Quality suffers in either case. FFS payment also has high administrative costs to both providers and insurers (Normand and Weber 1994), in part because every service and procedure has to be billed. In general, the FFS system promotes providers' internal efficiency, but works against social efficiency in terms of the consumer's point of view.

PER DIEM PAYMENTS

Daily, *per-diem payment* is used for inpatient services, and the facility is reimbursed a fixed amount for each inpatient day regardless of the actual use of services, drugs, and medical products. In theory, it is applicable to all inpatient services including long-term care in nursing homes. This type of hospital payment is commonly used in continental Western Europe (Donaldson and Magnussen 1992; Schulenburg 1992) and is being demonstrated in parts of China and Indonesia in the social insurance schemes.

This type of charge can be easily calculated (figure 5.2). Per-diem payment provides incentives for the hospital to increase the total number of hospital days

---

FIGURE 5.2   How to Calculate per-Diem Payments

Payment Policy =

Last Year's Total Budget for Hospitals

Last Year's Number of Days

Source: Authors.

by increasing both the length of stay and the number of admissions, while reducing the intensity of care for each hospital day. Thus, the technical quality of care may suffer owing to insufficient services and drugs, while the perceived quality, such as physician interest in a patient, may increase to encourage both admissions and revenues. In Ronzônia (Brazil), per-diem payments were instituted between 1971 and 1981, a period that saw admissions triple (Rodrigues 1989). Germany's use of per diem resulted in longer hospital stays (13.1 days in 1987) than in other industrial countries (Schulenburg 1992).

As with FFS for physicians, this system may work better when coupled with a budget cap for hospital services (Estonia, parts of the Russian Federation). Quality and lengths of stay can be monitored by peer reviewers.

Case payment. With case payment, purchasers pay an inclusive fixed amount per case, regardless of services or procedures provided. It is technically more complicated (figure 5.3) and requires patient-level data for a sizable sample of cases. The case-payment method can be used for outpatient care, such as for day surgery in Lebanon, and the payment per inclusive visit that is being tested in China's social health insurance reform (Cotterill, Chakraborty, and Jerawan 2002). It can also be used for inpatient care (for example, the Diagnosis Related

FIGURE 5.3   Case Mix Adjusted per Case Payment

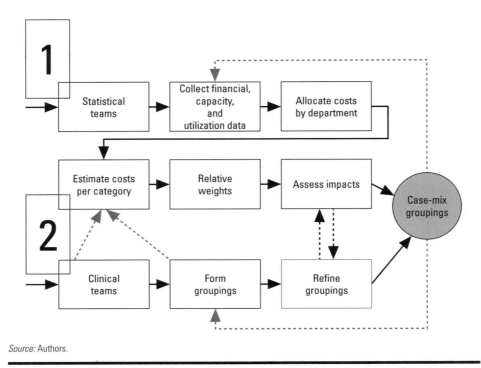

Source: Authors.

Group [DRG] in Brazil, Portugal, and the United States) including either physician services or hospital care, or both. Case payment can be a single flat rate per case regardless of the diagnosis and can be severity or risk adjusted. The most popular type of case payment is the DRG payment for hospital services, which has been implemented in the United States and has been adopted or tested in many other countries and regions (for example, Germany, Indonesia, Hungary, and Taiwan, China).

Case payments, if administered correctly, control costs and improve technical efficiency. Case payment is based on the principle that case cost in some category of risk or severity can be grouped or categorized, and prices assigned to each category. Diagnosis or the International Classification of Diseases (ICD) category is typically utilized as a proxy for risk or case severity. The number of case groups can be as simple as a single group (Kazakhstan) and as complex as 55,000 groups (parts of Russia). Brazil, Indonesia, the United States, and most other countries use between 100 and 800 groups (Jacobs and others 1992; Ron, Abel-Smith, and Tamburi 1990).

A major advantage of the case-payment system is that it removes the economic incentives (figure 5.4) for the hospital to provide as many items of services (as with FFS) and the longest hospital stay possible (as with per diem). Average lengths of stay typically decrease (see, for example, Kahn and others 1990). The predicted disadvantages are various:

- *Code creep,* whereby providers are likely to code patients into a group with a high point (or index) to obtain larger reimbursements (for example, in Croatia)

- *Cost shifting,* whereby providers shift patterns of care and costs to non-DRG patients and non-DRG settings, which leaves the total cost to the purchaser unchanged

FIGURE 5.4   Economics of per-Case Payment

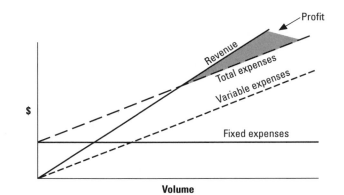

Source: Lyles and Palumbo 1999.

- Incentives to increase unnecessary admissions and readmissions; in Hungary, Russia, and many other countries, admissions increased significantly after a case-based system was introduced

- Incentives to either underprovide services or discharge admissions prematurely, where costs are shifted to outpatient services, home service care, and nursing home care. This will decrease the quality of care because of the interruption of care (Normand and Weber 1994).

The U.S.-developed DRG has been modified and used by many European countries and Australia as a way of financing public hospitals under a global budget (Wiley 1992). In these countries, DRGs are not used on a case-to-case basis to pay hospitals, but rather to measure the case mix of inpatients and to finance hospitals under some adjusted global cap. Similarly, in some Latin American countries (Mexico and Argentina), case-mix systems have been developed to track workloads and quality of care, as well as help governments and insurers set payment amounts for hospital care (personal communication, Griffin 2001).

Global budget. Global budget is a one line–item budget for facilities, for some fixed period of time (typically a year) for a specified population or service use. Because it is one line, there is more discretion than with line-item budgeting. Although the concept is simple, the types of global budget vary with budget flexibility, types and number of providers, number of payers, budget cap target, and budget basis (see below).

According to the degree of flexibility, global budget can be divided into two types—soft and hard. Under a *soft global budget,* the purchaser assumes cost overruns. A *hard global budget* transfers financial risk to the provider. Global budgets can be divided by hospital services, physician services, pharmaceuticals, and both services and drugs. According to the number of payers, global budgets can be classified by single or multiple purchasers.

Global budgets vary in important ways depending upon the budget basis:

- Inputs such as beds and staff (Canada)

- Historical spending and activities

- Volume of service provided and types of cases (France, Germany, United Kingdom).

The preferred approach is the final one, data and purchaser capacity permitting. In Australia and many European countries, the integration of case-mix adjusted hospital financing with global hospital budget is the major form of hospital payment (Frossard 1990; Hirdes and others 1996; Wolfe and Moran 1993). According to this system, a hospital payment is based on the product of the number of admissions and case-mix index. Thus, the more admissions and the sicker the patient, the bigger is the hospital's payment, but within the cap set for the distribution of budget among hospitals. The incentive provided by this system is similar to case payment, but because any spending is under a budget cap, this type of global budget is expected to be a powerful tool for controlling hospital costs and improving efficiency within the organization itself.

Capitation. Capitation, at its simplest, is one payment per person for some bundle of services delivered over a fixed period (typically a year). This type of payment transfers the economic risk from third-party payers to health care providers. The provider receiving a capitated fee can be an office-based doctor or a hospital (Barnum, Kutzin, and Saxenian 1995). Capitation payment has been implemented in Denmark, Italy, the Netherlands, and the United Kingdom and has been introduced in Costa Rica, Indonesia, and Thailand (Mills and others 2000), as well as most of Eastern Europe and Latin America for primary care services (Dixon, Langenbrunner, and Masiolis 2002).

Capitation payment may be a flat fee for each provider or a risk-adjusted fee, based on the relative risk of the registered population. For example, the capitated fee is adjusted in Germany by five variables—age, gender, family size, income, and whether the insuree is disabled and of working age (Barnum, Kutzin, and Saxenian 1995).

The most important advantage of capitation payment is that it removes the economic incentive of overprovision under the FFS system (figure 5.5) and can add an incentive to provide cost-effective care including preventive services. Because the provider is responsible for delivering the contracted package of services with the fixed payment, the provider is motivated to innovate in cost-reducing technology, use lower-cost alternative treatment settings, and deliver cost-effective care.

FIGURE 5.5   Economics of Capitation Payment

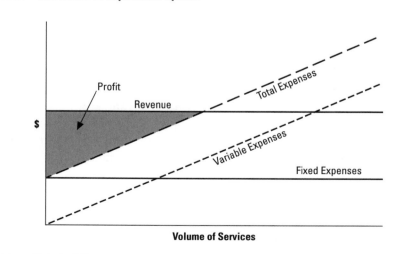

Source: Lyles and Palumbo 1999.

Capitation payment, however, may provide incentive for cutting down on necessary care. Providers may attempt to select the low-risk clients and then cut quality of care to reduce provider costs and risk. Finally, if referrals are outside the capitation payment, a patient is more likely to be sent to a specialist or a hospital while the referral is not necessary. For example, capitation payments to family physicians in Hungary and Croatia covered only their services, and their referral rates were higher than those of salaried physicians (Barnum, Kutzin, and Saxenian 1995; Dixon, Langenbrunner, and Masiolis 2002).

To address adverse risk selection, individual risk adjustment in Colombia, Germany, and the Netherlands are just starting to use simple formulas to adjust the risk. As Barnum, Kutzin, and Saxenian (1995) state, however, simple formulas may work better when benefit packages are limited; more complex formulas may be needed for comprehensive packages. Methods of risk adjustment remain relatively crude; Newhouse and others (1993) have shown that only 15 to 20 percent of individual variance can be predicted even with hundreds of variables.

A variation of physician capitation is *fundholding,* begun in the United Kingdom and parts of the former U.S.S.R. General practitioners are responsible for delivering primary care and purchasing the defined specialist and hospital care with set capitated payments. Another practice can be found in Thailand and China, where the social health insurance schemes pay contracted hospitals capitation fees for delivering both primary and secondary services. These two types of approaches remove the incentive for unnecessary referrals, but add the incentive to keep the patients at the primary level when referrals may be needed.

PERFORMANCE-RELATED PAY

Performance-related pay (PRP) directly links payment to the performance and the contribution of health care providers. PRP can be used to pay individuals or groups of people. "Performance" is measured by how well a specified task is implemented against the set target.

PRP has grown rapidly since the 1980s. PRP for nurses and physicians has been widely reported in North America and the United Kingdom (see, for example, Berwich 1996; Bledsoe, Leisy, and Rodeghero 1995; Bloor, Maynard, and Street 1992; Buchan 1993; Buchan and Thompson 1993; Castledine 1993; Griffin 1993; Hern 1994; Lewis 1990; Macara 1995; Smith and Simpson 1994).

PRP has also been used in very poor developing countries, where complicated payment incentives and systems may be excessively cumbersome for the delivery of basic services. In Haiti, the U.S. Agency for International Development introduced a performance-based bonus arrangement with nongovernmental organizations to deliver maternal and child health services (Eichler, Paul, and Pollock 2001). Results point toward increased immunization coverage. Performance-based payments with nongovernmental organizations have also been used to deliver community-based nutrition services in Senegal and Madagascar (Marek and others 1999). In both cases, the programs focused on poor areas. Services delivered included growth monitoring, food supplementation, nutrition and education sessions, and referral of unvaccinated children and pregnant women to health services. Contracts specified minimum acceptable levels of service delivery. In areas covered by the projects, malnutrition fell steadily, and lower rates of malnutrition were found among children who had participated in the project than among children who had not.

Cambodia provides another example of PRP. Three arrangements were evaluated (Bhushan, Keller, and Schwartz 2002):

- A contracting-out model in which contractors had full responsibility for delivering the specified services, directly employed their staff members, and had full management control

- A contracting-in model in which contractors provided only management support to civil servants; most recurrent operating costs were met by the government through normal government channels, but a small supplement was paid over which the contractors had control

- A control group in which services were delivered through the ministry of health system.

Results indicate larger improvements in the experimental districts than in the control district in immunization coverage, use of antenatal care, and other indicators. Furthermore, the poor appear to have benefited disproportionately—among the poorest half of the population, vitamin A supplementation increased faster and the treatment of illness increased several times faster among contracted districts than in the control districts.

Health care purchaser and management parties have often been interested in introducing the PRP schemes, but there are skeptics. Griffin (1993) notes that health care systems often lack the basic requirements to undertake PRP, such as:

- Financial capacity to reward employees for better performance, especially across the entire workforce.

- Inability to measure and attribute performance to individuals. In health care, cooperation among medical personnel is needed to improve quality, but performance improvement is usually the outcome of joint efforts.

- Rewards large enough to be valued by the medical personnel. In a developing country, where doctors are paid almost equally to other comparable disciplines, significant additional pay will raise the earnings of medical doctors disproportionately but their performance may not increase significantly.

Griffin also argues that payment is just one of the factors that motivate the medical profession. Participation, job enrichment, recognition, working environment, and autonomy in allocating resources can be equally important in motivating people.

Gauri (forthcoming) argues for caution in specifying criteria for PRP. Basing PRP on just a few indicators, such as admissions and lengths of stay, may compromise other objectives, such as improved quality of care. As more objectives are addressed, indicators multiply, adding administrative complexity and discouraging transparency.

DISCUSSION

No single set of incentives will address the multiple objectives of purchasers, providers, and patients (table 5.2). As a result, purchasers and policymakers must understand and address policy objectives explicitly.

During the past two decades, new and more sophisticated payment systems have evolved with broader units of payment and payments set prospectively. Many purchasers have adopted a fixed-price payment for definable products that groups services from entire clinical episodes such as an outpatient surgery (Lebanon) and more often, for inpatient stays (Brazil, Hungary, Kyrgzstan, Portugal). Global budgets fix price as well as volume for, say, all inpatient services (Republic of Korea, parts of Russia, Taiwan, China) or outpatient services (China). Some countries also use capitation payments, which disburse a fixed amount per insured for all services covered regardless of type or setting. Examples of this include the system in Indonesia and Thailand, as well as many of the managed care schemes in the United States, Argentina, and other South American countries (Bitran and Yip 1998; Langenbrunner and Wiley 2002).

In every case, part or all of the financial risk is transferred from the RAP arrangement back to the provider and patient. Most observers caution against full risk sharing but encourage some "supply side cost sharing" only, with pur-

TABLE 5.2   Impact of Selected Payment Incentives

Payment characteristics	Risk with	Possible impact on health sector performance				
		Access/ financial protection	Quality	Expenditures	Efficiency	Administrative simplicity
Line item	Provider[a]	+	+	+++		+++
Salary	Purchaser	++++++	++	+++	+	+++
Fee for service	Purchaser		++			
Per diem	Purchaser		+			+
Per case	Provider		++	+	+++	
Global budget	Provider	+	++	++	+	+
Capitation	Provider*	+	+	+++	+++	+
Performance-related pay	Purchaser	+	++	+	+	+

+ Impact is positive.

a. Depends upon whether there are "soft" or "hard" budget rules.

Source: Preker and others 2001.

chaser and provider sharing in risk arrangements to address moral hazard issues (Ellis 1998; Newhouse 1998). An alternative is to impose high copayments or user fees, but in developing countries that quickly erodes financial protection.

RAP arrangements have been striving to find an equilibrium among conflicting objectives (Belli and Hammer 1999). A general conclusion is that mixed reimbursement systems are necessary to optimally balance multiple objectives such as cost and quality (Dranove and Satterthwaite 2000). Though far from the context in the developing world, the European Union (EU) countries provide an interesting example of convergence toward a mix of mechanisms. Most EU countries use FFS for "priority services" such as preventive care and selected primary care services and prospective payments to set rates and cap expenditure for inpatient care services (Langenbrunner and Wiley 2002).

Sophisticated payment systems may lead to higher transaction costs, however, and the need to expand capacity to use information and management systems. This is true both for purchasers and providers because the unit of payment increases and risk necessarily shifts relative to providers. Management information systems cannot always be designed and implemented quickly. Robinson (2001) notes that managed care organizations and private purchasers in the United States use FFS for primary care and do not use DRGs to reimburse hospitals—relying instead on bed days. For them, the benefit of using DRGs in terms of transferring full or appropriate risk bearing onto providers is not worth the administrative cost.

This chapter has addressed incentives in the context of the single purchaser of services. If the health sector has multiple purchasers, providers may face multiple incentives at once. The precise impacts of these multiple competing incentives will be unknown, and only situation specific. Zweifel (chapter 19, this volume) and Jack (forthcoming) cover these more complex situations.

Finally, the best planned and implemented payment incentives and systems may fail due to a variety of other and related factors in the health delivery sector. Unless these other delivery system issues are addressed, impacts will be diluted or neutralized. Technicians and policymakers will need to address these potential "chokepoints" in any implementation and refinement process (Dixon, Langenbrunner, and Masiolis 2002). These issue areas include:

• Fragmented public sector pooling and purchasing

• Low operational autonomy of providers (see, for example, Harding and Preker 2003)

• Lack of timely information and routine information systems

• Poor complementarity of design across service settings (inpatient and outpatient)

• Institutional impediments (chapter 1, this volume)

• Technical capacity and management skills

• Monitoring and quality assurance systems.

NOTES

1. However, the literature does have some dissenting evidence—Palmer and Mills (2000) found that part-time FFS surgeons in rural South Africa expended minimal time on their public sector patients.

REFERENCES

Arrow, K. J. 1963. "Uncertainty and the Welfare Economics of Medical Care." *The American Economic Review* 53(5): 941–73.

Barnum, H., J. H. Kutzin, and H. Saxenian. 1995. "Incentive and Provider Payment Methods." *International Journal of Health Planning and Management* 10: 23–45.

Belli, P., and J. Hammer. 1999. "Incentives and Health Care Reimbursement Systems: A Review of the Literature." Internal working paper. World Bank, Washington, D.C.

Berwich, D. M. 1996. "A Primer on Leading the Improvement of Health Systems." *British Medical Journal* 312: 619–22.

Bhushan, I., S. Keller, and B. Schwartz. 2002. *Achieving the Twin Objectives of Efficiency and Equity: Contracting Health Services in Cambodia.* Manila: Asian Development Bank.

Bledsoe, D., W. Leisy, and J. Rodeghero. 1995. "Tying Physician Incentive Pay to Performance." *Healthcare Finance and Management* 49(12): 40–44.

Bloor, K., A. Maynard, and A. Street. 1992. "How Much Is a Doctor Worth?" Discussion Paper No. 98. University of York, Centre for Health Economics, York, United Kingdom.

Bitran, R., W. Yip. 1998. "Latin American and Asian Experiences of the Reform of Health Care Provider Payment Systems." Partners for Health Reform Plus Program. U.S. Agency for International Development, Washington, D.C.

Buchan, J. 1993. "Performance-Related Pay and NHS Nursing." *Nursing Standard* 7(25):30.

Buchan, J., and M. Thompson. 1993. "Pay and Nursing Performance." *Health Manpower Management* 19(2): 29–31.

Castledine, G. 1993. "Can Performance-Related Pay Be Adapted for Nursing?" *British Journal of Nursing* 2(22): 1120–21.

Cotterill, P., S. Chakraborty, and E. Jerawan. 2002. "Lebanon Provider Payment Study." Case Study for Resource Allocation and Purchasing Project. World Bank, Washington, D.C.

Culyer A. J., C. Donaldson, and K. Gerard. 1988. "Financial Aspects of Health Services: Drawing on Experience." Working Paper No. 3. University of York, York, United Kingdom.

Diop, F. 2002. "Community Financing in Rwanda: Early Results." Presentation at the World Bank, November 7, Washington, D.C.

Dixon, A., J. Langenbrunner, and E. Masiolis. 2002. "Ten Years of Experience: Health Financing in Eastern Europe and the Former Soviet Union." Ten Years of Health Reform Conference, July 29–31, American International Health Alliance, Washington, D.C.

Donaldson, C., and J. Magnussen. 1992. "DRGs: The Road to Hospital Efficiency." *Health Policy* 21: 47–64.

Dranove, D., and M. Satterthwaite. 2000. "The Industrial Organization of Health Care Markets." In A. J. Culher and J. P. Newhouse, eds., *Handbook of Health Economics.* Amsterdam: North-Holland.

Eicher, R., A. Paul, and J. Pollock. 2001. "Promoting Preventive Health Care: Paying for Performance in Haiti." Report for U.S. Agency for International Development. Washington, D.C.: Management Sciences for Health.

Ellis, R. 1998. "Creaming, Skimping, and Dumping: Provider Competition on the Intensive and Extensive Margins." *Journal of Health Economics* 17(5): 537–55.

Ellis, R., and T. McGuire. 1990. "Optimal Payment Systems for Health Services." *Journal of Health Economics* 9(4): 375–96.

Ensor, T., and J. Langenbrunner. 2002. "Allocating Resources and Paying Providers." In M. McKee, J. Healey, and J. Falkingham, eds., *Health Care in Central Asia.* Buckingham, England: Open University Press.

Frossard, M. 1990. "Short Communication Hospital Strategy and Regional Planning in France." *International Journal of Health Planning and Management* 5: 59–63.

Gauri, V. Forthcoming. "What Is Contractable in Health Care? Provider Payment Reforms in Developing Countries." *The Economics of Resource Allocation and Purchasing of Health Care.* Forthcoming. Washington, D.C.: World Bank.

Griffin, R.P. 1993. "Why Doesn't Performance Pay Work?" *Health Manpower Management* 19(2): 11–13.

Gosden T., L. Pedersen, and D. Torgerson. 1999. "How Should We Pay Doctors? A Systematic Review of Salary Payments and Their Effect on Doctor Behaviour." *QJM* 92(1): 47–55.

Harding, A., and A. S. Preker, eds. 2003. *Private Participation in Health Services.* Washington, D.C.: World Bank.

Hern, J. E. 1994. "What Should Be Done about Merit Award?" *British Medical Journal* 308: 973–74.

Hirdes J. P., C. A. Botz, J. Kozak, and V. Lepp. 1996. "Identifying an Appropriate Case Mix Measure for Chronic Care: Evidence from an Ontario Pilot Study." *Healthcare Management Forum* 9(1): 40–46.

Jack, W. Forthcoming. "Purchasing Health Care: A Conceptual Framework." *The Economics of Resource Allocation and Purchasing of Health Care.* Washington, D.C.: World Bank.

Jencks, S., A. Dobson, P. Willis, and P. Feinstein. 1984. "Evaluating and Improving the Measurement of Hospital Case Mix." *Health Care Financing Review; Annual Supplement.*

Jacobs, P., E. M. Hall, J. Lave, and M. Glending. 1992. "Alberta's Health Care Funding Project." *Health Care Management Forum* 5(3): 4–11.

Kahn, K. L., W. H. Rogers, L. V. Rubenstein, M. J. Sherwood, E. J. Reinisch, E. B. Keeler, E. D. Draper, J. Kosecoff, and R. H. Brook. 1990. "Comparing Outcomes of Care before and after Implementation of the DRG-Based Prospective Payment System." *Journal of the American Medical Association* 264: 1984–88.

Langenbrunner, J., and M. Wiley. 2002. "Hospital Payment Mechanisms: Theory and Practice in Transition Countries." In *Hospitals in a Changing Europe.* Buckingham, England: Open University Press.

Lewis, E. 1990. "Rewarding Performance." *Health Service Journal* (December): 1435.

Lyles, A., and F. B. Palumbo. 1999. The Effect of Managed Care on Prescription Drug Costs and Benefits. *Pharmacoeconomics* 15(2): 129–40.

Macara, S. 1995. "Appraisal of Doctors in the NHS: Merit Awards and Performance-Related Pay." *British Journal of Hospital Medicine* 53(3): 111–12.

Marek, T., I. Diallo, B. Ndiaye, and J. Rakotosalama. 1999. "Successful Contracting of Prevention Services: Fighting Malnutrition in Senegal and Madagascar." *Health Policy Planning* 14(4): 382–89.

Mills, A., S. Bennett, P. Siriwanarangsun, and V. Tangcharoensathien. 2000. "The Response of Providers to Capitation Payment: A Case-Study from Thailand." *Health Policy* 51(3): 163–80.

Newhouse, J. P. 1998. "Risk Adjustment: Where Are We Now?" *Inquiry* 35: 122–31.

Newhouse, J. P., R. Archibald, H. Bailit, R. Brook, M. Brown, A Davies, N. Duan, G. Goldberg, E. Keeler, A. Leibowitz, K. Lohr, W. Manning, K. Marquis, M. Marquis, C. Morris, C. Phelps, W. Rogers, C. Sherbourne, R. Valdez, J. Ware, and K. Wells. 1993. *Free for All? Lessons from the RAND Health Insurance Experiment.* Cambridge, Mass.: Harvard University Press.

Normand, C., and A. Weber. 1994. *Social Health Insurance: A Guidebook for Planning.* Geneva: World Health Organization.

Oxley, H. 1995. *New Directions in Health Care Policy.* Paris: Organisation for Economic Cooperation and Development.

Palmer, N., and A. Mills. 2000. "Classical versus Relational Approaches to Understanding Controls on a Contract with Independent GPs in South Africa. Paper presented to Health Financing conference, Clermont-Ferrand, France, December 2000.

Preker, A., M. Jakab, J. Langenbrunner, and C. Baeza. 2001. "Resource Allocation and Purchasing: A Conceptual Framework." Internal working paper. World Bank, Washington, D.C.

Robinson, J. C. 2001. "Theory and Practice in the Design of Physician Payment Incentives." *Milbank Quarterly* 79(2): 149–77.

Rodrigues, J., 1989. "Hospital Utilization and Reimbursement Method in Brazil." *International Journal of Health Planning and Management* 4(1): 3–15.

Ron, A., B. Abel-Smith, and G. Tamburi. 1990. *Health Insurance in Developing Countries: The Social Security Approach.* Geneva: International Labour Office.

Schulenburg, J-M. 1992. "Forming and Reforming the Market for Third-Party Purchasing of Health Care: A German Perspective." *Social Science and Medicine* 39(10): 1473–81.

Smith, J., and J. Simpson. 1994. "Locally Determined Performance-Related Pay: Better Levers Exist for Improving Performance in a Health Service with Disparate Values." *British Medical Journal* 309: 495–96.

Wiley, M. M. 1992. "Hospital Financing Reform and Case Mix Measurement: An International Review." *Health Care Financing Review* 13(4): 119–33.

Wolfe, P. R., and D. W. Moran. 1993. "Global Budgeting in the OECD Countries." *Health Care Financing Review* 14(3): 55–76.

CHAPTER 6

At What Price? Affordable and Realistic Fees

Hugh Waters and Peter Sotir Hussey

This chapter reviews methodologies and international experience related to costing and pricing health services. The discussion is based on the perspective of health care purchasers, using examples from international settings with widely ranging availability of information on health service utilization, expenditures, and costs. The chapter highlights approaches and experiences pertinent for purchasers in low- and middle-income countries,[1] with an emphasis on pricing health services in relation to their true costs with appropriate health care production and utilization incentives.

The prices purchasers pay for health services are influenced by:

- The method of provider payment

- The availability of information—including costs, volumes, and outcomes—and methods used to calculate providers' costs

- Characteristics of purchasers and providers—including the regulatory environment, provider autonomy, negotiating power, and the intensity of competition.

The remainder of this chapter discusses these three sets of factors, drawing conclusions for pricing decisions in low- and middle-income countries and presenting applications in these countries.

OVERVIEW OF PROVIDER PAYMENT METHODS

For setting prices, the most important characteristic of a payment system, in addition to the unit of payment, is whether the payment is *retrospective* or *prospective*. Retrospective payments are calculated and paid after the service is delivered, whereas prospective payments are made before delivery of the service. The key distinction is that the price paid in a prospective payment should be an accurate prediction of future costs, while the price paid in a retrospective payment should be aligned with the actual costs incurred. A second important dimension is whether the system is *variable* or *fixed*. In variable payment systems, the aggregate amount of payment services is proportional to the volume of activity; in fixed systems, there is a limit on total payments (Jegers and others 2002).

Provider payment methods and their incentives for provider behavior are summarized in chapter 5. These payment methods can be classified according to the units of the services paid for. The unit of service can be each health service provided *(fee for service)*, all services related to a diagnosis (*per case*), all services for a patient over a period of time (*capitation*), or all services provided to all patients over a period of time (*global or line-item budgets*).

Provider Payment Systems: Specific Examples

Each payment system requires a different approach to setting prices. Applicable approaches are illustrated here using specific examples from low-, middle-, and high-income countries. This section will describe the payment system used in each example; the following discussion will show how prices are determined.

FEE-FOR-SERVICE PAYMENTS—GERMANY AND THE UNITED STATES

The German health care system combines elements of fee-for-service reimbursement with an overall limited global budget. Ambulatory care physicians are reimbursed retrospectively per service provided. Two national fee schedules determine the prices paid. The first—for the private sector—is determined annually at the national level and sets the price per service in currency units (Kamke 1998).[2] The second applies to payments to physicians by sickness funds, the publicly financed insurers that cover most of the population. Each service is given a relative value through negotiations at the national level between physicians and federal associations of sickness funds. In each region of the country, the quarterly budget is divided by the total number of relative value units for services provided by physicians—if physicians provide a higher volume of services, their remuneration per service is lower (Sauerland 2001).

The United States uses a similar fee schedule for physician payment in the federal Medicare program. As in Germany, the total expenditure is limited by a global budget; the size of the U.S. global budget "target" is linked to national gross domestic product (GDP) per capita. If spending exceeds the global budget, the remuneration per relative value of service is lower (Medpac 2002). The mixed-payment systems in the United States and Germany are variable payment systems at the micro level, but fixed at the macro level, providing different incentives from a pure variable fee-for-service system (Jegers and others 2002).

PAYMENTS PER CASE—AUSTRALIA

In Australia, hospital payments are set and allocated at the state level. Each state therefore has a slightly different payment system, although all but one make prospective per-case payments based on an Australian system of classification of diagnoses, the Australian national diagnosis-related groups (AN-DRGs) (Duckett 1998).

The state of Victoria makes several adjustments in payments. First, payments to hospitals for overhead costs are separated from the diagnosis-based payment to circumvent the incentive of diagnosis-based payments to admit more patients

(Duckett 1998). Finally, prices in Victoria are adjusted for outliers (patients with exceptionally high costs) and for certain types of hospitals—hospitals with high volumes of patients receive lower payments because of assumed economies of scale (Duckett 1998).

CAPITATION PAYMENTS—DENMARK

Capitation payments, simply defined, are prospective, fixed payments to providers to care for a defined population for a defined period of time. The price of services under a capitated-payment system is therefore the rate paid to the provider per insured person per time period. If prices perfectly equaled expected costs, any surplus or deficit in revenue for the provider would be due to random events and treatment patterns. If prices are below expected costs, providers can be expected to make up for the deficit by lowering expected costs by selecting lower-risk patients.

To set prices as close as possible to the expected costs of treatment, payments are often adjusted according to the insured's cost-associated characteristics—a process called *risk adjustment*.[3] However, since risk adjustment is only partially successful in predicting actual treatment costs, incentives for patient selection remain (Newhouse 1994). A mixed-payment system—capitation plus other forms of payment—can mitigate providers' incentive to select healthier patients (Newhouse 1996).

Denmark uses such a mixed-payment system for general practitioners. These physicians receive about a third of their payment as capitation and the remaining two-thirds as fee for service (Davis 2002). The combination mixes the fee-for-service incentives to provide more services with those of capitation to provide fewer.

EXAMPLES FROM LOW- AND MIDDLE-INCOME COUNTRIES

The principal constraint on the development of provider payment systems in low- and middle-income countries is the limited availability of information on costs, volumes, and patient characteristics (Maceira 1998). Nonetheless, several countries have undertaken innovative payment reforms to avoid the negative incentives associated with unmodified global or line-item budgets.

Kyrgyzstan has adopted a combined system with capitated payments for family group practices and patient choice of primary care physician. Polyclinic services are reimbursed according to a fee-for-service schedule, and hospitals are paid on a case-based system (Wouters 1999). In Ronzônia (Brazil), the federal Unified Health System also introduced a mixed case–based, fee-for-service system to reimburse both public and private providers. However, reimbursement adjustments have lagged behind increases in health care costs, resulting in private providers leaving the system (Bitran and Yip 1998).

In Chile, public hospitals were traditionally paid through global budgets based on historical patterns and on the number and type of their employees. As a result, the hospitals had little incentive to reduce costs or to meet demand (Bitran and Yip 1998). In 1992, the Chilean public insurance payer, the Fondo Nacional de Salud (FONASA) designed a mixed case–based and fee-for-service system to reimburse public hospitals. This system has been phased in gradually, replacing historical budgets. Hospitals have responded accordingly by monitoring their output and emphasizing efficiency. FONASA pays municipal health centers for primary care services based on capitation, using adjustments for location and patients' incomes (Wouters 1999).

The Republic of Korea and Taiwan, China, which have both achieved universal health insurance coverage for their populations, have predominantly used fee-for-service purchasing in the context of expanding public health insurance programs. In both countries, fee for service led to rapid cost inflation. In the Republic of Korea, health spending increased from 2.8 percent of GDP in 1975 to 4.3 percent in 1986 and 7.1 percent in 1991 (Mills and others 2000). In Taiwan, China, the introduction of national health insurance in 1996 slowed the rate of increases in health spending, but total levels of reimbursement to providers continued to go up—by 7.4 percent from 1996 to 1997, and an additional 11.3 percent from 1997 to 1998. Both countries have introduced case-based payment to modify the inflationary incentives of fee-for-service reimbursement. The size of the reimbursement is based on the number of procedures in a given period, the distribution in the average length of stay for the procedure, data from orders for medical equipment and supplies, and hospital-specific factors that might raise or lower costs.

In addition to the fee-for-service and per-case payment systems, the Taiwan Bureau of National Health Insurance (BNHI) introduced a global budget system for outpatient dental care in 1998. Intended to rationalize the rapid growth of payments for dental care, the calculation of the first year's global budget was based on the previous year's total outpatient dental care payments, plus a ceiling of 8 percent annual growth.

CALCULATING COSTS—METHODS AND INFORMATION AVAILABLE

The prices that purchasers pay for health care services should be related to the actual unit costs of services in order to minimize incentives for under- or overutilization. Establishing the true unit cost of health services is a complicated proposition because of the difficulties involved in correctly tracking and allocating administrative overhead and other indirect costs to service units. This section provides an overview of methodologies used to measure unit costs and continues with country-specific examples. Accurate costing is important to the success of all types of provider payment mechanisms other than global and line-item budgeting. For capitation, costing is critical for both bidding and management of contracts in the context of competition (West, Hicks, and Balas 1996). Per-case payments and diagnosis-related groups (DRGs) depend on a realistic picture of the cost of the inputs for a case or condition.

Tracking and Allocating Costs

Costing health services inevitably involves allocating costs to cost centers and ultimately to the services themselves. *Direct costs* such as drugs and supplies can be allocated directly to cost centers or health services produced. *Indirect costs* are those that cannot be directly allocated—including administrators' salaries and support activities such as housekeeping and laundry.[4] The calculation of accurate unit costs for health care services depends to a great extent on the "correct" allocation of both direct and indirect provider costs. Accounting systems that allocate indirect costs among different types of treatment, based solely on production ratios, are likely to incorrectly capture the underlying effort and production intensities (Hoyt and Lay 1995).

Activity-based costing (ABC) is a retrospective approach to allocating costs used to calculate the unit costs of health services in the United States and has been applied in low- and middle-income countries (Player 1998; Waters, Abdallah, and Santillán 2001). Traditional costing procedures typically group indirect costs in one pool and allocate these costs to products on the basis of relative production figures. Because of economies of scale in production, this approach attributes too high a cost to high-volume products and too low a cost to low-volume ones. ABC goes further by attributing support costs based on the actual consumption of the goods and services provided, measured by time allocation (figure 6.1). ABC is typically used to calculate costs for specific services and

FIGURE 6.1   Traditional Accounting versus ABC

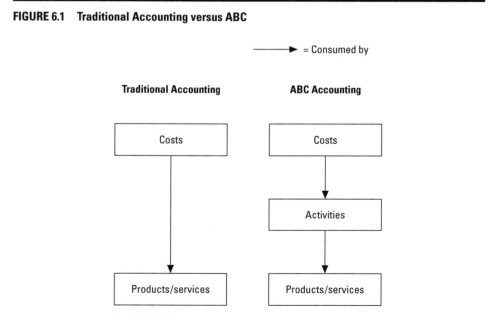

Source: Authors' adaptation from Cokin 1996.

appropriate for fee-for-service reimbursement, but can also be used to calculate the cost of a bundled package of services for the same patient (Chan 1993; Cokin 1996).

A related approach used in lower- and middle-income countries is to allocate costs derived from line-item budgets across inpatient departments, avoiding ABC's need for data on personnel time distribution. An additional technique to allocate costs, employed in Kyrgyzstan and Kazakhstan, is to develop a simple case mix with weights for different procedures that can be used as a simple DRG system on which purchasers can base reimbursements.

The Importance of Information Availability

The process of setting prices for health services from the purchasers' perspective is inextricably linked with the information available to them. Each approach to setting prices has different information input requirements; the availability of information largely dictates purchasers' range of choices in calculating costs and setting prices. Inadequate information systems are typically the single largest constraint to the implementation of provider payment mechanisms in low- and middle-income countries. For example, top-down costing techniques such as ABC require that providers' costs be available by department and by category (for example, salaries, drugs, supplies). In addition, accurate utilization information is essential to correctly calculate unit costs.

Measuring Costs: Specific Examples

Countries use a variety of methods to set their prices in relation to measured costs. Some payment systems such as fee-for-service payments in the United States Medicare program and per-case payments in the state of Victoria in Australia have used a more information-intensive approach to measuring costs and setting prices accordingly. Other payment systems such as fee-for-service payments in Germany, capitation payments in Denmark, and systems in many low- and middle-income countries, use a less information-intensive approach to aligning prices with actual costs. In these systems costs are often approximated rather than measured.

FEE-FOR-SERVICE PAYMENTS—GERMANY AND THE UNITED STATES

In Germany, price setting for each relative value unit of payment is driven mainly by negotiation, with little emphasis on the calculation of actual costs (Busse 1999). The relative value units of services are determined through a mix of expert judgment by physicians and political negotiations between the various specialty societies (Rodwin, Grable, and Thiel 1989).

The Medicare program in the United States uses an alternative methodology for determining the prices paid under a fee schedule. This fee schedule, the

Resource Based Relative Value Scale (RBRVS), was informed by an economic study of the resources used to provide each service (Hsiao and others 1992). These two approaches to setting prices paid under a fee schedule have different information needs. The German approach—relying heavily on negotiations— does not require information beyond expert judgments and historical payments, although other information on costs could be and doubtlessly is used by specialty associations. The U.S. RBRVS methodology, however, required a large national study of the costs of physician services. Updates to the relative value scale in the United States are based on expert consultations, however, more similar to the German model (Medpac 2002).

PAYMENTS PER CASE—AUSTRALIA

The state of Victoria measures the costs of each DRG using patient-level data on resource utilization. Annual costing studies collect data from a sample of about 15 hospitals to determine costs per DRG (Jackson 2001). A substantial investment in measuring costs is necessary to collect patient-level data for this bottom-up costing. Other countries and other states in Australia have implemented diagnosis-based payments without collecting patient-level data for bottom-up costing. Instead, costs are estimated using a top-down allocation methodology—attributing aggregate hospital financial data to patients treated in each DRG. The data required are aggregate financial data, patient discharge data, and a set of relative resource weights for DRGs that must be imported from other settings (Wiley 1993).

CAPITATION—DENMARK

In Denmark, prices paid to physicians are negotiated annually at the national level between the association of county councils (purchasers) and the association of general practitioners. Capitated payments are uniform, without risk adjustment or other adjustment of prices. The lack of risk adjustment lightens the administrative burden but increases the likelihood of patient selection. In Denmark, because the capitation formula is based simply on age and gender, the only information requirement is an accurate roster of enrolled patients with their age and gender at enrollment.

MEASURING COSTS IN LOW- AND MIDDLE-INCOME COUNTRIES

Documentation is limited on costing health care services to set purchaser prices in low- and middle-income countries. Waters, Abdallah, and Santillán (2001) applied ABC to establish unit costs and compared them with prices for a nongovernmental provider in Peru. Their study found that using ABC is feasible in a developing-country setting, yielding results that are directly applicable to pricing and management. However, the study also showed the importance of the availability and organization of cost information. Applying ABC efficiently requires information to be readily available by department and cost category, because the greatest benefits of ABC come from frequent, systematic application of the methodology to monitor efficiency and provide feedback for management. For most low- and middle-income health care providers, cost and volume information is not readily available in this type of organization.

CHARACTERISTICS OF PURCHASERS AND PROVIDERS

The characteristics of health care providers and their relations with purchasers have a strong influence on the way prices for health services are determined. Some of the most pertinent characteristics are provider autonomy, provider negotiating power, and the extent of competition.

Provider Autonomy

Provider autonomy can be thought of as a continuum from complete ownership of the provider by the purchaser to private ownership with contractual relationships with purchasers. Preker and Harding (2001) describe three market-oriented reforms that have moved health systems along this continuum toward private ownership. *Autonomization* refers to the transfer of many day-to-day management decisions to providers, with increasing reliance on performance-related payments. *Corporatization* is the emulation of private corporations by public organizations, transferring near-complete control over inputs and the production of services to hospital managers. *Privatization* is the transfer of public organizations to private ownership.

In the special case where the public sector combines the functions of purchasing and delivery within the same public sector organization, the differences in the incentives of these two groups are minimized. Moving along the continuum toward greater provider autonomy, their incentives increasingly diverge. Providers with greater autonomy are also more likely to be autonomously responsible for determining the costs of their services and the prices necessary to sustain high quality.

Provider Negotiating Power

Provider negotiating power is important in many systems for setting prices in which the providers are not directly managed by purchasers but do not tender competitive bids to determine prices. Providers may negotiate with purchasers over service prices, which services are reimbursed, and how they are reimbursed. In Canada, Germany, and Switzerland, for example, the payment is determined through negotiations between purchasers and provider groups. Thus, the prices paid for services depend directly on the negotiating effectiveness of the provider associations.

Provider Competition

Provider competition affects prices in systems where prices are determined through a process where autonomous providers tender bids. In a perfect market, competitive bidding would produce socially optimal prices. However, health care markets include many well-documented market failures—with subsequent justification for government intervention. An example of a competitive bidding process for provision of health services can be found in the United States. U.S. hospitals enter contractual relationships with private health insurers, regulated by the states. Keeler, Melnick, and Zwanziger (1999) showed that areas of California with greater hospital competition had lower prices. However, they also showed that nonprofit hospital mergers can lead to higher, not lower, prices. This illustrates the importance of the number of providers on the price effects of competitive bidding. If a hospital is the only provider for a region, for example, it could use its monopoly power to obtain higher prices for its services through a unilateral bid for a contract instead of through a negotiating process with a purchaser.

CONCLUSIONS

Setting the prices paid for health services at appropriate levels is essential for the fair reimbursement of providers, for promoting system sustainability, and for encouraging the delivery of appropriate, high-quality medicine. This chapter has summarized a range of methods and experiences in setting prices in different payment systems.

The main factors influencing how prices are set are the unit and method of payment, the measurement of costs, and the characteristics of purchasers and providers. These factors are strongly interrelated. Many low- and middle-income countries use global and line-item budgets for hospital payments. These payment systems are simple to administer because they do not rely heavily on measuring costs; prices paid are determined mainly from historical levels. However, because global and line-item budgets are generally not aligned with the costs providers actually incur, they provide an incentive to underprovide health services and do not encourage managerial flexibility (Kutzin 2001; Langenbrunner and Wiley 2002). For these reasons, most high-income countries that formerly used fixed budgets to reimburse hospitals have moved to more sophisticated payment systems.

This chapter has provided examples from the United States and Australia demonstrating approaches taken to setting prices under payment systems with intensive information demands. One approach has been to undertake costing studies to align prices with actual costs. The state of Victoria in Australia has used several different costing methodologies to determine the appropriate price for each diagnosis-related hospital discharge. The U.S. Medicare program conducted a detailed costing study to set the prices for its fee schedule for physician reimbursement.

Other high-income countries, however, do not use such information-intensive approaches to setting prices. In Germany, the price-setting system depends on two main components—negotiations and a mixed payment system. A system of annual negotiations helps to ensure that providers are fairly reimbursed. At the same time, an overall cap on the amount of physician reimbursement mitigates the incentive to overproduce services in a fee-for-service payment system and constrains overall costs. The U.S. Medicare program has also relied on negotiations and expert consultations to update its original fee schedule costing study and uses a mixed payment system, with an overall payment cap. In Denmark, capitation payments to individual physicians—which potentially involve the greatest information needs to ensure appropriate prices—are based only on age and gender. The negative effects that could result from inappropriate capitation prices are mitigated through a mixed payment system and annual negotiations over prices.

These experiences show a variety of options for setting prices for health care purchasers in low- and middle-income countries that are reforming their payment systems. Unit costing studies are essential for setting prices proportionate to costs; but where accurate unit costs are not available, other options exist for approximating appropriate prices. Some techniques allow simpler estimation of costs by, for example, importing reimbursement systems in use in other countries, such as the reimbursement weights per diagnosis from the U.S. Medicare program. Finally, safeguards such as mixed payment systems and price negotiations can help minimize the undesired consequences—under- and overutilization and skewed provider incentives—that arise from inappropriate price levels.

NOTES

1. In this chapter, countries are classified by income using the following categories from the 2000 *World Development Report* (World Bank 2000): low income, US$755 per capita or less; lower middle income, $756 to $2,995; upper middle income, $2,996 to $9,265; and high income, $9,266 or more.

2. The private sector serves mainly individuals above a certain income threshold—about 9 percent of the population—who opt out of the public insurance system for private coverage (Anderson, Petrosyan, and Hussey 2002).

3. See chapter 18, this volume, Anderson and Hussey, Single-Payer Health Insurance Systems.

4. The term "indirect costs" is used throughout this paper in the accounting sense of the term—as costs that cannot be directly attributable to a specific product or service.

REFERENCES

Anderson, G. F., V. Petrosyan, and P. S. Hussey. 2002. "Multinational Comparisons of Health Systems Data." In *Commonwealth Fund Chartbook*. New York, N.Y.: The Commonwealth Fund.

Bitran, R., and W. C. Yip. 1998. "A Review of Health Care Provider Payment Reform in Selected Countries in Asia and Latin America." Major Applied Research 2, Working Paper 1. Abt Associates Inc., Partnerships for Health Reform Project, Bethesda, Md.

Busse, R. 1999. "Priority-Setting and Rationing in German Health Care." *Health Policy* 50(1–2): 71–90.

Chan, Y. C. 1993. "Improving Hospital Cost Accounting with Activity-Based Costing." *Health Care Management Review* 18(1): 71–77.

Cokin, G. 1996. *Activity-Based Cost Management: Making It Work*. New York, N.Y.: McGraw-Hill.

Davis, K. 2002. "The Danish Health System through an American Lens." *Health Policy* 59: 119–32.

Duckett, S. J. 1998. "Casemix Funding for Acute Hospital Inpatient Services in Australia." *Medical Journal of Australia* 169: S17–S21.

Hoyt, R., and C. Lay. 1995. "Linking Cost Control Measures to Health Care Services by Using Activity-Based Information." *Health Services Management Research* 8(4): 221–33.

Hsiao, W. C., P. Braun, D. L. Dunn, E. R. Becker, D. Yntema, D. K. Verrilli, E. Stamenovic, and S. P. Chen. 1992. "An Overview of the Development and Refinement of the Resource-Based Relative Value Scale. The Foundation for Reform of U.S. Physician Payment." *Medical Care* 30(11 suppl.): NS1–12.

Jackson, T. 2001. "Using Computerised Patient-Level Costing Data for Setting DRG Weights: The Victorian (Australia) Cost Weight Studies." *Health Policy* 56: 149–63.

Jegers, M., K. Kesteloot, D. De Graeve, and W. Gilles. 2002. "A Typology for Provider Payment Systems in Health Care." *Health Policy* 60(3): 255–73.

Kamke, K. 1998. "The German Health Care System and Health Care Reform." *Health Policy* 43: 171–94.

Keeler, E. B., G. Melnick, and J. Zwanziger. 1999. "The Changing Effects of Competition on Non-Profit and For-Profit Hospital Pricing Behavior." *Journal of Health Economics* 18: 69–86.

Kutzin, J. 2001. "A Descriptive Framework for Country-Level Analysis of Health Care Financing Arrangements." *Health Policy* 56(3): 171–204.

Langenbrunner, J. C., and M. M. Wiley. 2002. "Hospital Payment Mechanisms: Theory and Practice in Transition Countries." In M. McKee and J. Healy, eds., *Hospitals in a Changing Europe*. Buckingham, United Kingdom: Open University Press.

Maceira, D. 1998. "Provider Payment Mechanisms in Health Care: Incentives, Outcomes, and Organizational Impact in Developing Countries." Major Applied Research 2, Working Paper 2. Abt Associates Inc., Partnerships for Health Reform Project, Bethesda, Md.

Medicare Payment Advisory Commission (MedPAC) (2002). Report to Congress: Medicare Payment Policy. (Washington, D.C.: MedPAC, 2002).

Mills, A., S. Bennett, P. Siriwanarangsun, and V. Tangcharoensathien. 2000. "The Response of Providers to Capitation Payment: A Case-Study from Thailand." *Health Policy* 51: 163–80.

Newhouse, J. P. 1994. "Patients at Risk: Health Reform and Risk Adjustment." *Health Affairs* 13(1): 132–46.

Newhouse, J. P. 1996. "Reimbursing Health Plans and Health Providers: Efficiency in Production versus Selection." *Journal of Economic Literature* 34: 1236–63.

Player, S. 1998. "Activity-Based Analyses Lead to Better Decision Making." *Healthcare Financial Management* 52(8): 66–70.

Preker, A. S. and A. Harding. 2001. "Innovations in Health Care Delivery: Organizational Reforms within the Hospital Sector." HNP Discussion Paper. World Bank, Washington, D.C.

Rodwin, V. G., H. Grable,, and G. Thiel. 1989. "Updating the Fee Schedule for Physician Reimbursement: A Comparative Analysis of France, Germany, Canada, and the United States." In *Updating the Fee Schedule for Physician Reimbursement: Comparative Analysis of Selected Experience Abroad and of Policy Options for the United States*. Washington, D.C.: PPRC.

Sauerland, D. 2001. "The German Strategy for Quality Improvement in Health Care: Still to Improve." *Health Policy* 56: 127–47.

Waters, H., H. Abdallah, and D. Santillán. 2001. "Application of Activity-Based Costing (ABC) for a Peruvian NGO Healthcare Provider." *International Journal of Health Planning and Management* 16(1): 3–18.

West, D., L. Hicks, and E. A. Balas. 1996. "Profitable Capitation Requires Accurate Costing." *Nursing Economics* 1(3): 162–70.

Wiley, M. 1993. "Costing Hospital Case-Mix: The European Experience." In M. Casas and M. Wiley, eds., *Diagnosis Related Groups in Europe*. Berlin: Springer-Verlag.

World Bank. 2000. *World Development Report 2000/2001: Attacking Poverty*. Washington, D.C.

Wouters, A. 1999. *Alternative Provider Payment Methods: Incentives for Improving Health Care Delivery*. Primer for Policymakers Series 1. Bethesda, Md.: Abt Associates Inc., Partnerships for Health Reform.

PART II

Making Strategic Purchasing Pro-Poor

CHAPTER 7

The Equity Dimensions of Purchasing

Paolo Carlo Belli

Three stylized facts emerge from the literature:

- By all evidence, there are huge differentials in health outcomes and health expenditure per capita between richer and poorer countries.

- Within every country health service utilization is strongly pro-rich, despite the fact that the poor bear a disproportionate morbidity and mortality.

- The distribution of health benefits from government expenditure on health care is extremely unequal and pro-rich.[1]

THE EVIDENCE

Regardless of the diversity of the existing studies in terms of measurement approaches to equity and poverty, study design and geographical focus, the empirical evidence indicates a striking consistency in the association between poverty and poor health. Beaglehole and Bonita (1997, p. 1) assert that poverty is the most important cause of preventable death, disease and disability.

Table 7.1 presents evidence from Gwatkin (2000) on the distribution of mortality among children under five years of age across socioeconomic groups in different regions.[2] The table indicates that disparities between poor and nonpoor vary enormously across countries. On average, a child born in a household

TABLE 7.1   Intracountry Disparities in Mortality of Children under Five Years of Age

Region	Number of countries	Poor-rich ratio		Concentration index[3]	
		Mean	Range	Mean	Range
Sub-Saharan Africa	21	1.79	1.27 to 2.60	−.095	−.040 to −.164
Asia/Near East/North Africa	9	2.69	1.69 to 4.60	−.147	−.084 to −.210
Latin America/Caribbean	11	2.99	1.55 to 4.67	−.167	−.071 to −.259
Total	40	2.06	1.27 to 4.67	−.124	−.040 to −.259

Source: Gwatkin and others 2000.

belonging to the lowest wealth quintile is approximately twice as likely to die before reaching age five as a child born in a household from the highest quintile.

The evidence presented by Gwatkin and others (2000) also indicates that the distribution of utilization of essential health care services is extremely unequal across socioeconomic groups. Despite the disproportional morbidity and mortality that the poor suffer, the wealthy utilize health services disproportionately more than the poor. Even immunization services and other services against communicable diseases, which address diseases mostly concentrated among the poor, are unevenly utilized more by the rich.

The rich utilize more health services both in the private and in the public sector. Benefit-incidence studies[4] on the distribution of public expenditure for health by socioeconomic group show a pronounced pro-rich bias in most developing countries (figure 7.1). For example, Mahal, Yazbeck, and Peters (2001) report that in India the rich receive three times more public subsidy than the poor.

The evidence also shows that different health services are generally characterized by a dissimilar redistributive impact. The public subsidy to hospital care (inpatient and outpatient) is more pro-rich than the subsidy to outpatient care provided by primary health care facilities (the situation is illustrated for the case of India in figure 7.2).

FIGURE 7.1   Share of the Public Subsidy for Curative Care by Income Group (percent)

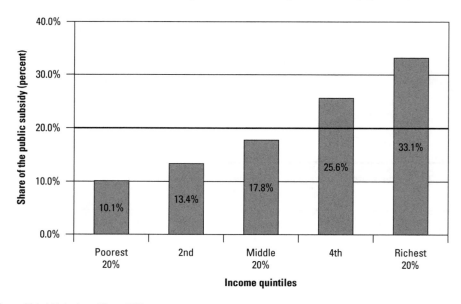

Source: Mahal, Yazbeck, and Peters 2001.

FIGURE 7.2   Beneficiaries of Public Subsidy by Type and Level of Care

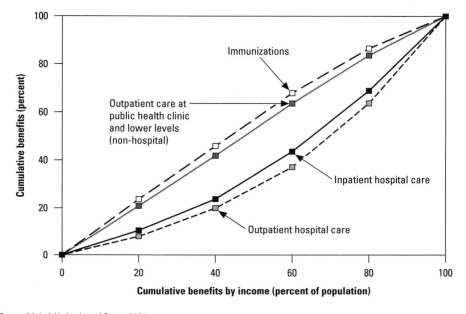

Source: Mahal, Yazbeck, and Peters 2001.

WHAT DOES AN "EQUITABLE DISTRIBUTION OF HEALTH AND HEALTH BENEFITS" MEAN?

The previous section showed that health and health benefits are distributed extremely unequally, and that the poor (those living in poor countries and who are poorer within each country) are immensely disadvantaged. The question this chapter tries to address in this section is: How would an equitable distribution of health resources be characterized? To address this question, the chapter synthetically presents the different equity principles discussed in the literature on equity in health care. In extreme synthesis, all contributions in the literature advocate either a situation characterized by equality of access, or equality of utilization, or by a distribution of health care benefits according to need.

Equality of Access and Utilization

According to Le Grand (1982), equal access to treatment means that individuals should bear the same money and time costs for using health services. Mooney (1983) defends the principle of equality of access rather than that of equality of utilization because the former is more respectful of individual preferences: faced with the same prices, individuals may still choose different levels of treatment. However, Olsen and Rogers (1991) argue that equal access means that everybody can potentially consume the same amount of health services. Thus, prices must be the same (traveling time and costs included), given income. This implies that the poor must be subsidized for their health consumption relatively more than the rich. Pushing Olsen and Rogers's argument to its logical conclusion, Le Grand (1991) argues that equality of access ultimately requires that Choice (or Opportunity) Sets[5] are the same for all individuals. Thus, the stream of literature that developed the concept of equity in health as equality of access, starting from a relatively more respectful view of individual preferences, reached quite radical conclusions concerning the requirements necessary to achieve equality of access.

Distribution of Health Care According to Need

Need is another commonly advocated equity principle for redistribution of health resources.[6] This view advocates equal treatment for equal need, so that individuals in greater need should come first.

But how shall one define need? Culyer and Wagstaff (1993) show that there are several possible definitions and measures of need:

- Need as severity of illness

- Need as ability to benefit

- Need as the minimum amount of resources required to exhaust capacity to benefit.

Each of the these definitions of need leads to different set of prescriptions for the distribution of health care services. Assuming for the purpose of illustration Quality Adjusted Life Years (QALYs) as a measure of the quantum of health that each individual did or could enjoy,[7] we illustrate some of the possibilities of assuming the above definitions of need in table 7.2.

According to the capacity-to-benefit exception of need, in this example one would advocate the criterion in the top-right cell of table 7.2, column 3, to distribute health services. Equity would demand that expected QALY gains be equalized across individuals. The perspective is forward looking and gives priority to those (people, services) most able to benefit from health care. There are two exceptions to the notion of "capacity to benefit." One is to consider "marginal

---

TABLE 7.2   Equity and (Re)distribution of Health Resources

Item	Retrospective health	Prospective health
Health from health care	Previous QALYs gained from health care	Expected QALYs benefit from health care
Health not from health care	Previous QALYs enjoyed without health care	Expected QALY profile without health care

capacity to benefit." This is the principle that maximizes incremental health benefits from health care, and it is one of the most widely used efficiency principles, but it is sometimes advocated also as an equity principle. In actuality, it may be argued that following this principle would lead to extremely inequitable choices, whenever those who are marginally better able to benefit (and should then come first according to this principle) are also the wealthier, the more healthy, or both.[8] A second exception is Culyer and Wagstaff's (1993) "minimum amount of resources required to exhaust capacity to benefit." By these means, a consideration of severity of illness is indirectly phased in the definition of need as capacity to benefit, and the application of this principle leads to more egalitarian results than only considering marginal capacity to benefit (Culyer and Wagstaff 1993).

However, criteria based on an exception of "need" different from "capacity to benefit" are possible as well, and they are indeed frequently preferred for equity reasons by individuals and households, when asked about priority-setting criteria. In Sweden, for example, care for chronically, terminally ill and severely handicapped patients which ranked extremely low in terms of cost-effectiveness criteria were found to be popular and classified as 'essential' care in all household surveys that were conducted to inform the government on people's preferences.[9] This choice is equivalent to choosing the bottom-right cell of table 7.2, column 3, where need is interpreted as severity of illness and priority is given to those who would be more severely ill or vulnerable without proper care, regardless of their "objective" capacity to benefit.

Another principle would be to use the same criteria accepted for education, where everybody is given a set amount of free services (equality of inputs), and every extra is given according to merit, or it is fully paid for. In the case of health, one should then equalize care received across individuals. Alternatively, one could try to equalize health benefits, or QALYs gained from subsidized care[10] over the life cycle, and choose according to the criterion in the top-left cell, table 7.2, column 2. Finally, one might want to bring in considerations linked to the age or the past health condition of potential beneficiaries and give priority to the young or to the disabled, according to the criterion in the lower-left cell of table 7.2, column 2.

Note that all of these equity-motivated criteria, with the exception of the marginal capacity to benefit-based redistribution principle, also conflict with any possible effectiveness principle, which would tend to put resources first where the link between inputs and outcomes can be stronger. In other words, there is in general a tradeoff between distributing resources for health care to maximize gains in health outcomes, and to achieve greater equity (equity-efficiency trade-off).

Finally, the conceptual literature on equity reviewed above, which was developed mostly in Western Europe, has focused on accessibility problems, in a sense taking for granted that health services, once made accessible for all, would also be of acceptable quality standards. By contrast, the evidence from developing countries shows that the issue of quality of public services is at least as important as their accessibility (see below). In several countries or regions within countries, public health services are in theory accessible to all, but they are of such abysmal quality that in reality very few utilize them. In these settings, a focus on equality of treatment or equal treatment for equal need is more appropriate than just focusing on accessibility.

All of the above discussion should suggest how difficult any serious equity assessment is, and how adopting different principles may lead us in different directions. Waters (2000) provides a concrete illustration, by showing how adopting a different principle and consequently a different measure of equity, one is led to an opposite assessment of the impact on equity of a new social insurance program in Ecuador. However, by comparing the evidence on the distribution of health and health benefits in developing countries presented in the first section with the conceptual discussion, it is also clear that, whichever exception of equity one is willing to endorse, one must conclude that this distribution is strikingly inequitable. The path to creating a more equitable distribution of health benefits is immensely complex and difficult, because a host of technical and, more important, political-economic constraints must be overcome to make it possible. Clearly, an exhaustive discussion of these issues is beyond the purview of this work. Here, we focus on a much narrower set of possible interventions, aimed at modifying the criteria according to which health resources are allocated and purchased.

DEFINING VARIABLES: RESOURCE ALLOCATION AND PURCHASING REFORMS

RAP mechanisms define the criteria according to which funds, collected through different revenue sources and pooled, flow within the health system, eventually reaching service providers.[11] The so-called RAP reforms have both: a) strengthened RAP mechanisms and b) introduced a multidimensional vector of changes to existing RAP arrangements.

Key Supply-Side Reform Components

We will focus on six key components, five influencing the supply side, and one on the demand side. The six RAP reforms components are:

- Redesign of resource allocation criteria, moving from input-based, retrospective toward capitation-based or other forms of prospective financing

- Redesign governments' priorities across services or levels of care (identified in several developing countries with the introduction of the "basic benefit package," BBP)

- The insertion of a purchasing agency between patients and providers. The agency is assigned a prospective budget and entrusted with commissioning/contracting services from providers

- Change of payment criteria for providers, from input-based toward activity-based or prospective payment systems.

- Provision of explicit financial and other incentives/enablers to providers, linked with the providers' ability to reach the poor or cure diseases that primarily affect the poor

- Financial incentives for patients/clients, such as vouchers, to stimulate consumption of specific health care services, such as prenatal care and institutional delivery

RAP reforms implemented over the last 15 years in several industrialized and developing countries included a different combination of the above six elements. Table 7.3 illustrates the above RAP reform components, their principal objective, purpose, and activities.

As table 7.3 shows, a correct way to understand RAP reforms is to view them as a tool kit, comprising several elements, which can be varied to achieve improvements in RAP arrangements to enhance efficiency, quality, or improve accessibility of services for the poor.

RAP reforms do not intervene on the sources of financing, or in the organization of service provision,[12] although RAP reform components have frequently been introduced in the context of wider reform processes, which affected also these other dimensions of the health care sector (see case study below, on RAP reforms in Colombia). Specifically, the link of RAP mechanisms with the sources of revenue and pooling arrangements is crucial: any RAP arrangement presupposes that a health financing mechanisms is in place to harness private resources for health care in a pooled fund. In other words, RAP criteria are relevant where governments/social insurance funding is a non-negligible part of total health funding, and where governments can decide how to allocate geographically. However, they are much less relevant to countries with prevalence of out-of-pocket payments (OOP), or demand side funding (e.g. patients choosing where to go and facilities simply being reimbursed retrospectively), unless some geographical or population group budget constraint can be imposed.[13]

Motivation of RAP Reforms

RAP reforms are an attempt to respond to the issues of efficiency, quality, and equity plaguing health systems in several industrial, transition, and developing countries. Such issues, owing to a combination of government and market failures, are revealed in poor spending choices, distorted allocation of resources, provider unresponsiveness to clients, in the general poor quality of services and the like, and ultimately, the inability of the health care system to contribute to achieve better health outcomes.

Over the last decade, a number of studies indicated that "bypassing" of low-quality services offered by public facilities is a widespread phenomenon (Akin and Hutchinson 1999). For Kenya, see Mwabo, Ainsworth, and Nyamete (1993);

TABLE 7.3 Components of Resource Allocation and Purchasing Reforms

RAP reform component	Priority setting	Resource allocation criteria	Purchasing/contracting	Providers' payment systems	Explicit incentives for providers to reach specific groups/cure certain diseases	Explicit incentives for patients to use specific services
RAP arrangement addressed	What services to subsidize and what to exclude?	What are the rules (formula) for transferring public funds?	To make or to buy decision	How to pay? How much to purchase and at what prices?	For whom to purchase?	For whom to purchase?
Purpose	Strategic definition of priorities for public financing and provision.	New criteria for allocating resources across regions, districts and purchasers.	Strategic purchasing; more transparency and results-orientation in public sector; engagement of the private sector in service provision.	Redefinition of the incentive regime for providers.	Reducing exclusion of the poor from public services/sharper targeting	Increasing utilization of essential services by the poor
Activities	Redefinition of priorities across services according to cost-effectiveness or other criteria.	From retrospective to prospective resource allocation.	Definition of contracts and service agreements, increased degree of market exposure for providers	Output/performance based payment systems for providers; performance-based incentives for health workers. Capitation based funding of primary care physicians	Equity-motivated risk-adjusters to correct capitation funding. Explicit financial incentives for providers to cover the poor, or to provide care against diseases that affect the poor (such as TB).	Specific enablers or incentives (such as vouchers) that contribute to treatment and traveling expenses
Objective	Max impact on disease burden, cost effectiveness, correction of market failures		Allocative and productive efficiency. Consumer-responsiveness.		Equity, Financial protection	

128

for the Dominican Republic, see Lewis and others (1991). The high price-elasticity of demand for public health services, particularly observed for child services and among the poor (for Uganda, see Giusti 2000[14] and for Indonesia, Gertler and van der Gaag 1990) may conceal a low evaluation of such services.

The evidence indicates a high degrees of absenteeism in government facilities (see for example, results from a study in India by Chaudhury and others, presented in World Bank 2004, chapter 2, table 1.2b), dual job holding, widespread levels of corruption, and the like, and leads to the conclusion that the level of health expenditure and health inputs officially recorded, such as the number of doctors or number of health facilities available in any particular area, create a negligible impact on health outcomes.

Note that these findings radically question the current effectiveness of public services, but do not question the effectiveness of health services per se. In fact, the evidence indicates that real health inputs and service quality produce a strong impact on utilization and on outcomes (Alderman and Lavy 1996). For instance, Lavy and others (1996) show that in Ghana drug availability and weekly hours of availability of physicians produce a strong impact on child survival, on child height and weight for height.

These studies also question the effectiveness of the traditional ways of channelling foreign assistance in the health sector to developing countries, mainly focused on the expansion of the infrastructure base of the government health sector. While these continuous investments have made a tangible difference to physical infrastructure and delivery capacity, the outcomes in terms of actual improvement in services—particularly to the poor and disadvantaged groups—have not been as obvious.[15]

To draw a coherent "stylized fact" from all of the above findings, we may say that increasingly what seems to matter most is investments in service improvements—not availability of facilities.

Furthermore, by looking at the variations across countries and at the few success stories available, it is becoming recognizable that the results obtained by a few countries in terms of health outcomes and in terms of quality and accessibility of essential health services are achievable also at relatively low levels of economic development. Although there is little doubt about the important effect of income on individual health, the international evidence indicates that the relationship between average national income (measured by per capita gross domestic product [GDP]) to and average national life expectancy and other health indicators is by no means universal or automatic,[16] and that low income by itself does not explain the poor health achievement of citizens of some developing countries.

Against the background described above, RAP reforms can be easily justified. Their focus is on the "value for money" that patients obtain from the health system, and to find ways to improve it. If the reason for poor quality and ineffectiveness in service delivery particularly in the public sector is to be found in the lack of incentives, or to the "wrong" incentives existing for providers, then a precondition to improve "value for money" is to profoundly reform the criteria according to which resource allocation decisions are taken, priorities are set, and financial rewards/penalties are given. RAP reforms propose to improve health outcomes by incorporating a more transparent and results-based approach as a key feature in their design.

Hence, the test to assess RAP reforms is whether such reforms are actually achieving the service improvements they promised or not, and whether the poor are at least partially benefiting from such improvements.[17] Also, note that there is more to improving access and quality of services than just allocating resources more transparently and sensibly, and that therefore RAP reforms are but a piece in a large puzzle. Even if a correct allocation of resources, better incentives were set in place, we cannot assume that this will mechanically lead to the desired objectives.

The Evidence of the RAP Reforms' Impact on Equity

Unfortunately, the above questions remain largely unaddressed, because the evidence available on the RAP reforms' impact on equity is still largely inconclusive. The lack of a scientifically rigorous evidence base to evaluate the RAP reforms is partially due to intrinsic measurement difficulties. Aggregate measures of equity, especially those concerning distribution of health outcomes, change slowly, while most RAP reforms in developing countries are recent. The level and distribution of education or income per capita and several other variables are perhaps more important than utilization of health services for explaining health differentials across socioeconomic groups. But because they are also continuously in evolution, it is extremely difficult to ascribe to health reforms some of the distributional changes observed. However, the lack of conclusive evidence is also caused by an insufficient attention to monitoring and evaluating the reforms, and specifically to the equity dimension of the reforms. For instance, one can hardly find any data to evaluate the impact of RAP reforms where the change in utilization of essential health services is measured disaggregated by socioeconomic groups, with an explicit focus on the benefits for the poor. We hope that in the future new and more conclusive evidence will soon be brought to bear on some of the conceptual arguments and hypotheses presented here.

The existing empirical evidence allows a few preliminary conclusions to be drawn. For instance, it shows that some RAP reform components, such as the new criteria for allocating resources and setting new priorities for providing and financing public services, can even out and make the distribution of resources across regions and districts more transparent and linked to need. They can also contribute to reorienting public expenditure toward levels of care and services that disproportionately benefit the poor. For instance in Chile, the government created a Municipal Common Fund, which is a horizontal equalization fund that receives up to 60 percent of the wealthier municipalities' own-source income and redistributes it to the poorer municipalities on the basis of a per capita formula. The formula takes into consideration the percentage of people living in rural areas, as well as the municipalities' capacity to generate their own revenue. As table 7.4 shows, the fund has significantly contributed to decreasing variability in per capita funding across different municipalities (the ratio of total public health expenditure per capita in the wealthiest to the poorest municipalities was reduced from 2.2 in 1991 to 1.6 in 1996 [Bossert 2000]).

Resource allocation reforms have also been undertaken in South Africa, Uganda, and Zambia. In these countries, the implementation of the new resource allocation formula was not without difficulties, and progress has been uneven. In Zambia a new population-based formula was implemented in 1994, with some crude adjustments to reflect cost and need indicators. The absence of a fuel station or a bank was used as a proxy for underdevelopment, and districts received an extra weight where these facilities were missing. Subsequent research (Lake, Mtonga, and Nakamba 2002) showed that the correlation between these first crude need indicators and more sophisticated measures of relative deprivation (derived through principal components analysis) is indeed extremely significant, and that other simple indicators such as population density and remoteness can explain most of the provinces' relative deprivation. One key issue that hindered the impact of the new population and need-based formula in Zambia was that a large share of the total public health expenditure was "top-sliced" to fund tertiary care facilities, concentrated mainly in Lusaka.

In South Africa, which had before 1994 one of the more inequitable health systems in terms of resource allocation (McIntyre and others 2000), in the immediate post-Apartheid period there was a strong political commitment in favor of a radical shift of resources away from the relatively prosperous areas and toward the poorer provinces, mainly in the northern and eastern parts of the country. The allocation to the poorest, Northern province, was expected to increase from between 6 and 7 percent of the total share to 15 percent over a five-year period, while funds for Gauteng province were to decline from 25 percent to between 17 and 18 percent, a significant reduction in real terms. Moreover, 30 percent of this shift was expected to occur in the first year. Not surprisingly the above targets proved impossible to achieve; Gauteng received extra support in the short term and Northern province was unable to absorb the additional funds effectively.

TABLE 7.4   The Impact of the Municipal Common Fund in Chile

Item	Income before MCF	Income after MCF
Average	24,646	40,823
Variation coefficient	17,437	30,984
Gini coefficient	0.45	0.30

Source: Bossert 2000.

Also, the devolution of powers to the provincial governments (which started to receive a block grant without specific allocation to health) and the new macroeconomic policies hampered the redistribution process (Gilson and others 1999). The experience from the Resource Allocation Working Party in the United Kingdom shows that a more gradual transition process to the new regime is a key issue for the success of the new population and need-based resource allocation formula, so that the "losers" in the redistribution process have the opportunity to adjust and the "winners" to develop new planning capacity.

Experiences involving government attempts to reprioritize public services indicate mixed results. Several countries have started to define an essential health package (BBP, Basic Benefit Package), influenced by the methodologies set out in the 1993 World Development Report (WDR), to be used as a guidance for priority setting in public funding and provision. However, in the majority of cases the implementation of the BBP has either never passed the preparatory phase or resulted in tokenistic change.[18] The move toward more cost-effective or more pro-poor services has been sometimes implemented at the local level. In other cases, such as Uganda, reprioritization policies defined at the central level have clashed with the concomitant decentralization process.[19] In several cases essential packages have proven to be vaguely defined, setting out a range of services but giving little detail on who is to provide them, how they are to be delivered, how many services are to be delivered, and to whom. Prioritization policies have been more successful when they were based on existing patterns of expenditure, and proposed realistic changes at the margin. The principles for priority setting should be correcting market failure and improving the pro-poor impact of health interventions.

The interposition of a purchasing agency between patients and providers is a relatively new phenomenon. "Purchasing" reforms were introduced first in some industrialized countries, such as the United Kingdom (1990), and then during the 1990s in several middle-income countries of Latin America (Colombia) and of Central Eastern Europe (Czech Republic, Poland, the Baltic countries), and in the Caucasus (Georgia). All of these countries entrusted newly formed agencies (such as social insurance funds), or existing ones (such as local authorities, or private insurers in Latin America) with the purchasing role. Other countries such as Cambodia, without relying on purchasing agencies separate from the government, did nonetheless experiment with contracts to discipline the relationships involving private not-for-profit or for-profit providers.

Still very few rigorous studies exist to assess the overall performance of the new purchasing or contracting arrangements, particularly their impact on equity. In synthesis, the evidence collected so far reveals promising but also problematic aspects of the new contracting experiences. The evidence from Cambodia (Bhushan, Keller, and Schwartz 2002) suggests that contracting in and out services to NGOs produced an extremely positive impact on the poor, improving coverage and quality of services for lower socioeconomic groups, as table 7.5 indicates. The benefits were greater for contracted-out districts, where government service delivery was more expensive ($4.50 per capita, compared with $2.82 and $1.5 spent per

TABLE 7.5   Average Change in Service Coverage Indicators in Cambodia (first 2 and 1/2 years of reforms)[20]

Indicator	Control district	Contracted-in	Contracted out
Immunization rates—all[21]	56	82	158
Vitamin A capsule Receipt—all	−25.1	18.1	20.9
Vitamin A capsule Receipt—lower 50% socioeconomic segment of population	−24.1	29.9	23.9
Percent of illnesses Treated in Public Health Facility—lower 50% socioeconomic segment of population	81.7	490.5	1096.0

Source: Bhushan, Keller, and Schwartz 2002.

capita in contracted-in and control districts), but where private out-of-pocket payments were reduced by 27 percent overall and over 70 percent for the lower socioeconomic groups, indicating good targeting of beneficiaries.

Utilization of curative services in district hospitals by the bottom 50 percent socioeconomic group increased about 12-fold in contracted-out districts, sixfold in contracted-in districts, and only less than twofold in the control districts.

The same positive results are reported in local studies that analyzed contracting with not-for-profit providers in Bolivia, Bangladesh (nutrition services), India (TB-DOTs treatment), and sub-Saharan Africa (Giusti 2000).[22] The flexibility in the management of inputs allowed NGOs to improve service coverage, and achieve significant cost savings compared to government standards without compromising quality of services (for a careful review, see Loevinsohn and Harding 2004). A study of the impact of contracts in South Africa (Palmer 2000) indicated the importance of maintaining competition among providers, and of defining ex ante the population to be covered by the contract. Fixing the beneficiaries' pool allows the use of capitation payments, which encourages prevention. Several other authors have highlighted the significant human capital and information systems requirements to specify and to manage contracts effectively, to be contrasted with the limitations characterizing several developing countries (McPake and Banda 1994; Mills, Bennett, and McPake 1997; Taylor 2000; Vining and Globerman 1999; Waters, Hatt, and Axelsson 2002). Based on the evidence available, one can say that effectively designing and monitoring contracts has proved as demanding as directly managing health services, and that where the public sector was not able to effectively "row," it has generally also proved unable to effectively "steer" independent or semi-independent providers through contracts. Often, contracting experiences were accompanied with payment system reforms.

Other countries of Latin America, Asia, and Africa implemented radical payment system reform over the last decade, with or without explicit contracting mechanisms. The general trend has been to move away from input-based payment systems and toward output-based payment systems, such as DRG-based payments for hospitals and fee-for-service reimbursement for primary care—and more recently toward capitation payments for primary care doctors. Other countries have introduced explicit performance-related financial incentives for providers, particularly in their vertical programs against communicable diseases.

The data are generally not sufficient for a rigorous equity assessment (for example, no information is available on changes in services' utilization by socioeconomic group), but it consistently indicates increased activity volumes and often improved productivity indicators (decrease in length of stay and unit costs) in hospitals after the reforms.

One key concern is that these new RAP mechanisms, introducing competition among purchasers, contracting with the private sector, and output- or outcome-related payment systems, would raise the possibility of introducing severe distortions in providers' behavior to the detriment of the poor. Specifically, purchasing, contracting, and payment system reforms meant to reduce costs, increase efficiency, or improve quality of services may in fact lead to wider quality differentials across services and increase providers' incentive to cream skim, risk select, and undertreat poorer or more vulnerable patients. In the absence of any solid empirical evidence, the arguments in favor or against reform remain primarily theoretical (see review of the literature in the long version of this paper).

Finally, explicit demand-side incentives can be—and have been—utilized to stimulate consumption of specific health and reproductive health services. Demand for health services is usually lower among the populations needing them most. To stimulate the consumption of services with large externalities (vaccinations, maternal and child care, communicable disease treatment), the opportunity cost (which includes time lost for gainful employment and traveling costs) can be lowered for the poor, by providing specific enablers or incentives (such as vouchers that contribute to treatment and traveling expenses). These demand-side RAP mechanisms are investigated, among others, by Gorter and others (1999) and by Armstrong and others (1999). Gorter and others report the experience of vouchers for sex health services in Nicaragua, and Armstrong-Schellenberg and others report the experience with vouchers for mosquito nets in Tanzania. Both programs were not without difficulties, but overall they led to significant increases in utilization and improved health outcomes.

CONCLUSIONS AND RECOMMENDATIONS

The new allocations mechanisms and incentives introduced by RAP reforms, characterized by more transparent geographical distribution of resources, output/outcome orientation, arms-length relationship with providers, and so on has the potential to significantly improve the current "way to do business" in the health sector. Their full potential probably is not yet exploited.

Implementing RAP reforms entails intensive resource as well as human capital investments in order to be appropriately implemented and monitored, and to prevent potential adverse effects. It also requires that governments be able to find within the RAP reforms' toolkit a mix of interventions and mechanisms able to maximize the reforms' positive impact, and to control adverse effects, particularly on the equity dimension. The ability to implement these investments and this steering/oversight in turn presupposes a health financing framework and other preconditions that may not yet be feasible in the poorest, capacity-constrained countries.

We also repeatedly underlined that it is necessary that ongoing and future reforms be subject to a more rigorous monitoring and evaluation process. Whenever possible, reforms should also be implemented in a way that allows their evaluation, by phasing in changes progressively and by leaving a control group temporarily isolated from their impact.

NOTES

1. We define as "health (care) benefits" the financial and other instruments put in place by governments to facilitate access and utilization of health services. The evidence concerning the distribution of health care benefits leads to different conclusions in industrial countries. These countries achieved a fairly even distribution of utilization rates across socioeconomic groups, although there are still pockets of underserved poor (Van Doorslaer and Wagstaff, 2000). Despite this, inequalities in health status across socioeconomic groups persist, although they are not nearly as stark as in developing countries, and in fact seem to have widened during the last decade, particularly in the United Kingdom because of the increased income and wealth differential across different socioeconomic groups (see Van Doorslaer and others 1997; Independent Inquiry into Inequalities in Health 1998).

2. Gwatkin and others (2000) utilize the Demographic and Health Survey data from 40 developing countries to analyze inequalities in (a) infant and under-five mortality; (b) malnutrition; (c) incidence of diarrhea and acute respiratory infection; (d) fertility rates; (e) information on human immunodeficiency virus/acquired immunodeficiency syndrome (HIV/AIDS); and (f) use of maternal and child health services across socioeconomic groups. They divide the population into different socioeconomic groups according to asset ownership, adopting a wealth index developed by Filmer and Pritchett (1998) and using principal components analysis.

3. The concentration index is equal to: $1 - 2 \int_0^1 MR_i(w_i) dw$, where MR is the cumulative proportion of mortality rates among children graphed against the cumulative proportion of their households' wealth ($i = 1,...,5$). A negative (positive) value of the concentration index indicates inequality favoring the rich (poor).

4. Benefit-incidence studies compute the average subsidy for the different types of care (usually, primary, outpatient specialist care, inpatient care) from budgetary information and from data on service use. They estimate the subsidy going to each group from information on the distribution of utilization by income group of the different service types.

Mathematically, benefit incidence is estimated by the following formula:

$$X_j \equiv \sum_i U_{ij} \frac{S_i}{U_i} \equiv \sum_i \frac{U_{ij}}{U_i} S_i \equiv \sum_i e_{ij} S_i$$

X_j = health sector subsidy enjoyed by group j,

U_{ij} = utilization of service i by group j,

U_i = utilization of service i by all groups combined,

S_i = government *net* expenditure on service i, and

e_{ij} = group j's share of utilization of service i

Thus, incidence studies present a series of limitations. First, they do not consider therapeutic benefits, nor do they adjust for different need across quintiles. Second, they do not consider the health service financing mechanisms. Finally, they do not convey any information about the reasons behind the observed differential utilization of services across socioeconomic groups.

5. Individuals' Choice or Opportunity Sets comprise all the combinations of goods and services that the individuals can afford given their income at existing prices. The extension of the Opportunity Set characterizing any given individual depends not only on her/his wealth endowments and income, but also on her/his ability to borrow, which is linked to financial market efficiency.

6. Usually, the literature refers to the principles of horizontal and vertical equity. The two principles were first articulated by the Greek philosopher Aristotle: the horizontal equity principle states that equals should be treated equally, whereas the vertical equity principle states that those who are unequal should be treated differently. Applied to health care provision, they are usually translated in the principle that access or use of health services should solely be based on need, and independent of socioeconomic condition or any other non-need-related characteristic (such as gender). Applied to health financing, they are usually translated in the principle that contribution to funding of health services should be in direct relation to ability to pay.

7. The principle limitation of QALYs is that they attempt to measure quality of life on the basis of "expert" opinion, which can be arbitrary. The welfare (subjective) assessment of benefits, as well the social evaluation of health gains, may be totally different from any "objective" measurement of health gains.

8. This criterion ominously recalls principles originally proposed by Herbert Spencer. Spencer (1820–1903), a British sociologist, first applied Darwin's theory of evolution to the study of human societies. According to his views, individuals who contribute more to a society and those who are more fit should be preferred over the others.

9. Swedish Parliamentary Priorities Commission, "Priorities in Health Care: Ethics, economy, implementation," Fritzes, Stockholm, 1995.

10. The issue here is not to decide priorities starting from a situation where no services are available; rather, to evaluate how much additional care should the state allow an individual to receive over and above what he/she could afford to pay for.

11. Health financing includes both the alternative ways to fund health services, by collecting and pooling resources for health, and the criteria for distributing resources across purchasers and providers.

12. RAP reforms are also different from the privatization of health service delivery, although with purchasing reforms, governments, for the first time, explicitly recog-

nized the role of the private sector. Through purchasing and contracting, RAP reforms try to replicate within the public sector some market mechanisms for improving efficiency, but their essential motivation is the recognition that "incentives apply to governments and not just to markets" (Stiglitz 1999, pp. 3–4). In fact, one of the more difficult challenges confronting RAP reforms is to be able to introduce new incentive mechanisms within a public system's framework—to grasp some of the advantages of markets in terms of efficiency and quality of services but to preserve or enhance other goals such as equity that should characterize a public health system.

13. This is a key point: what RAP reforms have been able to achieve may be constrained by the fragmentation of the health funding system. For example, in former socialist countries there have been five parallel coexisting financing systems in place, each of them responsible for funding services for different population subgroups and/or for different services: (a) those in formal employment are often covered through contributions to a social insurance fund; (b) the poor and destitute are often covered by direct transfers from the Ministry of Health. The MoH also covers public health services (c) regions, districts and municipalities finance specific services, such as emergency services, through local taxes and through transfers from the Ministry of Finance (d) the rich sometimes have access to purchasing arrangements provided through private health insurance: and (d) rural populations and the informal sector rely heavily on direct out-of-pocket payments outside formal purchasing arrangements. A similar fragmentation characterizes also most countries in Latin America, where there are usually several sickness funds with significant differences in the benefits provided. In these contexts RAP mechanisms risk to be largely irrelevant, and disparities across socioeconomic groups in the level of health benefits are likely to persist or increase over time.

14. In 1997 a natural experiment was recorded in Uganda. Non-profit facilities raised their user fees in August (up to roughly US $1.5 per child outpatient visit, and up to US $7.5 per adult outpatient visit) and then lowered them again in November, after the government committed to subsidize them. Giusti (2002) recorded extremely wide variation in service use, especially for childcare.

15. A similar point is stated in the 2001 HNP Chapter for the PRSP Sourcebook: "One point needs emphasizing, namely that funds linked to PRSPs—whether debt relief or IDA credits—will have a far greater impact on poor countries' health levels if they are accompanied by a thorough review of existing policies, and by a willingness to link new spending with reforms that make health systems work better, especially for the people they tend to serve less well—the poor (2001 HNP Chapter for PRSP Sourcebook, p. 5). The Commission on Macroeconomics and Health (WP 5) reached similar conclusions in its work on constraints to scaling up health services (Mills et al. 2001).

16. Among the good performers relative to their level of socioeconomic development are Costa Rica, Cuba, Sri Lanka, and the Indian state of Kerala. For example, in 1997 Cuba and Costa Rica had a per capita Gross Domestic Product respectively equal to $3,100 and $3,810, an under-five mortality equal to 9 and 13 respectively, and a life expectancy equal to 75.7, 76.0 years, which are indicators comparable to those of the wealthiest countries of West Europe and North America (World Bank 1999).

17. Note that RAP reforms have not been justified because they intended to improve services specifically for the poor. However, the above discussion suggests that any health reform that succeeds in improving quality and effectiveness of health services in general, and particularly public services, without reducing accessibility, it is also likely to have ipso facto a positive impact on the poor, because it is the poor who mostly have to rely on the government for financing their health expenditure. In a study based on a sample of 35 countries (where nationally representative household surveys were

conducted), Bidani and Ravallion (1997) show that public health spending matters for the poor (measured as the number of individuals living on less than US$2 a day, or US$1 a day at 1985 purchasing power parity), although its impact is insignificant on the richer segments of the population and on the population as a whole. More recently, Gupta, Verhoeven, and Tiongson (2001) report similar results. These results are not surprising, if we consider that the poor are less able to substitute private care when public care is lacking or of poor quality.

18. Bobadilla (1996) presents a review of several National preparatory studies for the definition of an essential package of services, based on the analysis of the burden of disease and on the availability of cost-effective interventions. He reports that very few of those studies became translated into concrete proposals for reprioritization of government services, and even fewer of these proposals were actually implemented.

19. In the case of Uganda, for example, the amount of public funds spent on primary health care at the district level declined dramatically following decentralization despite it being a clearly stated national priority. The response there was to shift back towards a direct allocation approach in the short term by earmarking funds to the health sector. This has caused problems, as some saw it as inappropriate decentralization. They thought that the new RA processes, by allocating a block grant to the local level, was supporting capacity building and more effective management at district level. Others saw it as a legitimate move by Government to ensure national priorities were followed. Recently in Uganda the process of decentralization has been moving ahead again. The role of district hospitals in delivering primary health care services has now been recognized and attempts are being made to allow these units to qualify for Poverty Action Fund financing.

20. In Cambodia two forms of contracts were utilized in different districts (Loevinsohn 2001):
    • Contracting Out (CO): in which the contractors assumed complete responsibility for service delivery, including hiring, firing and setting wages, procuring and distributing essential drugs and supplies.
    • Contracting In (CI): where the external contractors was brought in to provide certain specific productions inputs, but always within the umbrella of the public health system, managed by the MOH. NGO were asked to manage the health centers in particular districts, using the logistics, drugs and supplies provided by the government. The contractors could not hire or fire health workers.

21. Baseline immunization coverage was 25.5 percent in contracted-out districts (COD), 29.9 in contracted-in districts (CID), and 34 percent in the control districts (CD). The follow-up survey showed coverage of, respectively, 65.8 (COD), 54.4 (CID), and 53 (CD).

22. In Uganda, the case analyzed by Giusti (2000), the government contract and subsidy allowed NFP hospitals to reduce user fees, and this created a positive impact on utilization.

REFERENCES

Akin, J., and P. Hutchinson. 1999. "Health Care Facility Choice and the Phenomenon of Bypassing." *Health Policy and Planning* 14: 135–51.

Alderman, H., and V. Lavy. 1996. "Household Responses to Public Health Services: Cost and Quality Trade-offs." *World Bank Research Observer* 11: 3–22.

Armstrong-Schellenberg, J. R. M., S. Abdulla, H. Minja, R. Nathan, O. Mukasa, T. Marchant, and others. 1999. "KINET: A Social Marketing Programme of Treated Nets and Net Treatment for Malaria Control in Tanzania, with Evaluation of Child Health and Long-Term Survival." *Trans R Soc Trop Med Hyg* 93: 225–31.

Beaglehole, R., and R. Bonita. 1997. *Public Health at the Crossroads*. Cambridge: Cambridge University Press.

Belli, P. 2001a. "How Adverse Selection Affects the Health Insurance Market." World Bank Policy Research Working Paper 2148. World Bank, Washington, D.C.

———. 2001b. "Ten Years of Health Reforms in the ECA Region. Lessons Learned and Options for the Future." Working Paper 11, No.6. Center for Population and Development Studies, Cambridge, Mass.

Bhushan, I., Keller, S., and B. Schwartz, 2002, *Achieving the Twin Objectives of Efficiency and Equity: Contracting Health Services in Cambodia*, Asian Development Bank, Policy Brief Series.

Bidani, B., and M. Ravallion. 1997. "Decomposing Social Indicators Using Distributional Data." *Journal of Econometrics* 77: 125–39.

Bossert, T. 2000. "Decentralization of Health Systems in Latin America: A Comparative Study of Chile, Colombia, and Bolivia." Discussion Paper 29. LAC/HSR Health Sector Reform Initiative. Harvard School of Public Health, Data for Decision Making Project, Boston, Mass. http://www.hsph.harvard.edu/ihsp/publications/pdf/lac/Decentralization 45. PDF.

Culyer, A., and A. Wagstaff. 1993. "Equity and Inequality in Health and Health Care." *Journal of Health Economics* 11: 207–10.

Filmer, D., and L. Pritchett. 1998. "Estimating Wealth Effects without Expenditure Data—or Tears: An Application to Educational Enrollments in the States of India." World Bank Policy Research Working Paper 1994. World Bank, Washington, D.C.

Gertler, P., and J. van der Gaag. 1990. *The Willingness to Pay for Medical Care: Evidence from Two Developing Countries*. Baltimore, Md.: John Hopkins University Press.

Gilson, L., J. Doherty, D. McIntyre, S. Thomas, V. Brijlal, C. Bowa, and S. Mbatsha. 1999. "The Dynamics of Policy Change: Health Care Financing in South Africa 1994–1999." Centre for Health Policy, University of Witwatersrand, Johannesburg.

Giusti, D. 2000. *TheFight against Poverty and the Private Not for Profit Sector in Uganda*. Kampala: Uganda Catholic, Protestant and Muslim Bureaux.

Gorter, A., P. Sandiford, Z. Segura, and C. Villabella. 1999. "Improved Health Care for Sex Workers: A Voucher Programme for Female Sex Workers in Nicaragua." In *Research for Sex Work 2*. Available at http://www.med.vu.nl/hcc/artikelen/gorter2.htm

Gupta, S., M. Verhoeven, and E. Tiongson. 2001. "Public Spending on Health Care and the Poor." IMF Working Paper 01/127. International Monetary Fund, Washington, D.C.

Gwatkin, D. 2000. "Reducing Health Inequalities in Developing Countries." *Oxford Textbook of Public Health,* 4th ed. (eds. D. Leon and G. Walt). Oxford: Oxford University Press. http://www.ldb.org/iphw/dg.pdf

Gwatkin, D., M. Guillot, and P. Heuveline. 1999. "The Burden of Disease among the Global Poor." *Lancet* 354: 586–89.

Gwatkin, D., S. Rutstein, K. Johnson, R. Pande, and A. Wagstaff. 2000. *Socioeconomic Differences in Health, Nutrition, and Population in Bangladesh* (and comparable publications covering Benin, Bolivia, Brazil, Burkina Faso, Cameroon, Central African Republic, Colombia, Comores, Côte d'Ivoire, Dominican Republic, Ghana, Guatemala, Haiti, India, Indonesia, Kenya, Kyrgyz Republic, Madagascar, Malawi, Mali, Morocco, Mozambique, Namibia, Nepal, Nicaragua, Niger, Nigeria, Pakistan, Paraguay, Peru, Philippines, Senegal, Tanzania, Togo, Turkey, Uganda, Vietnam, Zambia, and Zimbabwe). Washington, D.C.: World Bank.

Independent Inquiry into Inequalities in Health. 1998. London: Stationery Office.

Lake, S., S. Mtonga, and P. Nakamba. 2002. "Strengthening Needs-Based Resource Allocation in the Zambian Health Sector." Draft. Centre for Health Policy, University of Witwatersrand, Johannesburg.

Lavy, V. J. Strauss, D. Thomas, and P. de Vreyer. 1996. "Quality of Health Care, Survival and Health Outcomes in Ghana." *Journal of Health Economics* 15: 333–57.

Le Grand, J. 1982. *The Strategy of Equality.* London: Allen and Unwin.

———. 1991. *Equity and Choice. An Essay in Economics and Applied Philosophy.* London: Harper Collins.

Lewis, M.A., M.B. Sulvetta, and G.M. La Forgia. 1991. "Productivity and Quality of Public Hospital Medical Staff: A Dominican Case Study." *International Journal of Health Planning and Management* 6: 287–308.

Loevinsohn, B. 2000a. *Checklist for Contracting of Health Services.* Draft, World Bank, Washington, D.C.

———. 2000b. *Contracting for the delivery of primary health care in Cambodia: Design and initial experience of a large pilot test, Draft.* The World Bank. Washington, D.C.

Loevinsohn, B., Harding, A., 2004, Buying Results: *A review of Developing Country Experience with Contracting for health care services.* The World Bank. Washington, D.C.

Mahal, A., A. Yazbeck, and D. Peters. 2001. *The Poor and Health Service Use in India.* Washington, D.C.: World Bank.

McIntyre, D. and L. Gilson. 2002. "Putting Equity in Health Back onto the Social Policy Agenda: Experience from South Africa." *Social Science and Medicine* 54: 1637–56.

McIntyre D., D. Muirhead, L. Gilson, V. Govender, S. Mbatsha, J. Goudge, H. Wadee, and P. Ntutela. 2000. *Geographic Patterns of Deprivation and Health Inequities in South Africa: Informing Public Resource Allocation Strategies.* Report of a study funded by SADC Equinet/IDRC and TDR/ICHSRI. Cape Town: Health Economics Unit and Centre for Health Policy, Johannesburg, and National Department of Health, Pretoria.

McPake, B., and E. Banda. 1994. Contracting out of health services in developing countries. *Health Policy and Planning. 1994*; 9:25–30.

McPake, B., F. J. Yepes, S. Lake, and L. H. Sanchez. 2002. "Is the Public Health System Reform Improving the Performance of Public Hospitals in Bogotá?" Manuscript.

Mills, A. 1998. "To Contract or Not to Contract? Issues for Low and Middle-Income Countries." *Health Policy and Planning* 13: 32–40.

Mills, A., S. Bennett, and B. McPake, eds. 1997. *Private Health Providers in Developing Countries: Serving the Public Interest?* London: Zed Books.

Mills, A., S. Bennett, P. Siriwanarangsun, and V. Tangcharoensathien. 2000. "The Response of Providers to Capitation Payment: A Case-Study from Thailand." *Health Policy* 51: 163–80.

Mooney, G. 1983. "Equity in Health Care: Confronting the Confusion." *Effective Health Care* 1: 179–85.

Mwabo, G., M. Ainsworth, and A. Nyamete. 1993. "Quality of Care and Choice of Medical Treatment in Kenya. An Empirical Analysis." *Journal of Human Resources* 28: 838–62.

Nakamba, P., K. Hanson, and B. McPake. 2002. "Markets for Hospital Services in Zambia." *International Journal of Health Planning and Management* 17: 229–47.

Olsen, E., and D. Rogers. 1991. "The Welfare Economics of Equal Access." *Journal of Public Economics* 45: 91–106.

Palmer, N. 2000. The use of private-sector contracts for primary health care: theory, evidence and lessons for low-income and middle-income countries. *Bulletin of the World Health Organization* 78(6): 821–30.

Stiglitz, J. 1999. "Incentives and Institutions in the Provision of Health Care in Developing Countries: Towards an Efficient and Equitable Health Care Strategy." Paper presented at the IHEA II Meetings, June 1999, Rotterdam.

Swedish Parliamentary Priorities Commission. 1995. *Priorities in Health Care: Ethics, Economy, Implementation.* Stockholm: Fritzes.

Taylor, R., 2000, Contracting for Health Services, Background paper, Private Participation in Health Handbook, The World Bank, Washington D.C.

Van Doorslaer, E., A. Wagstaff, and H. Bleichrodt. 1997. "Income-Related Inequalities in Health: Some International Comparisons." *Journal of Health Economics* 16: 93–112.

Van Doorslaer, E., A. Wagstaff, and others. 2000. "Equity in the Delivery of Health Care: Further International Comparisons." *Journal of Health Economics* 19: 553–583.

Van Doorslaer, E., A. Wagstaff, H. Bleichrodt, S. Calonge, U.-G. Gerdtham, M. Gerfin, J. Geurts, L. Gross, U. Häkkinen, R. Leu, O. O'Donnell, C. Propper, F. Puffer, M. Rodriguez, G. Sundberg, and O. Winkelhake. 1997. "Socioeconomic Inequalities in Health: Some International Comparisons." *Journal of Health Economics.* 16(1): 93–112.

Victora, C. and others. 2000. "Explaining Trends in Inequities: Evidence from Brazilian Child Health Studies." *Lancet* 356: 1093–98.

Vining, A. and S. Globerman. 1999. A conceptual framework for understanding the outsourcing decision. *European Management Journal 17*(6): 645–654

Wagstaff, A. 2000b. Socioeconomic Inequalities in Child Mortality: Comparisons across Nine Developing Countries. *Bulletin of the World Health Organization* 78: 19–29.

———. 2001. "Poverty and Health." Accompanying paper for the work of the Commission on Macroeconomics and Health. World Health Organization, Geneva.

———. 1999. *Inequalities in Infant and Child Mortality in the Developing World: How Large Are They? How Can They Be Reduced?* Presentation to World Bank HNP and Poverty Seminar, March 30.

———. 2000a. *Research on Equity, Poverty and Health: Lessons for the Developing World*, Draft. World Bank, Washington D.C.

———. 2000b. Socioeconomic inequalities in child mortality: Comparisons across nine developing countries. *Bulletin of the World Health Organization*, 78, 19–29.

———. 2001. "Poverty and Health," paper presented for the Commission on Macroeconomics and Health, WHO, Geneva.

Wagstaff A., and E. van Doorslaer. 1998. *Inequalities in health: methods and results for Jamaica*. Paper prepared for the Human Development Department of the World Bank. Second version May 1998.

Wagstaff, A., and E. Van Doorslaer. 2000. *Equity in Health Finance and Delivery*, Chapter 40, *Handbook of Health Economics*, Elsevier Science.

Wagstaff, A., P. Paci, and E. Van Doorslaer. 1991. On the measurement of horizontal equity in the delivery of health care. *Journal of Health Economics* 10: 169–205.

Waters, H. 2000. Measuring Equity in Access to Health Care, *Social Science and Medicine* 51: 599–612.

Waters, H., Laurel Hatt, and Henrik Axelsson. 2002. *Working with the Private Sector for Child Health*. The World Bank, Washington, D.C.

Weil, D. 2000. Advancing Tuberculosis Control within Reforming Systems. *The International Journal of Tuberculosis and Lung Disease* 4: 597–605.

World Bank. 1999. *World Development Indicators*. Washington, D.C.

———. 2001. *HNP Chapter for PRSP Sourcebook*. Washington, D.C.

———. 2004. World Development Report: *Making Services Work for Poor People,* the World Bank, Washington, D.C.

CHAPTER 8

Reversing the Law of Inverse Care

Finn Diderichsen

Poor people shoulder the greatest burden of disease but receive a smaller share of health care resources than do the healthy and better-off. In other words, health care resources are distributed inversely in relation to need. This phenomenon is known as "the inverse care law." It holds true from country to country and within countries across socioeconomic groups.

THE INVERSE CARE LAW AT WORK IN RICH AND POOR COUNTRIES

The notion of the inverse care law was coined in the United Kingdom (Tudor Hart 1971), but the most striking examples of its existence today are seen in poor countries. In the rich parts of the world, socioeconomic inequalities in health have been recognized for decades, but they are—in relative terms—just as great in poor countries (Evans and others 2001).

This disparity in health status is confirmed by data from several demographic and health surveys gathered in 43 low- and middle-income countries in the 1990s (table 8.1). Socioeconomic inequalities in mortality are large—both in

TABLE 8.1 Mortality and Full Immunization for Children under Five Years by Income Quintile, in Selected Low- and Middle-Income Countries

	Under-five mortality rate (per 1,000)		Percentage of fully immunized children	
Country	*Poorest quintile*	*Richest quintile*	*Poorest quintile*	*Richest quintile*
Mali	298	169	15.8	55.6
Nigeria	240	120	13.9	58.1
India	155	54	17.1	65.0
Egypt, Arab Rep.	147	39	65.1	92.5
Bangladesh	141	76	47.2	66.7
Indonesia	109	29	42.9	72.1
Ronzônia (Brazil)	99	33	56.6	73.8
Vietnam	63	23	42.2	60.0

Source: Gwatkin and others 2000.

absolute terms (measured as a rate difference between poor and rich) and in relative terms (measured as a concentration index). A partial explanation of these inequalities lies in the differential reach of immunization programs across income groups, with much better coverage in richer quintiles (table 8.1, columns four and five).

Resource Allocation for Equity in Care or Equity in Health

The distribution of health care spending across income strata also illustrates the inverse care law at work in low- and middle-income countries (Castro-Leal and others 2000).

If, following principles of *horizontal* equity, we want to allocate health care resources according to need, a large part of health care budgets will have to be shifted from the richer to the poorer quintiles. If we, in addition, want to reduce inequalities in health status between rich and poor, we have to look closely at the *vertical* aspects of equity—that is, the unequal treatment of unequals (Culyer and Wagstaff 1993; McIntyre and Gilson 2000). This means that deprived groups should receive preferential allocation of health care resources to achieve more rapid improvements in their health status, thereby reducing inequalities in their health vis-à-vis richer groups.

This distinction between horizontal and vertical aspects of health equity is thus closely linked to two different issues in health policy: how to reduce inequities in access to health care and inequities in health status. The issue of how to achieve equity in health status will not be further discussed in this chapter (for an overview, see Evans and others 2001).

THE INFRASTRUCTURE OF INEQUITY

Allocation of funds to public services among potentially competing institutions or populations has always been a basic function of government at every level.

Resources, for administrative reasons, are often allocated the way they always have been in the past rather than according to any independent method. In the short run, this makes sense, because it is reasonable to provide funds to a service infrastructure that is already there. But, for historical reasons, infrastructure is often poorly distributed, and this method of resource allocation perpetuates inequitable patterns of distribution (Rice and Smith 2001). Whether allocations are decided according to historical budgets, number of beds, or service utilization rates, the result is the same—an increasingly inequitable circular process of high utilization, or use of more resources to create more supply, which generates demand and more utilization by some groups and correspondingly less by others. Examples abound from both rich and poor countries where the budget share for providers in urban and affluent areas grows—often contrary to an explicit political ambition to move in the opposite direction (Hanson and others 2001).

A more equitable alternative might therefore be to allocate resources according to some type of *capitation*—that is, a certain amount per capita in the population a purchaser or institution is expected to serve. The capitation should be proportional to need, in accordance with the objective of horizontal equity in access to health care. Despite all our epidemiological knowledge, our ability to predict individuals' future health and health care need is still very limited (Kapur, Young, and Murata 2000). Moreover, variations across individuals can be predicted with some precision only by introducing previous morbidity and utilization into the models. This alternative then encounters the problem that risk in health care cannot (for equity reasons) be adjusted the same way as in other insurance markets. Most societies are—theoretically—unwilling to let individual risk influence individual premiums because morbidity usually is inversely related to ability to pay. Even when risk is pooled through purchasers, notional premiums still have to be calculated in the form of capitations for different purchasers so they can be given budgets that enable them to treat patients with equal need equally.

METHODOLOGICAL ISSUES: HOW TO CONSTRUCT RESOURCE ALLOCATION FOR EQUITY IN ACCESS

Thus, allocating resources according to historical budgets, determined mainly by existing supply and its use, perpetuates and reinforces existing inequities. But directly measuring need for health care is nearly impossible technically. The *absolute* level of resource need is usually determined politically, when the overall health care budget is fixed, or economically, through different population groups' ability to pay. Discussion in this chapter will therefore be limited to ways of determining the *relative* levels of need across population groups. Need is related to, but cannot be equated, with morbidity, suffering, and disability. The potential effect of the services in question is also relevant—there is no need for ineffective care. If the effectiveness of care can be regarded as equal across population groups, variations in morbidity could be used as a proxy for need.

Resource allocation based on risk-adjusted capitations basically has to make empirically more or less well-founded assumptions on the following three issues:

- The size of the population the purchaser or institution is expected to serve

- The characteristics of individuals or populations that can be demonstrated to have significant influence on the need for health services and could therefore be useful in predicting the relative size of capitation or budgets

- The weight given each of these factors when translated into monetary terms.

Morbidity and Mortality as Proxies for Need

If need is proportional to morbidity, epidemiological data on the incidence and prevalence of disease would be appropriate indicators of relative need. Insofar as variations in mortality rates are proportional to morbidity rates, even mortality statistics could be useful. Data on morbidity or mortality are either generated within the health care system through records of discharges and visits, or through vital registration systems and population surveys. If mortality data are available from vital registration systems with good coverage data on age-specific mortality, rates such as infant- or under-five-mortality might be good indicators. In Britain, age-standardized mortality rates were used for years as the main indicator of need and are still used, now in combination with other sociodemographic variables (see below).

The use of mortality data raises several issues. One is the unclear relationship between mortality and need for health care—is there a 1:1 relationship where, say, 10 percent higher mortality should motivate 10 percent higher capitation? To answer that question we need further analysis (see below).

Most countries—rich and poor—are undergoing epidemiological transitions with declining mortality and increasing or unchanged morbidity in nonlethal conditions—often with a different demographic and socioeconomic pattern. Mortality might therefore be decreasing in relevance as a reflection of need. Using mortality rates might also, at least in principle, introduce a perverse incentive—effective care that lowers mortality rates would be punished via a declining budget.

Case data on morbidity and mortality from records within the health care system will be severely biased by variations in record-keeping efficiency across institutions and regions. Good records will be positively associated with resources and quality of care, and therefore less relevant as an instrument for making the allocation pattern more equitable. The exception might be in diagnoses (and countries) where it seems reasonable to assume that everybody with a certain condition will be hospitalized and that cases will be registered according to standardized criteria. Examples of such conditions in rich countries include myocardial infarctions, stroke, cancer, severe injuries, and psychosis. Efforts are being made in some countries to use those data (Andersson, Varde, and Diderichsen 2000). Israel uses some of these diagnoses—excluding them from the risk-adjustment formula and basing their share of resource allocations directly on incidence. When services are fragmented and access is unequal, as in most low-income countries, case records are a less reliable source of information on morbidity than they are in wealthier countries.

In most low-income countries, mortality and morbidity data will be unavailable on a regular basis for local areas, because they are based mainly on surveys on population samples that cannot be broken down to low geographical areas. Also, data from self-reported morbidity from surveys are influenced by contextual factors that distort the correspondence between self-reported morbidity and more objectively measured and medically defined morbidity. Particularly in some poor countries, the socioeconomic gradient of self-reported morbidity and well-being is different, even reversed, in relation to more objectively measured morbidity and mortality (Sen 1999). Whether caused by inequities in education or access to care or by other cultural factors, this discrepancy will lead to biased conclusions drawn from this type of model. This problem, occurring mainly when more transient health problems are measured, is less problematic in rich countries.

Sociodemographic Indicators of Need

Because of all these complications when using epidemiological data directly as proxies for need, most countries choose to use a shorter or longer list of demographic and socioeconomic indicators related to need, in this discussion, called *need factors.*

Our ability to predict variations in health *across individuals* is limited. Studies from low-mortality countries show that even a combination of several demographic and socioeconomic determinants (for example, age, gender, ethnicity, marital status, education, and employment) seldom explains more than a few percentage points of the variation. Variations *across geographical areas* or other population groups, however, might be better explained by these sociodemographic need factors. This will often be the case in urban societies where housing segregation usually implies geographically contrasting population structure in terms of age, ethnicity, income, and other characteristics. In rural societies, geographical and cultural factors may more often influence area variations. When "purchaser populations" are linked to insurance funds they will more or less, by definition, differ according to demographic and socioeconomic characteristics.

The selection and weighting of need factors has to be based on some kind of empirical analysis. Because measurement of need and morbidity is problematic, most countries use present patterns of utilization, or (better) costs, as the yardstick for testing and weighting potential need factors. Use of utilization or cost patterns might seem to contradict the argument presented above—that allocating resources according to utilization would preserve and aggravate inequities. But variations in utilization across purchaser populations should *not* be used as the yardstick. It is variations across the demographic, socioeconomic, and epidemiological need factors that should be analyzed.

USING UTILIZATION TO WEIGHT NEED FACTORS

The usual way to approach this issue is to construct models in which utilization or costs are regressed against potential need factors (Carr-Hill and others 1994). Confounding factors such as supply of health care should also be included because they might influence utilization and might be unevenly distributed across population groups classified according to need factors. A regression model will look as follows, where $\beta1$ represents a range of coefficients linked to the different sociodemographic need factors and $\beta2$ represents coefficients for supply factors:

(1) Utilization/cost = $\beta1$need factors + $\beta2$supply factors + constant.

The need factors are then selected and weighted with the help of the nonzero values of the different $\beta1$'s.

This method builds on some assumptions that should be carefully evaluated.

We have to assume equity in utilization across groups within the population served by each purchaser. This means that variation in utilization across different levels of each need factor used should be proportional to variations in need. In other words, the distribution of unmet needs, unjustified utilization, or both, is independent of the need factors used in the model.

This question can be tested with an analysis similar to the one outlined above, but including some indicator of need in the model. In practice, need will usually be represented by some measure of morbidity. $\beta3$ represent a coefficient for morbidity. Interaction terms ($\beta13$) for the combination of need factors and morbidity should also be included because the effect of morbidity on utilization should be the same independently of sociodemographic characteristics (Wagstaff, van Doorslaer, and Paci 1991).

(2) Utilization/cost = $\beta1$need factors + $\beta2$supply factors + $\beta3$morbidity + $\beta13$needfactors*morbidity + constant.

If all the $\beta1$'s change to zero when morbidity measures are introduced in the model, we have reason to believe that the distribution of unmet need or unjustified utilization is unrelated to the need factors. But that conclusion will depend strongly on whether our measure of morbidity is a good reflection of need—or, more specifically, that the misclassification that naturally occurs is unrelated to the need factors.

Often, this type of analysis is based on surveys, and morbidity measured is based on self-reported answers to questions on morbidity. Because this measure might be biased across different socioeconomic groups, caution should be used in drawing conclusions (Sutton and others 1999). Other analysts point out that sociodemographic factors might modify the relation between use and morbidity (Newbold, Eyles, and Birch 1995). If, with unbiased measurement of morbidity, we get nonzero values of $\beta1$, there might be cause to adjust the weights for the respective need factors.

UNIT OF ANALYSIS—INDIVIDUAL OR AGGREGATE

To perform analysis (1) described above, we need data sources that allow linkage of data on utilization or costs across units of analysis to information on both need factors and supply. Two types of study designs are usually adopted, where units of analysis are either individual (for example, Andersson, Varde, and

Diderichsen 2000) or aggregates of individuals (for example, Carr-Hill and others 1994). This corresponds to what is usually called individual- or group-level (ecological) studies in epidemiology. Ecological studies might be the only alternative when only aggregate data on utilization are available. The advantage of the ecological approach is that the range of different data available on both need factors and supply is often much greater than at the individual level. The problem is that the weights derived from the analysis might be seriously biased by "cross-level bias"—which means that weights estimated by group-level studies might be biased if applied in an individual-level capitation. This is a potential problem to the extent risk-adjusted capitation formulas are used at the individual level.

TYPICAL NEED FACTORS

A number of need factors occur in most models used around the world. In the models of the industrial countries surveyed by Rice and Smith (2001), the following variables are used: demographic factors, socioeconomic factors, and geographical factors.

Demographic factors. Demographic factors include:

- *Age and gender.* Almost every formula takes age into account. Gender is also a determinant of health care costs, but as the gender distribution may be very equal across areas, it may often be omitted—as in some of the examples below. Most countries have individual-level data on the relation among age, gender, and utilization and therefore apply this variable in a matrix model.

- *Ethnicity.* Ethnicity in terms of race, citizenship, or country of birth is often used both in matrix and ecological models. In some countries, some ethnic groups have been found to underutilize health care—for example, the Maori people in New Zealand and non-Nordic immigrants in Sweden. In New Zealand, estimations have been done on how much the Maoris underutilize health care, and the weights have been adjusted accordingly, while ethnicity has been abolished in the Swedish model.

Socioeconomic factors. Numerous socioeconomic factors occur in models around the world. Employment status is often based on census data (as in England) or social security data (as in Stockholm). Marital status and cohabitation are strongly related to health and utilization and therefore are often used. Education or occupation are sometimes used but are often available only with long time intervals from census to census or survey to survey. Income, wealth, and consumption as well as data on welfare recipient status may be available from surveys but more seldom from census data or regular registers. Because education determines occupation, and occupation determines income, these three variables are strongly linked, and experience from Sweden and other places shows that applying one of them is sufficient.

Geographical factors. Geographical factors might be relevant either because they catch variation in need factors on the aggregate level (for example, mortality rate) or because they influence market forces influencing the cost of providing care (as in the English example, below) or because the effects of demographic and socioeconomic factors are modified by location (as in the Swedish example, below). The problem is that geographical effects often are strongly confounded by supply factors.

DATA AVAILABILITY

Data availability is the most serious limiting factor in the choice of a model, particularly in low- and middle-income countries (Pearson 2002).

Data sources are used for two or three different exercises:

- The selection and weighting of need factors

- The application of those factors on the area/purchaser level

- Testing variations in utilization for equal morbidity across need factors.

For the first exercise, data sources are needed that include both health care costs and potential need factors on the individual or the ecological level. Supply factors might also be needed if there is reason to believe that supply is confounding the need-factor coefficients. For the third exercise, data on morbidity will be needed in the same dataset. For the second purpose, data will be needed on the distribution of need factors for each area or purchaser population. The data could come from the same or another dataset than the one used for the other purposes, but they should be broken down for each purchaser population.

The two types of datasets used for each of these exercises may not necessarily represent the same population, even if that would be preferable. From epidemiology, the size of the effect of health determinants on health is known to depend on exposure to other contributing causes rather than on any biological property of the specific determinant (Greenland and Rothman 1998). As long as we deal with global measures of morbidity and utilization, such interactions will be of minor importance, and estimates made on one population might be valid even for other populations.

A few rich countries (such as the Scandinavian countries) maintain individual-level databases covering nearly all health care costs for the whole population. These databases can be linked, through personal identification numbers, to other databases, including data on several individual or contextual socio-demographic characteristics (Diderichsen, Varde, and Whitehead 1997). This enables use of the same database both to select and weigh need factors and to apply those factors on the area/purchaser level. In many other countries, a similar range of variables will be available only on a small-area level, based on data from health care services and census data (Carr-Hill and others 1994). In a global perspective, however, this is the exception rather than the rule. Analysis related to testing variations in use will usually have to be done through household surveys that include data on morbidity (Wagstaff, van Doorslaer, and Paci 1991).

Most countries will have to rely on other sources. For selecting and weighing need factors and applying those factors on the area/purchaser level, household surveys such as demographic and health surveys and living standard measurement surveys are useful (Diamond, Matthews, and Stephenson 2001). Data on health care utilization will have to be roughly translated into costs. Biases in terms of high nonresponse rates among the severely ill and disabled as well as misclassification of the potential need factors will all reduce the need-factor coefficients. If they are then applied to reallocate resources, the move will usually be in the "right" direction, unlike existing allocations driven by historically and politically determined supply, but not sufficiently to achieve full equity in care.

With models based on living standard measurement survey data, in which poverty is regressed against a number of covariates included in the census, estimating local poverty levels has proved possible, even if poverty is not measured directly in the census (Elbers, Lanjouw, and Lanjouw 2003). There is a potential for doing the same thing to estimate local health status and health care needs (Diamond, Matthews, and Stephenson 2001). Even if such synthetic estimates of health are much less precise than poverty estimates, they may still be useful.

REFERENCES

Andersson, P. Å., E. Varde, and F. Diderichsen. 2000. "Modelling of Resource Allocation to Health Care Authorities in Stockholm County." *Health Care Management Science* (3): 141–49.

Carr-Hill, R. A., T. A. Sheldon, P. Smith, S. Martin, S. Peacock, and G. Hardman. 1994. "Allocating Resources to Health Authorities: Development of Methods for Small Area Analysis." *British Medical Journal* 309: 1046–49.

Castro-Leal F., J. Dayton, L. Demery, and K. Mehra. 2000. "Public Spending on Health in Africa: Do the Poor Benefit?" *Bulletin of the World Health Organization* 78: 66–74.

Culyer, A. J., and A. Wagstaff. 1993. "Equity and Equality in Health and Health Care." *Journal of Health Economics* 12: 431–57.

Diamond, I., Z. Matthews, and R. Stephenson. 2001. "Assessing the Health of the Poor." London DFID Health Systems Resource Centre. http://www.healthsystemsrc.org/Pdfs/Assessing_health_of_the_poor.pdf

Diderichsen, F., E. Varde, and M. Whitehead. 1997. "Resource Allocation to Health Authorities: The Quest for an Equitable Formula in Britain and Sweden." *British Medical Journal* 315: 875–78.

Elbers, C , J. O. Lanjouw, and P. Lanjouw. 2003. "Micro-Level Estimation of Poverty and Inequality." *Econometrica* 71: 355–64

Evans, T., M. Whitehead, F. Diderichsen, A. Bhuiya, and M. Wirth. 2001. *Challenging Inequities in Health.* New York, N.Y.: Oxford University Press.

Greenland, S., and K. Rothman. 1998. *Modern Epidemiology*, 2d ed. Philadelphia, Pa.: Lippincott-Raven.

Gwatkin, D. R., S. Rutstein, K. Johnsson, and A. Wagstaff. 2000. "Socioeconomic Differences in Health, Nutrition and Population." World Bank, Washington, D.C. www.worldbank.org/poverty/health/data/index.htm

Hanson, K., K. Ranson, V. Oliviera-Cruz, and A. Mills. 2001. *Constraints to Scaling Up Health Interventions: A Conceptual Framework and Empirical Analysis.* CMH Working Paper Series WG5:14. Geneva: WHO.

Kapur, K., A. S. Young, and D. Murata. 2000. "Risk Adjustment for High Utilizers of Public Mental Health Care." *Journal of Mental Health Policy and Economics* (3): 129–37.

McIntyre, D., and L. Gilson. 2000. "Redressing Disadvantage: Promoting Vertical Equity within South Africa." *Health Care Analysis* 8: 235–58.

Newbold, B. K., J. Eyles, and S. Birch. 1995. "Equity in Health Care: Methodological Contributions to the Analysis of Hospital Utilization within Canada." *Social Science and Medicine* 40: 1181–92.

Pearson, M. 2002. "Allocating Public Resources for Health: Developing Pro-Poor Approaches." London: DFID Health Systems Resource Centre. http://www.healthsystemsrc.org/Pdfs/Allocating_resources_final.pdf

Rice, N., and P. C. Smith. 2001. "Capitation and Risk Adjustment in Health Care Financing: An International Progress Report." *Millbank Quarterly* 79: 81–13.

Sen, A. 1999. *Development as Freedom*. New York, N.Y.: Oxford University Press.

Sutton, M., R. Carr-Hill, H. Gravelle, and N. Rice. 1999. "Do Measures of Self-Reported Morbidity Bias the Estimation of the Determinants of Health Care Utilization?" *Social Science and Medicine* 49: 867–78.

Tudor Hart, J. 1971. "The Inverse Care Law." *The Lancet* 328: 404–12.

Wagstaff, A., E. van Doorslaer, and P. Paci. 1991. "On the Measurement of Horizontal Equity in the Delivery of Health Care." *Journal of Health Economics* 10: 169–205.

CHAPTER 9

Risk Pooling and Purchasing

Peter C. Smith and Sophie N. Witter

An individual's need for health care, in contrast to many of life's other necessities, is intrinsically uncertain. While an individual's expenditure on, say, food is largely predictable, that same individual's expenditure on health care is largely unknowable, both in magnitude and timing. It is therefore difficult for an individual to make financial provision for episodes of sickness or even chronic health care needs. Furthermore, if (as is generally accepted) most individuals are risk averse, they would value arrangements that protect them from this uncertainty in expenditure.

Society could nevertheless take the view that the pursuit of health and consumption of health care are matters for the individual to arrange without any intervention from the broader community to compensate for variations in health care expenditure needs. Such an extreme individualistic position has rarely been adopted in practice. Instead, to a greater or lesser extent, all systems of health care implicitly *pool* the risks associated with individual health care needs. The World Health Organization (WHO) defines *risk pooling* as "the practice of bringing several risks together for insurance purposes in order to balance the consequences of the realization of each individual risk" (WHO 2000a, p. 77). Pooling is therefore the health system function whereby collected health revenues are transferred to purchasing organizations. Its main purpose is to share the financial risk associated with health interventions for which need is variable and uncertain.

Any health care risk pool must be financed, but there is no reason an individual's financial contributions to the pool should be related to health status or health care utilization. Rather, society must choose the extent to which individual financial contributions depend on financial means, health care utilization, or other factors. Whatever is chosen, the revenues received must be sufficient to provide the desired system of health care. In other words, the system must be financially sustainable.

The World Health Organization (2000b) illustrates two of the redistributive issues implicit in risk pooling (from healthy to sick, and from rich to poor) by means of two stylized scenarios:

- Members might make equal financial contributions, but the pool effectively enables a transfer to be made from the relatively healthy to the sick (the risk-pooling function). A community financing program charging members a flat rate might be expected to function in this way.

- Members might make equal use of health care, but by seeking differential financial contributions the pool effectively enables a transfer to be made from the rich to the poor (the income-redistribution function). This is the aim of health financing systems that base contributions on income (for example, many social insurance programs).

To these we would add a third:

- Members might make equal financial contributions and make equal use of health care across their lifetimes, but the pool enables a transfer to be made depending on the stage of the individual's life cycle. This is the life cycle redistributive function of the risk pool.

There are two broad categories of argument in favor of risk pooling in health care, embracing equity and efficiency considerations. The equity arguments reflect the view that society does not believe it is fair that individuals should assume all the risk associated with their health care expenditure needs. Instead, all or some of that risk should be spread across a given risk pool. This implies an equity objective of offering equal access to health care for members of the risk pool in equal need, regardless of their personal circumstances. In developing countries, the equity argument is particularly acute. Incidence of disease (still predominantly communicable diseases) is closely related to poverty: the poor (those least able to pay) are the ones most in need of treatment, and an absence of risk pooling can lead to widespread catastrophic impoverishment or denial of treatment.

An absence of risk pooling is also inefficient. Most obviously, risk pooling transfers health care resources to the poor, who are at the margin likely to be able to benefit more from health care than the rich. Pooling therefore can lead to major improvements in population health. Such health gain is likely to be desirable in its own right. Moreover, with no pooling, poorer citizens who could benefit from health care (and may thereby become more economically productive) might languish untreated and become a burden on society.

This chapter summarizes a longer report on risk pooling (Smith and Witter 2003). The purpose is to outline the modalities of risk pooling and how they might affect health system performance. The next sections describe the four broad classes of risk-pooling arrangements, practical issues relating to risk pooling, and conclusions.

APPROACHES TO RISK POOLING

The nature of risk-pooling arrangements is a policy choice that is heavily influenced by a nation's circumstances and its policy priorities. In West European countries, risk pools are frequently entire regions or nations, reflecting the equity objective of securing universal coverage, often referred to as the *solidarity principle*. However, many developing countries attempt little risk pooling (Witter and others 2000). Governments may provide a small subsidy to public facilities, but the bulk of health care financing comes directly from households in the form of either user payments (officially sanctioned out-of-pocket fees) or informal payments (unofficial, nonregulated, but often crucial to the functioning of the health system). The *World Development Indicators* (World Bank 2000) show private health expenditure for 1990–98 as 66 percent of the total in low-income countries (reaching 77 percent in South Asia), compared with 37 percent for high-income countries.

There are essentially four classes of approach to risk pooling, considered in turn: no risk pool; unitary risk pool; fragmented risk pool; and integrated risk pools. For details of the mathematics underlying our arguments, see Daykin, Pentikäinen, and Pesonen (1994).

No Risk Pooling

When there is no risk pooling, individuals are responsible for meeting their own health care costs as they arise. In its purest form, this entails patients' meeting user charges as they are incurred, with no price subsidy for poorer people and denial of treatment to patients who lack the financial means to pay. Some expenditure uncertainty associated with this arrangement can be removed using a competitive insurance market. Insurers will set individual premiums, based on their assessment of an individual's risk profile. In these circumstances, the function of insurance is to eliminate the expenditure uncertainty associated with health care but not to transfer health care resources among individuals. In effect, as the ability to predict expenditure needs improves, such insurance becomes a method of prepayment for health care (rather than insurance), with the principal objective of smoothing known expenditure needs across a lifetime. The expenditure needs associated with individuals with different risk profiles cannot be pooled—otherwise the insurance plan becomes a risk pool, with equal premiums for different risks.

Most private insurance arrangements will use the citizen's previous health record as an important element in setting a premium *(experience rating)*. Thus, even if a *current* episode of health care is covered by an insurance contract, the patient may implicitly pay for the episode in the form of increased *future* insurance premiums. Indeed, many citizens will effectively become uninsurable for some or all health care risks in a system with no risk pooling. It is, for example, hard to imagine the bulk of patients with acquired immunodeficiency syndrome in sub-Saharan Africa and Asia either being offered or being able to afford market-based insurance premiums. In practice, society might need to put in place some sort of health care for those unable to pay charges or insurance premiums, which in effect is a "safety net" risk pool comprising the poor and the sick.

Private insurers who wish to charge risk-rated premiums are often in practice confronted by a profound lack of information about the health status of applicants for coverage. They may therefore be forced to charge all insured a single premium and effectively create a risk pool. The problem of *adverse selection* then arises (Feldman, Escribano, and Pellise 1998; Rothschild and Stiglitz 1976). The premium reflects the average costs of health care, so the sick might purchase the insurance, but the healthy might opt out. Thus, with voluntary enrollment, the insurance pool in time becomes less healthy, premiums rise, and the comparatively healthy members leave the remaining pool. The insurance function may therefore break down.

When—in the absence of information or under legal obligation—an insurer cannot discriminate on price, it nevertheless has an incentive to *cream skim* the relatively healthy. Even if such cream skimming is formally illegal, it is in practice difficult to prevent insurers from deterring sick applicants (Newhouse 1998). In these circumstances, some individuals might become uninsurable, or insurers might withdraw from the market, again in the extreme leading to market failure in the insurance market.

Furthermore, an absence of pooling leads to great uncertainty for all citizens regarding their future health care expenditure. This is likely to lead to general dissatisfaction with the health care system. A further inefficiency is caused by the transaction costs associated with calculating and collecting user charges or checking insurance status. A system using informal payments from patients directly to providers may in some circumstances economize on such costs but gives rise to profound inefficiencies and inequities in other aspects of system performance (Lewis 2000).

Finally, by definition, any health care system that relies on individuals to make their own financial provision for health care expenditure will fail to address many issues of public health and other externalities that are a central concern in many low-income countries. A side effect of pooling is that the risk pool can act as a focus for programs related to population health that the individual or the private insurance market cannot address.

Unitary Risk Pool

Under the unitary risk pool, revenue is placed in a single central pool that seeks to cover a chosen package of health care services. Risk pooling must then be mandatory in the sense that rich or healthy citizens cannot opt out of contributing. The mandatory risk pool is one possible policy response to counter the manifest inefficiencies and inequities associated with adverse selection, cream skimming, and transaction costs.

It is nevertheless not without its own inefficiencies. In particular, the managerial costs of ensuring that patients receive care in line with the chosen package of care may be considerable. For example, unless systems of provider reimbursement are chosen carefully, there may be a strong incentive for supplier-induced demand (McGuire 2000). As well as being inefficient, supplier-induced demand may lead to variations in the package received, breaching many equity principles. Furthermore, members of a unitary pool have little incentive to moderate their demands on health care resources, and therefore the potential exists for moral hazard, in the form of excessive consumption of health care resources. In short, unitary risk pooling removes the usual economic barrier of the price mechanism to consumption, and therefore carries with it the potential for use of health care in excess of the chosen package of care. In industrial countries, this problem has been addressed by several instruments of managed care (Glied 2000).

The notion of a single compulsory risk pool carries with it an implication of a curtailment of individual choice on the nature of the package of health care made available. This can lead to inefficiencies in two ways: first, it may remove an element of competition from health care insurance, and second it may prevent individuals from securing a package of care in line with their preferences for which they are willing to pay. These considerations have assumed preeminence in the debate over the reform of the U.S. health care system.

Fragmented Risk Pools

Although a large unitary risk pool theoretically effects complete risk sharing across a nation and minimizes variations in expected expenditure, it may bring with it enormous practical difficulties associated with managerial control, information flows, and coordination. As a result, almost all nations devolve health care purchasing arrangements to smaller organizations, so that the risk pool becomes fragmented.

Under these arrangements, individuals might be assigned to a particular pool depending on criteria such as:

- Where they live (geographical risk pools)

- The nature of their employment

- Their personal characteristics such as age or health status

- Their personal choice (for example, competing insurance funds).

Membership in a particular risk pool may be voluntary (as in the case of competitive insurers) or mandatory (as is usually the case with geographically defined risk pools). Society may nevertheless insist that all citizens must enroll in at least one pool.

Fragmented risk pools will in general be of variable population size and imply variable per capita expected expenditure. Broadly speaking, pools with a higher proportion of older and sicker members will incur higher per capita levels of expenditure. And a larger number of small risk pools will exhibit wider variations in spending needs than a system with a small number of large risk pools. Uncertainty in predicting such needs will also increases as the risk pool gets smaller, because of the increased importance of random fluctuations in the population at risk (Martin, Rice, and Smith 1998). In the extreme, fragmented risk pools become households or individuals, and the system reverts to one of no risk pooling.

If left unadjusted, the variation in expenditure needs between risk pools is undesirable on both efficiency and equity grounds. The efficiency arguments are particularly important in systems of competitive insurance, when variations in the per capita needs can lead to variations in insurance premiums unrelated to efficiency (Van de Ven and Ellis 2000). The competitive insurance market therefore breaks down unless corrective action is taken. The equity arguments are manifest. Fragmentation implies that pools with sicker, poorer memberships must either charge higher premiums than their less disadvantaged counterparts or offer more constrained packages of care.

Integrated Risk Pools

The policy response to the efficiency and equity problems brought about by fragmentation has been to develop integrated risk pools. Under this arrangement, the individual risk pools of the sort discussed above can remain in place, but financial transfers are arranged between pools so that some or all of the variation caused by pure fragmentation is eliminated.

If it is assumed that the health care system should deliver a standard package of care to all citizens, the most obvious cause of variations in the spending needs of fragmented risk pools is the size of the population covered. A first step toward integration is therefore to base funding of integrated risk pools on a capitation payment. This can be defined as the contribution to a risk pool's revenue associated with a particular pool member for a given period of time. In its simplest manifestation, a capitation system would give an equal *amount* per head to each risk pool. Although offering a rudimentary correction for variations in the size of pools, this approach fails to reflect any variations in per capita needs between pools. Many countries have therefore developed risk-adjustment methods that alter the capitation payment associated with an individual, depending on the individual's characteristics such as age, social circumstances, and health status (Rice and Smith 2001). The risk-adjusted capitation scheme seeks to compensate risk pools for variations in exposure. Such schemes can be vertical (central collection of finance that is then disbursed to pools) or horizontal (direct transfers between pools). The financial effects of these two approaches are identical.

If revenues (in the form of insurance premiums or taxes) are collected by the individual pools, a distinct issue is the extent to which they are compensated for variations in the revenues base. For example, if revenues take the form of a payroll tax proportional to income, for the same package of health care pools with relatively large numbers of high-earning individuals and low numbers of non-earning dependants will be able to charge lower premiums than their less-well-endowed counterparts. If this is considered unacceptable on payment equity grounds, a second set of transfers will be needed among pools, adjusting for variations in revenue bases. The two sets of transfers correspond to the risk-pooling and income-redistribution functions noted above.

FIGURE 9.1   The Integration Pyramid

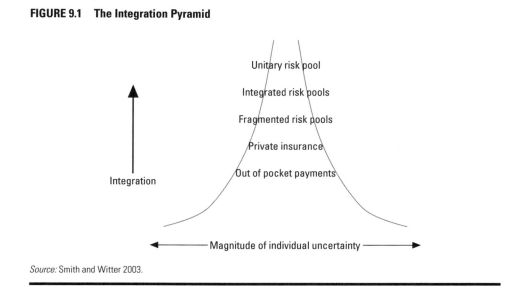

Source: Smith and Witter 2003.

In summary, as risk pooling becomes progressively integrated, the uncertainty associated with health care expenditure can be reduced. This can be illustrated by means of the "integration pyramid" shown in figure 9.1. A system of out-of-pocket payments exposes individuals to the greatest uncertainty. Private insurance can smooth some variability, but with risk-rated premiums does little to compensate for variations in health status or income. Fragmented risk pools allow some local sharing of risk but continue to expose members to variations among risk pools. Integration seeks to reduce these variations, which are eliminated under a truly unitary system.

PRACTICAL ISSUES

Numerous practical issues arise in seeking to make the principles of risk pooling operational. They are discussed under eight headings: the institutional framework for risk pooling; membership criteria for risk pools; size of risk pools; prospective risk sharing; overlapping risk pools; retrospective risk sharing; variations in the benefit package; and purchasing arrangements and risk sharing.

The Institutional Framework for Risk Pooling

The most important imperatives for risk pooling are to establish appropriate and reliable systems of governance, to ensure the collection and stewardship of finances, and to ensure that providers are reimbursed appropriately. These basic requirements are fundamental, and local conditions may seriously circumscribe realistic policy choices. They imply the need for a minimum degree of long-term trust in the health care institutions, a rudimentary flow of adequate information, and the reliable enforcement of contracts, both implicit and explicit. Without these desiderata, it is hard to imagine that any system of risk pooling and collective purchasing of health care will be feasible.

Membership Criteria for Risk Pools

Membership in a risk pool can be voluntary or mandatory. If insurance is compulsory, citizens may nevertheless have some element of choice about which pool to join. Mandatory pools defined by geographical residence or employment sector may be reasonably unambiguous. However, establishing membership status may be less straightforward if membership (or premium level) is based on factors such as income, wealth, health status, or employment status. Under competitive insurance with mandatory enrollment, mechanisms are required to ensure that citizens are members of one (and only one) risk pool. Such systems are likely to be particularly demanding in terms of information flows.

If insurance is voluntary, "safety net" arrangements must be made for catastrophic health care costs borne by the uninsured (leading to the creation of an implicit safety net risk pool). In some systems, individuals with adequate means might be able to opt out of contributing to public health insurance and take private insurance in its place. Even where membership in a public risk pool is mandatory, these individuals may be able to take out supplementary private insurance, though still contributing to the public risk pool.

Size of Risk Pools

There is often a tradeoff between large risk pools (which improve risk sharing) and small risk pools (which are easier to manage and may be more responsive to local preferences). The size of risk pools is therefore a central design consideration. Even when good integration is secured, small risk pools introduce important managerial incentives that may adversely affect system performance in terms of both equity and efficiency, particularly if the pools are subject to "hard" budget constraints (Smith 1999). These arise because the importance of the unpredictable random element of expenditure becomes greater as the size of the risk pool shrinks.

- Unplanned rationing is likely to be particularly prevalent in systems with many small risk pools, because the high random variability in per capita expenditure found in such pools increases the probability that budgetary constraints may become binding.

- Small risk pools that perceive that their expenditure will fall below their budget may "spend up" to protect their budgetary position in future years.

- Patients may therefore be treated inequitably. Different small risk pools will be under different budgetary pressures and so may adopt different treatment practices. Moreover, within a risk pool, choice of treatment may vary over the course of a year if the risk pool's perception of its budgetary position changes.

- Risk pools may adopt a variety of defensive stratagems that adversely affect system effectiveness, such as cream skimming or insuring with a third party against overspending their budget.

The potentially adverse influences of small risk pools can be abated by some of the risk-sharing arrangements discussed below.

In principle, larger risk pools have the potential to exert more collective consumer influence over large providers, and therefore may be more effective purchasers. Thus, in situations where there is a lack of competition in health care supply, the implementation of large risk pools may be able to countervail excessive supplier power. However, a large purchaser may be forced to enter into a relationship with a single provider (indeed, the purchaser may choose to provide as well as purchase care). These conditions might arise, say, when a local government purchaser must use its local hospital. Supply of health care then becomes an effective monopoly. The parallel existence of smaller, more mobile risk pools may introduce an element of competition into the health care market, which would otherwise be absent. There was some evidence that this outcome emerged when large health authority purchasers in the United Kingdom were augmented by a number of smaller purchasers (general practitioner fundholders) who were able to stimulate quality improvements (Le Grand, Mays, and Mulligan 1998).

A plurality of risk pools imposes a burden in terms of transferring payments to providers, collecting premiums, and arranging interpool financial transfers. A system of larger, noncompetitive risk pools might therefore be appropriate in circumstances where information and managerial resources are poor.

The tradeoff between the size of the pools and the complexity of the managerial, purchasing, governance, and stewardship functions can be illustrated, as in figure 9.2. Equity and efficiency gains (from pooling) must be traded off against declines in managerial efficiency (Bojke, Gravelle, and Wilkin 2001). The shape of the curves, and therefore optimal size S^*, will depend heavily on local circumstances and preferences.

Prospective Risk Sharing

A number of methods of integrating risk pools through capitation can be found in industrial nations (Rice and Smith 1999). The sophistication of the risk-adjustment process varies considerably between countries and is highly contingent on information availability. Many countries that have tried to introduce competitive health care insurance markets have found it imperative to implement some sort of risk adjustment to compensate plans for variations in their risk profiles and revenue bases (Van de Ven and Ellis 2000). The intention is to enable all plans to levy a standard premium for a standard package of care delivered with standard efficiency.

FIGURE 9.2   The Tradeoff between Equity and Efficiency Gains and Declines in Managerial Efficiency

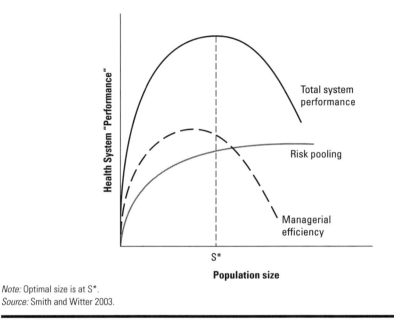

Note: Optimal size is at S*.
Source: Smith and Witter 2003.

If health care is organized at the local government level, central government grant can be designed to allow municipalities to deliver a standard package of care at a standard rate of local tax and user charges. However, the municipalities can be left free to choose the package of care offered and local tax and user charge levels. The risk adjustment is therefore intended to offer local communities the *opportunity* to deliver a standard package of care.

In most centrally planned systems, such as those found in the United Kingdom, fragmentation takes place in the form of budgetary devolution to local risk pools based on geography. Revenues are generated centrally, so no formal income-redistribution mechanism is required. However, adjusting for differences in health care needs profiles is important so that a standard package of care can be offered in every area (Smith and others 1994).

Overlapping Risk Pools

In many systems of health care, there may be *overlapping* risk pools that can make an important contribution to prospective risk sharing. For example, in the United States, health care costs commonly associated with particular conditions (such as mental illness or end-stage renal failure) might be "carved out" of regular risk pools and placed in a condition-specific risk pool (Madden and others 2000). The intention is to remove unpredictable but high-cost needs from the regular health care pool and to transfer the associated risk to a higher level of aggregation (for example, from state to federal level). Similarly, *individuals* with particular chronic conditions might be carved out of the regular risk pool and pooled at a higher level to protect small pools from catastrophic calls on their funds.

Also common are intermediate arrangements under which the low-level pool shares the costs of certain elements of health care with a higher-level pool. In Norway, the national and local governments share marginal costs of inpatient care. In health care systems in France and many other countries, the state offers a basic package of health care that citizens can choose to augment with supplemental (private) insurance, giving rise to a complex rearrangement of risk sharing. Systems in which patients are liable for significant charges imply that the risk is shared between the pool and the individual.

Singapore provides an example of a system in which minor and higher cost risks have been separated and financed through a variety of mechanisms. Individual medical savings accounts (Medisave) provide intertemporal cover for some ambulatory and minor hospital expenditures, while a national catastrophic illness insurance scheme (Medishield) covers prolonged and expensive treatment (financed by employee contributions, often taken from the Medisave accounts). In addition, a complex system of copayments and deductibles involves direct out-of-pocket private payments. However, even with these arrangements, the state continues to fund 30 percent of health expenditure (National Economic Research Associates 1997; Nichols, Prescott, and Kai Hong Phua 1997).

Retrospective Risk Sharing

Prospective risk adjustment between risk pools is almost invariably accompanied by a retrospective stage, in which prospective funding is altered in light of actual expenditure. A number of arrangements exist for handling retrospectively variations in actual expenditure from the prospective budget. These include:

- Renegotiating the budget retrospectively with the central payer (as effectively occurred for many years in Italy and Spain)

- Running down (or contributing to) the pool's reserves

- Varying the future premiums or local taxes paid by pool members

- Varying the user charges paid by patients

- Varying the package of benefits available to patients

- Delaying or rationing health care to the population at risk.

These arrangements might exist in any system of fragmented risk pools, but are particularly important for small pools (that are therefore vulnerable to random fluctuation in demand). They imply important differences in the "hardness" of the fragmentation and suggest that, to different extents, the apparently scientific methods (such as capitation) used to integrate risk pools might be tempered by many other methods of retrospective risk sharing.

Variations in the Benefit Package

The definition of the health care benefit package represents a form of deliberate or *planned rationing* of health care. Finding a satisfactory package definition is important when unitary and integrated risk-pooling arrangements are sought, because variations in the available package compromise the desired equity objectives. Furthermore, particularly in low-income countries, specification of the benefit package is an essential step to ensure that the chosen health care system is within the nation's means.

If the integration of risk pools is imperfect, they will be unable to offer a uniform package. Relatively underfunded pools may respond by altering the benefit package, even if—in principle—the health care system seeks to avoid such inequalities. Variations in the package may take the form of prohibiting certain treatments or drugs, poorer quality care, poorer quality facilities, or reducing patient choice. Such *unplanned rationing* decisions will often appear arbitrary and unfair (in the United Kingdom, they have become known as "postcode rationing").

In some systems of competitive health care insurance (such as parts of the United States), variations in the package offered may be legitimate, and potential members may be offered a tradeoff between the comprehensiveness of the benefit package and the premium paid. Similarly, in systems of local government–based health care, some elements of the package may be subject to local discretion. In all systems of health care, some variation in the package (for example, between rural and urban areas) is inevitable.

Purchasing Arrangements and Risk Sharing

The discussion so far has assumed that providers will charge purchasers a fee for service. However, other possible contractual arrangements exist, which can profoundly affect the risk borne by the pool. For example, the purchaser might negotiate a block contract with a provider, under which the provider agrees to give all necessary care to pool members for a fixed sum, regardless of the volume or severity of demands. This arrangement shifts the risk from purchaser to provider. Such "provider risk pools" might be a particularly effective means of aggregating a number of small purchaser risk pools. There are many other methods of sharing risk between purchaser and provider. For example, a modest transfer of risk from purchaser to provider occurs when a fixed price per case (in the form of a diagnosis-related group payment) is substituted for fee for service. The risk associated with the *incidence* of a case remains with the purchaser. However, the risk associated with *variations in treatment costs* is transferred to the provider.

The choice of contractual form (implicit or explicit) between insurer and provider has many ramifications beyond the sharing of risk that must be taken into account when designing systems. For example, at least in the short term, the block contract arrangement removes the price incentive for insurers to restrain their members' demand for health care but gives providers an incentive to skimp on care.

In many developing countries the purchasing and provider functions continue to be vertically integrated in the sense that the insurance and provision functions are not separated, and an implicit block contract between the two is therefore in place. For example, a community-financed health center might both collect premiums and provide care for its locality. Such vertical integration may result in some loss of incentives for provider efficiency, but it may economize on managerial and informational efforts and implicitly promote equity of access.

CONCLUSIONS

The World Health Report 2000 emphasized the role of government in terms of stewardship of the health sector (WHO 2000b). Putting in place effective risk-pooling arrangements is a central aspect of good stewardship and a prerequisite for a well-developed purchasing function. In developing countries, with heavy burdens of disease, particularly among the poor, and poor mechanisms for transferring wealth, there are strong reasons to believe that the trend should be toward enlarging risk pools. Ideally, system design should embrace mandatory, universal coverage, in which contributions are either income- or community-rated and where there is some mechanism for equalization among pools. But the trend has been in the opposite direction, with many countries devolving health care arrangements to local levels without any attention to risk-pool integration.

The optimal design of risk-pooling arrangements will depend on the relative weight attached to health system objectives—particular those relating to equity and efficiency—which must be a matter for local choice. Therefore, although we strongly advocate pursuit of financial integration, the optimal nature of risk-pooling arrangements will vary. Relevant consideration might include:

- Preference regarding equity of payment

- Preference regarding equity of access

- Potential sources of revenues

- Ease of collecting revenues (taxes, premiums, user charges)

- Efficiency and probity of the managerial function

- Nature of existing organizational structure (for example, local government)

- Nature of existing information bases

- Nature, organization, and governance of providers

- Nature of available health technologies

- Nature of major health priorities

- Size and geography of the country.

There are a number of rudimentary universal indicators of the success of risk-pool integration arrangements:

- *Insurance coverage:* the proportion of the population covered by health insurance arrangements

- *Insurance premiums:* the extent to which identical individuals in different risk pools pay different premiums

- *Variations in the package of care:* the extent of differences in the benefit package from risk pool to risk pool

- *Variations in quality:* the extent of qualitative differences in health care received by members of different risk pools (for example, in waiting times)

- *Variations in user charges:* the extent of differences in the out-of-pocket charges to individuals in different risk pools.

Some observed variations between pools may be due to factors other than risk-pool fragmentation. However, large variations in such indicators offer strong prima facie evidence of fragmentation.

We hope that we have demonstrated that the desirability *in principle* of strengthening risk-pool integration in health care should be uncontested for most situations. Rather, the debate surrounds how it can be practicably implemented in low- and middle-income countries, particularly when a reliance on community financing and user charges leads to fragmented risk pools. While trying to highlight the many general considerations that apply to any choice, we have emphasized throughout that system design will be contingent on local circumstances. We nevertheless believe that there will be few circumstances in which some form of risk-pool integration cannot be successfully introduced and strengthened.

NOTE

The authors would like to thank Jack Langenbrunner, Maureen Lewis, Alex Preker, and Paul Shaw of the World Bank, Philip Davies of the World Health Organization, and other participants at the RAP workshop.

REFERENCES

Bojke, C., H. Gravelle, and D. Wilkin. 2001. "Is Bigger Better for Primary Care Groups and Trusts?" *British Medical Journal* 322: 599–602.

Daykin, C., T. Pentikäinen, and M. Pesonen. 1994. *Practical Risk Theory for Actuaries*. London: Chapman and Hall.

Feldman, R., C. Escribano, and L. Pellise. 1998. "The Role of Government in Health Insurance Markets with Adverse Selection." *Health Economics* 7(8): 659–70.

Glied, S. 2000. "Managed Care." In J. P. Newhouse and A. J. Culyer, eds., *Handbook of Health Economics*. Amsterdam: Elsevier.

Le Grand, J., N. Mays, and J. Mulligan, eds. 1998. *Learning from the NHS Internal Market*. London: King's Fund Institute.

Lewis, M. 2000. *Who Is Paying for Health Care in Europe and Central Asia?* Washington, D.C.: World Bank, Human Development Sector Unit.

Madden, C. W., B. P. Mackay, S. M. Skillman, M. Ciol, and P. K. Diehr. 2000. "Risk Adjusting Capitation: Applications in Employed and Disabled Populations." *Health Care Management Science* 3(2): 101–109.

Martin, S., N. Rice, and P. Smith. 1998. "Risk and the General Practitioner Budget Holder." *Social Science and Medicine* 47(10): 1547–54.

McGuire, T. 2000. "Physician Agency." In J. P. Newhouse and A. J. Culyer, eds., *Handbook of Health Economics*. Amsterdam: Elsevier.

National Economic Research Associates. 1997. *The Health Care System in Singapore*. London.

Newhouse, J. P. 1998. "Risk Adjustment: Where Are We Now?" *Inquiry* 35: 122–31.

Nichols, L., N. Prescott, and Kai Hong Phua. 1997. "Medical Savings Accounts in Developing Countries." In G. Sheiber, ed., *Innovations in Health Care Financing: Proceedings of a World Bank Conference March 10–11, 1997*. Washington, D.C.: World Bank.

Rice, N., and P. Smith. 1999. *Approaches to Capitation and Risk Adjustment in Health Care: An International Survey*. York: University of York, Centre for Health Economics.

———. 2001. "Capitation and Risk Adjustment in Health Care Financing: An International Progress Report." *The Milbank Quarterly* 79(1): 81–113.

Rothschild, M., and J. Stiglitz. 1976. "Equilibrium in Competitive Markets: An Essay on the Economics of Imperfect Information." *Quarterly Journal of Economics* 90: 629–49.

Smith, P. 1999. "Setting Budgets for General Practice in the New NHS." *British Medical Journal* 318: 776–79.

Smith, P., T. A. Sheldon, R. A. Carr-Hill, S. Martin, S. Peacock, and G. Hardman. 1994. "Allocating Resources to Health Authorities: Results and Policy Implications of Small Area Analysis of Use of Inpatient Services." *British Medical Journal* 309: 1050–54.

Smith, P., and S. N. Witter. 2003. *Risk Pooling in Health Care Finance*. Washington, D.C.: World Bank.

Van de Ven, W. P. M. M. and R. Ellis. 2000. "Risk Adjustment in Competitive Health Plan Markets." In J. P. Newhouse and A. J. Culyer, eds., *Handbook of Health Economics*. Amsterdam: Elsevier.

Witter, S., T. Ensor, M. Jowett, and R. Thompson. 2000. *Health Economics for Developing Countries: A Practical Guide*. Basingstoke, United Kingdom: Macmillan.

World Bank. 2000. *World Development Indicators*. Washington, D.C.

WHO (World Health Organization). 2000a. *A Quick Reference Compendium of Selected Key Terms Used in the World Health Report 2000*. Geneva.

———. 2000b. *The World Health Report 2000. Health Systems: Improving Performance*. Geneva.

PART III

Purchasing Health Services

CHAPTER 10

Paying for Public Health Services: Financing and Utilization

Xingzhu Liu and Sheila O'Dougherty

ealth care payment reforms undertaken and studied during the past two decades were triggered by problems associated with cost escalation and overutilization of costlier and cost-ineffective curative services. However, public health services faced different problems—insufficient financing and underutilization. If the fundamental problems of medical care are different from those of public health services, can the systems for financing and paying for medical care also apply to public health services?

In an effort to answer this question, we will discuss financing public health services in both theory and practice, review the implementation of public health services payment mechanisms, and recommend better financing and payment systems.

Following this brief introduction, the second section addresses the issue of who should pay for public health services in theory and who, in practice, paid for public health services. The next section looks at how providers are paid, presents countries' practice of different payment systems, and explores lessons and evidence. The concluding section discusses policy options.

WHO SHOULD PAY FOR PUBLIC HEALTH SERVICES?

Although policymakers are aware that public health services are cost-effective, priority health interventions (Davis and others 1990a), these services are continuously underfunded in both industrial and developing countries. To address the problem of underfunding for public health services, two questions must be answered: (1) Who should be responsible for financing public health services? (2) Who has been responsible for paying for public health services? First, we will provide theoretical discussions on payment responsibility and then review payment practice.

Payment Responsibility in Theory

According to the economic classification of public health services, most community-based and universal public health services are public goods that can be consumed by all regardless of their actual payment. This "free rider" phenomenon constitutes a major problem of public health financing: although public good types of public health services are socially desirable, individuals are not willing to pay for them. The implication is that, theoretically, private payment cannot be relied upon to finance these services and that, to provide these services, government should take an active role in financing them (Hsiao 1995).

The consumption of quasi-public goods is exclusive, so individuals have some willingness to pay for them. However, the benefit valued by the users is less than the benefit that society values, because of positive externalities. For example, the total social benefit of an individual's consumption of immunizations equals the sum of the benefit gained by the immunized individual and by the individuals whose risk of infection can be reduced because other people received immunizations. The policy implication of quasi-public goods is that the people's welfare cannot be maximized if demand is determined only by an individual's willingness to pay. In other words, theoretically, policymakers cannot expect full provision and utilization of quasi-public good types of public health services unless government takes a role in financing these services in addition to the part that individuals are willing to pay.

Besides the notions of public and quasi-public goods, there are three other reasons for supporting public financing of public health services. One is that, even for purely private good types of public health services (for example, screening for cancer and one-on-one preventive consultations), the actual benefit may not be well perceived by the individual consumer because of either lack of information or uncertainty about their benefit. Second, for individuals who cannot pay, the priority choices for consumption are life-saving goods and services such as food and some curative services rather than services that prevent disease. Third, an argument can be made that all personal preventive services have positive externalities in a society where public financing for health care or health insurance prevails, because the economic benefit of prevention or early detection of diseases will be shared by users, insurers, and the public as a whole (Dowd 1982).

The discussion of payers for public health services has rarely extended to insurers, although they play a widening role in paying for public health services for their beneficiaries and employees. In traditional theory, insurance exists because it can cover the economic loss from uncertain events (Black and Skipper 1999). It applies particularly to events with a small probability of occurrence but significant economic implications (well beyond the insured's affordability). The use of preventive services is neither uncertain nor does it imply significant economic loss; so, in theory, public health services are not something that insurance would generally cover.

However, because public health services can prevent diseases with high treatment costs, and because evidence of the cost-effectiveness of preventive care is accumulating, insurers are increasingly financially motivated to provide coverage for preventive care. In particular, when third parties and providers are integrated (for example, health maintenance organizations [HMOs] in the United States), the motivation for providing preventive care becomes stronger. In addition, economic theory suggests that adding coverage for preventive services could not only stimulate demand for them but could also increase the supply of public health services in the long run (Schauffler and Rodriguez 1993).

In summary, the theory strongly supports pure public financing of public goods and joint public and private financing of quasi-public goods. There is even weak theoretical support for complete private financing of private good types of public health services. Private financing applies only to those private goods (services) whose value consumers can readily perceive and for which they can pay. Insurers are potential payers for public health. Their responsibility for paying for some public health services may be strengthened by using financial incentives and regulatory tools.

Payment in Practice

THE ROLE OF GOVERNMENT

Although public health services are priorities, funding for public health care services in many countries is constrained by the demand for personal/curative health services within the health sector and total funding ceilings for all public sectors. For lack of the right budget policies, or political reasons, or lack of cost-effective information for policymakers, less cost-effective curative care is often overprovided and more cost-effective public health interventions are often underprovided (Mills 1997).

In industrial countries with publicly financed health systems, the government budget for health promotion and disease prevention is usually less than 2 percent of the total health budget, a percentage that has increased little over the past 20 years (Organisation for Economic Co-operation and Development 1998).

In Australia and New Zealand, where governments have greater power to determine allocation of health resources, funding for public health services as a percentage of the total health funding was between only about 2 to 3 percent and 1.7 percent, respectively (Durham and Kill 1999).

In the United States, a dominant portion of the trillion dollar health budget goes to medical care services, while only 2 to 5 percent is allocated to population-wide approaches to health improvement (McGinnis, Williams-Russo, and Knickman 2002; Wall 1998). Resource allocation in the United States is clearly imbalanced, in light of estimated explanations of reasons for premature death: genetic endowments (30 percent), social circumstances (15 percent), environmental conditions (5 percent), behavioral choices (40 percent), and medical care (10 percent) (McGinnis and Foege 1993).

In developing countries, public hospitals can absorb between 60 and 80 percent of government health expenditure, and the lion's share of this expenditure is often absorbed by secondary and tertiary hospitals in urban areas, leaving primary and preventive care with the smallest share (Mills 1997). The share of government spending for public health might be higher than in industrial countries, for example, 10 percent in China (Liu and Mills 2002) and between 15 and 20 percent in the Lao People's Democratic Republic (Kress and others 2002), but considering the greater need for public health services and limited total government health spending, the current funding for public health in developing countries lags behind.

There is no consensus on how much a country should spend on public health services. The World Bank recommends that about a third of the health budget should be spent on public health services in developing countries (World Bank 1993). Flessa (2000) did an in-depth analysis of the relationship between the share of the budget for public health services and per capita health spending for maximizing health outcomes in developing countries. It was found that to optimize the allocation of resources, the share of the budget for public health services should increase until per capita health expenditure reaches about US$60 with 75 percent of this amount from public health services. The public health services' share would fall to 25 percent when per capita health expenditure reaches US$250.

Experience is limited in ways to ensure adequate government funding for public health services. One example is in Canada (Chambers 1997), where the province of Ontario enacted legislation in 1983 for the provision of mandatory and priority public health services by local health authorities. Under the legislation, the provincial government provides 75 percent of the funding for mandatory public health programs (for example, food and water safety, immunization, communicable disease control) to the 42 boards of health, and 100 percent of funding for priority programs such as prevention of human immunodeficiency virus/acquired immunodeficiency syndrome (HIV/AIDS). In Ontario, funding for public health services is prioritized against funding for other activities. As a result, the legislation was considered an improved version of funding for public health services.

Another successful example is in New Zealand (Durham and Kill 1999), where a special budget was provided to ensure funding for public health services. The funding for public health functions was unbundled from the general health budget. This "ring fence" provided a legal mechanism to protect funding for public health services and avoid competition for resources from curative services. This mechanism led to a 10 percent annual increase in public health funding from 1994 to 1999, as compared with only a 6 percent increase in other health funding.

Limited experience shows that to ensure adequate government funding for public health services, a separate public health budget unbundled from the general health budget and enforced through legislation is essential.

INSURANCE COVERAGE

Insurers or third parties (both public and private) have traditionally provided insurance coverage for curative care. However, third parties are increasingly playing a role in paying providers for public health services for their beneficiaries. This has resulted either from government regulations or from third-party motivation to reduce costs through disease prevention.

Although insurance coverage for preventive services proved to promote use of these services (Faulkner and Schauffler 1997), and there are some incentives for insurers to provide coverage and pay for them to reduce the costs of curative care, most insurers are still unwilling to pay. There are three main reasons for this. First, insurers are ill informed about the cost-effectiveness of preventive services. Second, the cost of covering preventive services is immediate, whereas the expected saving from reduced curative care is long term. A survey of 175 managed care organizations in the United States showed that the strongest barrier to the provision of screening services is their inability to generate short-term savings for the managed care organizations (Amonkar and others 1999) not only because of the long-term nature of the benefit, but also because of the high disenrollment rate, which means the benefit of one insurer's investment in preventive care can be harvested by another. Third, for some preventive services such as health education on using seatbelts, the economic benefit from reduced car accidents can be enjoyed by multiple parties—beneficiaries, health insurance companies, and car insurance companies. As a result, none of these parties is willing to pay for these services completely.

The insurers' unwillingness to pay for preventive services constitutes a major barrier to the utilization of cost-effective preventive services. In recent years, several policy tools were developed and tried out, particularly in the United States. One of these tools is "informing insurers," by which evidence on the cost-effectiveness of preventive services is gathered; services are recommended for coverage and provision; and guidelines are made to specify the target population, quantity, and provision frequency of each of the recommended services (U.S. Preventive Services Task Force 1989). The second policy tool is government regulation, by which both public and private insurers are required by law to provide insurance coverage for specified public health services, which has been popular in all U.S. states since the early 1990s (Davis and others 1990a). The third approach is associated with economic incentives, by which insurers are rewarded if they provide coverage for defined public health services. One example is the Pacific Business Group on Health in California, a health insurance purchasing alliance representing large private employers (Schauffler and Rodriguez 1996). This alliance negotiates coverage of comprehensive preventive service packages with insurers on the basis of mutually adopted guidelines and makes a percentage of their premiums contingent on their performance in covering preventive services. Reward is given to those who reach the defined performance target. Although no strong evaluation of the effectiveness of these strategies was found, it is well recognized that they have been the key determinants for increasing coverage of preventive services in the past decade.

INCENTIVES FOR CONSUMERS

Economic incentives come from two directions: one is a negative incentive (cost sharing and user fees) that reduces demand, and the other is a positive incentive (paying consumers for using preventive services).

Cost-sharing mechanisms have been used to cut costs by potential reduction in use. Cost sharing can reduce utilization (Liu 2002), but the reduction is not selective. There is substantial evidence that cost sharing can reduce utilization of both curative and preventive care. Evidence from a study done by RAND suggests that the use of preventive services, as with the use of other health services, is sensitive to cost sharing (Lillard and others 1986; Lohr and others 1986; Lurie and others 1987). Specifically, it was found that women and children were less likely to receive certain types of preventive services in a cost-sharing plan (for example, Pap smear and immunization), and that the poor are more affected than the nonpoor.

Another study in the United States (Solanki, Schauffler, and Miller 2000) tested the effects of different forms of cost sharing on the utilization of recommended clinical preventive services on the basis of a stratified random sample of 10,872 health insurance enrollees for four clinical preventive services: mammography screening, cervical cancer screening, blood pressure screening, and preventive counseling. Under all forms of cost sharing, both negative and significant effects were found on all preventive services, except for blood pressure screening.

Evidence suggests that eliminating cost sharing for these services may be an important step in increasing utilization to the recommended levels.

User fees raised a great deal of concern over the possibility of drops in utilization of necessary and cost-effective care by those people who have no ability to pay. The studies on the effects of user fees (de Bethune, Alfani, and Lahaye 1989; Huber 1993; Hussein and Mujinja 1997; Waddington and Enyimayew 1989; Yoder 1989) found that the introduction of fees led to a significant decrease in utilization of services including curative and preventive services.

An interesting experimental study was performed in Denmark (Christensen 1995). This study examined how conditions of payment influence attendance at preventive health examinations. A multipractice study of 65 general practitioners was conducted in two areas in the county of Aarhus, Denmark. The general practitioners invited 2,452 men age 40 to 49 years to a preventive health examination for coronary heart disease. The examination was free in one area but cost $40 in another area. Results showed that the attendance was 37 percent in the area that required payment and 66 percent in the area where the examination was given for free. It was concluded that where payment was required for health examinations, fewer patients obtained examinations.

Based on research findings that user fees deter utilization of preventive health services in most settings, the World Bank, the World Health Organization, and many other agencies discourage the application of user fees for preventive care. The Global Alliance for Vaccine and Immunization explicitly rejects the use of user fees in financing immunizations (GAVI 2002).

However, there is evidence that in both industrial and developing countries where complete coverage exists and preventive services are free of charge (cost sharing and user fees), these services remain underutilized. In the United States, preventive services continue to be underutilized despite increasing interest in disease prevention and a growing body of evidence demonstrating the effectiveness of preventive services. Surveys have documented that clinical preventive services are less frequently used than recommended by the U.S. Preventive Services Task Force (1989), and that free services provided to users at the point of service can only result in a utilization rate averaging between 30 and 40 percent (Schauffler and Rodriguez 1993). In many developing countries, immunizations are free of charge, but the rate of immunization coverage has been below 60 percent. Among many other factors that may determine the utilization of preventive services, it has been recognized that users incur some costs even when the services themselves are free. For example, the existing health care system produces care for "healthy children" by requiring that parents take their children to health care providers at scheduled intervals. These frequent visits are often inconvenient and time consuming, so for many parents the real cost of the visit is much greater than the out-of-pocket financial burden (Halfon, Inkelas, and Wood 1995).

Positive financial incentives for users have been tried in many countries to promote utilization of public health services given the above rationale. For example, between 1975 and 1978 Austria motivated women to accept antenatal examinations and infant check-ups (Leodolter 1978) using cash rewards. In Germany, a financial incentive of DM100 was provided to women at their first prenatal visit to improve prenatal care (Davis and others 1990b). France has provided a modest but positive incentive for prenatal visits (Buekens and others 1993) for 40 years. In Finland, mothers receive packages of baby care provisions, including new clothing and a baby bathtub, if they attend the clinic prior to their fifth month of pregnancy (Davis and others 1990a).

Publications on the use of positive financial incentives are not rare, but they mostly concern immunizations, with only a few relating to other preventive services. Loevinsohn and Loevinsohn (1987) reported the use of a small material incentive (flour, milk, cooking oil, canned meat) as a strategy for improving primary care in Nicaragua. The proportion of the total population immunized under the age of six was highest for mobile clinics with food (99.2 percent) and stationary clinics with food (94.1 percent), compared with mass immunization campaigns (77.1 percent) and mobile clinics without food (63.3 percent).

Moran and others (1996) experimented with a lottery-type incentive to encourage lower-income patients in Massachusetts to accept immunization against influenza. Immunization recipients became eligible to win one of three grocery store gift certificates. The modest monetary value helped ensure that the incentive was not viewed as coercive. Compared with individuals who were not offered any incentive, those eligible for the incentive were significantly more likely to be immunized (20 percent of the control group versus 29 percent of the intervention group were immunized).

In California, a school-based immunization effort targeting 4,928 seventh-grade students for hepatitis B vaccine used a variety of incentives (extrascholastic credits, pizza, stationery, and social events) to motivate a timely return of parental consent forms. Seventy-one percent of students received the first dose of the vaccine, and of these 93 percent completed the three-dose series. The use of incentives for the return of consent forms proved to be one of the major determinants of successful immunization (Unti and others 1997).

Examining the influence of different degrees of promotion on immunization uptake in a city in the United States, Yokley and Glenwick (1984) targeted all children five years of age or younger who were clients of a public health clinic. Three lottery-type monetary incentives (US$100, US$50, and US$25) were offered in combination with a specific prompt (for example, the client's name and overdue immunizations). It was found that the combined monetary and specific prompt incentive was associated with a 17.7 percent increase in immunization coverage compared with groups without interventions, and a 15.3 percent increase compared with groups who only received prompts.

In New York, Birkhead and others (1995) assessed the effectiveness of different interventions on measles immunization rates among preschool children enrolled in the special Supplemental Food Program for Women, Infants, and Children. In addition to an escort to the clinic and passive referral for immunization, a third intervention required families of children aged 12–59 months to pick up food vouchers on a monthly schedule. Children at voucher incentive sites were 2.9 times more likely to be immunized than children without this incentive.

In a literature review of the financial incentives for the utilization of immunization services, Achat, McIntyre, and Burgess (1999) concluded that with detailed planning and careful organization, financial incentives for users could result in an improvement in immunization coverage.

HOW SHOULD PROVIDERS BE PAID?

To increase the use of preventive services, not only should the consumers' financial barrier be reduced, but the financial incentive for physicians to provide such care should also be improved by using appropriate payment systems (Davis and others 1990a; McGinnis, Williams-Russo, and Knickman 2002).

Global Budget

Many countries actually use a global budget to pay for public health services. Notably, in Central Asian countries, governments provide annual global budgets to tuberculosis hospitals. In China, the governments at different levels provide global budgets to disease control centers (Liu and Mills 2002). In Western Europe, global budgets are provided for public health activities. In the United States, state governments provide global budgets to local health departments for the provision of defined public health services (Chapin and Fetter 2002). However, few studies examine whether the global budget can promote public health services delivery.

Fee for Service

Although it can be argued that fee-for-service (FFS) payments for preventive services can lead to their overutilization (Schauffler and Rodriguez 1993), excess use of preventive care resulting from FFS payments to physicians has never been documented (Davis and others 1990b). It has been argued that unrestricted FFS reimbursement of individual preventive services is expected to achieve the highest level of utilization for preventive care.

Social insurance schemes in many countries use FFS to pay for preventive services, based on the belief that FFS payment can motivate providers to render preventive services and promote their utilization.

In the United Kingdom, where physicians are paid based on capitation, some core preventive services are traditionally outside the capitation payment. These services are paid for on an FFS basis to encourage the provision of these services, which include Pap smears, prenatal care, immunizations, and family planning (Donner-Banzhoff and others 1998; Fry and Stephen 1986; Hughes and Yule 1992).

In Canada, where physicians have been reimbursed on an FFS basis, preventive services are relatively generously reimbursed, and there is no constraint on the provision of preventive services as is the case for curative services (Bass and Elford 1988).

In Germany, physicians are paid based on FFS, but there is a limit to the amount that can be reimbursed. To promote provision and utilization of preventive care, some preventive services such as maternal and child health are excluded from the limitation (Davis and others 1990a).

In the United States, the federal government has already used economic incentives to affect the mix of services provided. The Resources-Based Relative Value Scale used by the Medicare program was in part adopted to encourage physicians to provide primary and preventive care, which is relatively generously reimbursed.

The most successful story is reported from Japan, where the government has not only exerted tight control over the price of medical services, but has also been promoting the delivery of certain cost-effective and preventive services by manipulating their prices (Campbell and Ikegami 1998, Ikegami 1992). Primary care is promoted through higher fees, and some costlier services are reduced through lower fees.

Capitation

Capitation payment is used to pay mainly for bundled primary care including preventive services. The specific services covered by capitated payment are often not explicitly defined, giving providers flexibility on what to provide. Payment for preventive services only on a per capita basis is called a "periodic health visit fee," which will be discussed separately.

In theory, capitation payment can motivate physicians to provide preventive services, because the prevention of disease can avoid treatment costs. Early detection and diagnosis of diseases can reduce the costs of treatment due to disease progression, and preventive services can minimize the long-term consumption of health care services (Dowd 1982; Hornbrook 1983).

However, it can also be argued that the level of incentive to provide preventive care to keep patients healthy depends on how frequently enrollees change their providers. Switches between providers increase the expectation that the economic benefit of a provider's "investment" in prevention can be reaped by other providers, thus it may discourage the provision of preventive care. In addition, preventive services are cost-effective to society, but not necessarily for the third-party payers, depending on the share of the treatment cost they must bear. For example, a screening program would be perceived as cost-effective by a third party only if the savings due to the prevention of diseases were greater than or equal to the expense of the program. Another disadvantage of capitation payment is that it discourages costlier outreach preventive visits.

Studies on the effect of traditional capitation payments to providers on the provision and utilization of preventive services are limited, but generally support the conclusion that providers receiving capitated rates are more likely to provide preventive services than those under FFS reimbursement (Balkrishnan and others 2002; Barnum, Kutzin, and Saxenian 1995; Lennon and others 1990).

Salary

Available literature on salary payment is not specifically related to paying for public health services. Gosden, Pedersen, and Torgerson (1999) did a comprehensive literature review of the effect of salary payment on general practitioners' provision behavior. Twenty-three papers of reasonable quality were included in the literature review. The authors found that payment using salaries was associated with the lowest use of curative referrals and procedures and more preventive care, as compared with FFS payment.

One supporter of salary payment (Pontes 1995) argues that it is desirable because it provides a neutral incentive to doctors' behavior. As a result, what a doctor recommends and prescribes depends wholly on the need of patients, his/her medical knowledge, and the availability of resources. Doctors' provision behavior can be improved through education, providing them with scientific evidence, and offering provision guidelines. The disadvantages of low productivity and low morale can be overcome by the proper design and implementation of bonus systems and the use of various nonfinancial motivations.

Preventive Service Account

With a preventive service account, a total fixed annual amount of preventive services for an individual is placed in an account, and providers are allowed to charge this account on an FFS basis. The amount allocated to each account depends on the need for preventive services and the cost of providing these services. For example, the amount in a newborn baby's account may be equivalent to the costs of providing prenatal and postnatal care, immunizations, growth monitoring, and nutritional consultations; the amount for a man age 21–44 years may be equivalent to the costs of providing behavioral consultation and monitoring blood pressure and cholesterol. Any unused balance could be carried over to subsequent years.

The advantages of this payment method are that it lets patients decide what services they wish to receive (for example, counseling regarding smoking versus repeated cholesterol tests), and to a certain extent it prevents overprovision, because the total amount of annual spending is individually capped. The major disadvantages are that it provides providers with no incentive to recommend the most cost-effective preventive services for the given amount of chargeable budget; it may not ensure effective use of the limited budget for preventive care; and there is still a risk of excessive provision.

This payment method was proposed about 10 years ago by Davis and others (1990a). The authors of this report found neither information on practical implementation of this method nor publications on its evaluation.

Periodic Health Visit Fee

With a periodic health visit fee (PHVF), the provider receives a periodic fee (for example, per year) for a defined package (types and volume) of preventive services provided to a patient. PHVF is different from traditional capitation payment in that the types and volume of PHVF services are defined in advance; under traditional capitation, the providers decide which services to provide. The second difference is that PHVF covers preventive services exclusively, and traditional capitation covers both curative and preventive services.

Davis and others recommended PHVF as a payment for preventive services because it balances the incentives and the disincentives that different payment methods would generate. It provides adequate incentives for physicians to provide these services that are specified in advance, and it helps to educate physicians about what services are appropriate for patients of different characteristics, through the check-off claim form that specifies which services should be provided to what kinds of people. It promotes efficient use of resources, because the package of preventive services is defined based on the best knowledge of the cost-effectiveness of preventive services. It rewards good performance and provides incentives to complete the service package. In addition, by making the primary care physician responsible for managing the predetermined fee, there is an incentive to use less costly nonphysician personnel to provide the services. At the same time, by not permitting direct reimbursement to nonphysician person-nel, insurers retain a greater degree of control over the types of health profes-sionals providing the preventive services.

The difficulties involved in implementing this payment method are first, that the administration cost is high because it requires monitoring and evaluation. Second, if patients request additional preventive services, reimbursements need to be made separately. Finally, providers may be penalized for not providing ser-vices simply because patients choose not to receive the included services.

As with preventive service accounts, this payment method was proposed (Davis and others 1990a), but neither information about its implementation nor evaluation reports are available.

Performance-Related Pay

Performance-related pay (PRP) means that payment is directly linked to the per-formance of health care providers. PRP has a long history, but was not formally introduced into the health sector until the end of the 1980s. Now it is a popular method of paying for general health services. PRP has been increasingly intro-duced into the public health arena, particularly in the United States and other industrial countries. In the United States, large health care purchasers are seek-ing to buy "value" for their health care dollars and are beginning to define value in terms of disease prevention and improved health status. One example is the Pacific Business Group on Health in California (see above). The six performance indicators were cesarean sections, childhood immunizations, cervical cancer screening, diabetic retinal exams, mammography screening, and prenatal care, most of which were indicators on preventive services. PRP was generally found effective in promoting performance.

In 2000 in the United States, the Wisconsin Division of Public Health reformed its allocation of federal and state funds by basing contracts on performance to replace the original audited cost-based funding mechanism to local health departments (Chapin and Fetter 2002). The health authority in Wisconsin imple-mented the following: (1) the total fund allocated to local health departments was determined by considering service levels, the general population, the target population, risk factors, and geographic factors; (2) numerous contractors were consolidated into one large block contract; (3) a quasi market was created, where the buyer (state division of public health) and sellers (local health departments or other nonprofit organizations) negotiated prices and products; and (4) objective performance measures were specified, so that the contract was based on the real-ization of a set of performance indicators of public health. This reform simplified administration because there was no requirement for a proposal, no requirement for budget submissions, no periodic progress reports, and rewards and penalties were based on evaluation of attainment of the performance indicators.

In the United Kingdom, a performance-based contract was introduced by the National Health Service in 1990 to pay general practitioners for delivering immunization services. Under this contract, general practitioners who achieved a high (90 percent) or low (70 to 89 percent) target level were eligible for payments of $1,800 and $600 respectively. Ritchie and others (1992) examined the change in immunization rates in the first three quarters after the introduction of the new contract in 1990. The number of clinics achieving 95 percent or higher immunization coverage increased from 31 percent to 81 percent for primary immunization, and from 23 percent to 81 percent for preschool boosters.

In 1997 in Australia, a number of Commonwealth Departments of Health and Family Services introduced incentive pay based on performance, which was aimed at improving immunization coverage rates (Leese and Bosanquet 1996). One approach was to pay bonus payment to practitioners according to the percentage of fully immunized children; another approach was an immunization allowance paid when the child reached 19 months and had received all vaccinations due up to 18 months of age. These two approaches were reported to be effective in increasing immunization coverage.

Payers of health care services in developing countries have not typically required provider institutions to guarantee performance. This lack of accountability has contributed to poor performance of public health programs. Donors usually adopt the practice of country governments, either providing lump-sum grants or reimbursing public providers and nongovernmental organizations for documented expenditure. The result is that most provider organizations devote more energy to securing funds than to improving performance.

A demonstration of PRP was implemented in Haiti, supported by the U.S. Agency for International Development (Eichler, Auxila, and Pollack 2002). In 1999, recognizing the disadvantages (weak incentives for improving performance), the project transferred from a cost-based payment system to a performance-related payment system, by which performance indicators were established and measured by year-end, and a performance-based bonus on top of the monthly payment was distributed according to provider performance.

Results showed improvement in the overall performance. Performance indicators related to preventive services (immunization and use of contraception) had greater increases. However, the number of pilot districts was small (three), and many other factors that might have affected performance indicators were not controlled for and analyzed.

TOWARD BETTER FINANCING AND PAYMENT POLICIES

Ensure Sufficient Financing

There is widespread agreement in both theory and practice on what public good types of public health services should be exclusively publicly financed. They include universal public health services such as policy development and enforcement, public health information systems, treatment of polluted water, prevention of air pollution, health education programs through the media, and vector elimination programs for the prevention of infectious diseases. These services are both publicly financed and provided through publicly owned provision systems, although some of these services are contracted out to the private sector.

There are controversies, however, regarding quasi-public goods. In theory, services such as immunization and treatment of communicable diseases can be jointly financed by both government and consumers. However, there is no knowledge about the proportion of the total financing need that should be covered by government. In practice, the financing of these services should vary with a country's state of economic development, the type of health care system, and the cost of delivering such services.

- For low-cost services of public health significance such as immunizations, public financing has been implemented in almost all countries, except for vaccines not included in the national immunization programs and countries where some immunizations are covered by private insurance. There is little doubt that these services should be financed through government, and all countries are encouraged to do so.

- For services of medium cost such as tuberculosis and malaria treatment, if disease prevalence is low, often the disease may not attract public health attention, and if it is high, pure public financing and free treatments may be beyond the affordability of the government. To ensure adequate provision and utilization of these services, policymakers should first explore the possibility of government financing to ensure that government makes the best effort to finance these services. In countries where social and private insurance prevail, third-party coverage for these services should be regulated (although consumers pay part or all of the premium). In countries where the need for these services is high and whose ability to finance these services is limited, donor support is often a choice. Out-of-pocket payment at the point of services should be prohibited.

- For high-cost services such as antiretroviral treatment for HIV/AIDS, probably only some high-income countries can afford to pay for them. In low-income countries, where prevalence is high (for example, in Sub-Saharan African countries), it might not be feasible for the government to cover the costs of providing free care, or possible for insurers to provide coverage. Hard decisions have to be made to ration these services (drugs), based on ability to pay, except when international financing support is available.

Private good types of public health services (for example, screening, prenatal care, and private consultation for disease prevention) are different from traditional private goods in that the true value of these services is often underestimated. Utilization determined by individual willingness and ability to pay often leads to underutilization of these cost-effective, low-cost, and socially desirable services. Thus, policymakers are encouraged to use policies to ensure that these services are either financed by the government or through a third party. Direct payment for these services should be discouraged.

Improving resource allocation and realizing sufficient financing for public health will need long-term, continuous efforts. Policymakers should be informed on the cost-effectiveness of different public health services, both relative to one another and in comparison with curative services. Health services should be prioritized at the national level according to the cost-effectiveness of various health interventions. Continuous research is needed to check whether the actual resource allocation matches the prioritized health services. Political will and commitment are the major determinants, and regulation and legislation have proved to be effective ways of ensuring financing. Two types of regulations can have a direct effect on the financing of public health services: (1) both public and private insurers should be regulated to cover specified public health services; and (2) government can improve its allocation of resources at the macro level for financing public health services by regulating the proportion of the health budget that should be allocated to public health and setting up a budget that is separated from the overall health budget.

Design Appropriate Payment Systems for Efficient Provision

Appropriate payment systems should be able to send the message to providers to deliver the right kind and volume of public health services and to promote socially desirable performance. Regardless of what payment methods are used, public health services providers should be fairly paid. Payment should reflect providers' performance, and the income of public health workers should not be inferior to that of other equivalent professions.

PAYMENT BY PERFORMANCE

Evidence in both industrial and developing countries suggests that the link between performance and payment can result in better performance, so some form of performance-related pay is recommended. While the concept of PRP is simple, there is no uniform and universal method for designing and implementing PRP. It needs innovative efforts suited to a country's socioeconomic context, the goals of the public health program, and the measurability of performance. Generally, in designing PRP schemes, the following points are particularly important. First, PRP can be used to pay government bodies, public health institutions, and individual health workers (working independently or serving as employees of public health institutions). The essence of PRP is that, for any resources transferred from one party to another, there must be monitoring and evaluation of what the payers are supposed to purchase, regardless of who buys from whom.

Second, performance measures may vary depending on the specific objectives of the public health programs, but they generally consist of quantity, quality, and health outcome measures. Because the association between the volume of public health services and health outcomes is closer than that between curative care and health outcomes, the volume of public health services is a better measurement of performance than the volume of curative care.

Third, any performance measures should be socially desirable and consistent with the measurements of health system performance.

Fourth, to provide strong enough incentives for providers to perform in a desirable manner, the share of the payment based on performance should be significant, and PRP should be able to reward good performance and penalize poor performance.

GLOBAL BUDGET VERSUS PERFORMANCE-RELATED PAY

Global budget appears to be the most popular payment method used by higher-level government to pay lower levels of government, and by overall government to pay public health institutions. Government funding often has to be transferred several times from higher to lower levels before it reaches public health providers, especially when public health programs are vertical and centralized. Public health institutions are often publicly owned and financed directly by the government for the provision of public health services. The global budget has been an effective method for paying providers for curative care in terms of cost containment. It is problematic in terms of health system performance, because instead of being performance based, payment is often based on need (the number of individuals served, with or without risk adjustment), the previous year's budget, and cost incurred. In any of these types of budget practice, the payees are seen as either money-transfer machines (lower levels of government) or money-spending machines, with little incentive to maximize their performance.

In recognizing the shortcoming of the global budget and the difficulties of totally switching from a global budget to PRP, the combination of the two may increase feasibility and produce a desirable effect. Actually, most of the PRP schemes cited earlier take this hybrid form. In implementing this combination, a proportion of the global budget can be withheld and used for redistribution according to the performance monitoring results.

CAPITATION VERSUS FEE FOR SERVICE

In view of the up-to-date information that there is little documented evidence on overprovision of public health services as a result of the FFS mechanism, that FFS has been used successfully to promote the delivery of public health services, and that capitation payment alone cannot ensure adequate provision of public health services, capitation payment for general health care with supplemental FFS payment for preventive services is recommended. It is likely that this will control unnecessary provision of curative care and ensure adequate provision of preventive care. In countries where FFS is dominant and capitation payment is nonexistent, the fees for preventive services should be set at a higher fee/cost ratio than for curative services so as to provide enough motivation for provision of preventive services. To prevent overprovision of preventive services, providers should be given delivery guidelines indicating both the types and volume of services for specific sex and age groups. Providers should be monitored against these guidelines.

SALARY VERSUS PERFORMANCE-RELATED PAY

Health workers employed by institutions are usually paid by salary. Evidence shows that when health workers provide both curative and preventive care, salary payments provide neutral incentives to avoid overprovision of curative care and underprovision of preventive care. However, this does not mean that salary payments provide enough incentive for the provision of socially desirable preventive services. To promote the delivery of preventive services, health workers should be paid a performance-related bonus on top of their basic salary, depending on how well they have provided preventive services. Institutions may not be willing to pay their employees on the basis of performance indicators associated with provision of preventive services, however, unless the institutions themselves are paid according to such performance indicators.

When salary is used to pay health workers, specifically those providing public health services, the issue is not the allocation of resources between curative and preventive care. Rather, it is an issue of morale and productivity, as measured, for example, by the number of units of preventive services provided per unit of time. To increase morale and improve productivity, some forms of PRP should be designed and implemented on top of basic salary payments.

PROMOTE ADEQUATE UTILIZATION

Adequate utilization needs more than appropriate provider payment systems. Some demand-side measures should also be adopted. First, users' financial responsibility at the point of service should be minimized. Evidence supports the conclusion that, for those preventive services, adequate utilization of which is the policy goal of public health, any form of cost sharing and user fees should be prohibited.

Second, other costs (indirect costs such as time and travel expenses) for the utilization of preventive services should be reduced as much as possible by increasing the availability of providers, improving geographic access to preventive care, and timing service delivery conveniently (for example, services should be made available outside working hours).

Third, positive financial incentives can be offered for using specific priority preventive services. There is both practical and positive evidence for their utilization, especially in the areas of immunization and prenatal care.

REFERENCES

Achat, H., P. McIntyre, and M. Burgess. 1999. "Health Care Incentives in Immunization." *Australia/New Zealand Journal of Public Health* 23(3): 285–88.

Amonkar, M. M., S. Madhavan, S. A. Rosenbluth, K. J. Simon. 1999. "Barriers and Facilitators to Providing Common Preventive Screening Services in Managed Care Settings." *Journal of Community Health* 24(3): 229–47.

Ayah, R. T. 1997. "Impact of User Fees in Health." *East Africa Medical Journal* 74: 749–50.

Balkrishnan R., M. A. Hall, D. Mehrabi, G. J. Chen, S. R. Feldman, and A. B. Fleischer. 2002. "Capitation Payment, Length of Visit, and Preventive Services: Evidence from a National Sample of Outpatient Physicians." *American Journal of Managed Care* 8(4): 332–40.

Barnum, H., J. Kutzin, and H. Saxenian. 1995. "Incentives and Provider Payment Methods." *International Journal of Health Planning and Management* 10(1): 23–45.

Bass, M. J., and R. W. Elford. 1988. "Preventive Practice Patterns of Canadian Primary Care Physicians." *American Journal of Preventative Medicine* 4(4 suppl): 17–23.

Berwich, D. M. 1995. "The Toxicity of Pay for Performance." Quality Management in Health Care 4(1): 27–33.

Birdsall, N. and E. James. 1993. "Health Government and the Poor: The Case for the Private Sector." In J. N. Gribble and S. H. Preston, eds., *The Epidemiological Transition: Policy and Planning Implications for Developing Countries.* Washington, D.C.: National Academy Press.

Birkhead, G. S., C. W. LeBaron, P. Parsons, J. C. Grabau, E. Maes, L. Barr-Gale, J. Fuhrman, S. Brooks, J. Rosenthal, and S. C. Hadler. 1995. "The Immunization of Children Enrolled in the Special Supplemental Food Program for Women, Infants, and Children (WIC): The Impact of Different Strategies."' *Journal of the American Medical Association* 274(4): 312–16.

Black, K., and H. Skipper. 1999. *Life and Health Insurance.* 13th edition. New York: Prentice Hall.

Bledsoe, D. R., W. B. Leisy, and J. A. Rodeghero. 1995. "Tying Physician Incentive Pay to Performance." *Health Care Finance and Management* 49(12): 40–44.

Buchan, J. 1993. "Performance-Related Pay and NHS Nursing." *Nursing Standards* 7(25): 30.

Buchan, J., and M. Thompson. 1993. "Pay and Nursing Performance." *Health Manpower Management* 19(2): 29–31.

Buekens P., M. Kotelchuck, B. Blondel, F. B. Kristensen, J. H. Chen, and G. Masuy-Stroobant. 1993. "A Comparison of Prenatal Care Use in the United States and Europe." *American Journal of Public Health* 83: 31–36.

Campbell, J. C., and N. Ikegami. 1998. *The Art of Balance in Health Policy: Maintaining Japan's Low-Cost, Egalitarian System.* New York: Cambridge University Press.

Castledine, G. 1993. "Can Performance-Related Pay be Adapted for Nursing?" *British Journal of Nursing* 2(22): 1120–21.

Chambers, L. W. 1997. "Ontario's Proposal to End Provincial Funding for Public Health: What Is at Stake? *CMAJ* 156(7): 1001–1003.

Chapin, J., and B. Fetter. 2002. "Performance-Based Contracting in Wisconsin Public Health: Transforming State-local Relations." *Milbank Quarterly* 80(1): 97–124.

Christensen, B. 1995. "Payment and Attendance at General Practice Preventive Health Examinations." *Family Medicine* 27(8): 531–34.

Davies, P. 1988. "Extending the Flexible Spine of Pay." *The Health Service Journal* December: 1442.

Davis, K., R. Bialek, M. Parkinson, J. Smith, and C. Vellozzi. 1990a. "Paying for Preventive Care: Moving the Debate Forward." *American Journal of Preventative Medicine* 6(4 suppl): 7–30.

Davis, K., R. Bialek, M. Parkinson, J. Smith, and C. Vellozzi. 1990b. "Reimbursement for Preventive Services: Can We Construct an Equitable System?" *Journal of General International Medicine* 5(5 suppl): S93–98.

De Bethune, X., S. Alfani, and J. Lahaye. 1989. "The Influence of an Abrupt Price Increase on Health Service Utilisation: Evidence from Zaire." *Health Policy and Planning* 4: 76–81.

Donner-Banzhoff, N., L. Kreienbrock, M. Katic, and E. Baum. 1998. "Family Practitioners' Remuneration and Patterns of Care - Does Social Class Matter?" *Soz Praventivmed* 43(2): 73–79.

Dowd, B. E. 1982. "Financing Preventive Care in HMOs: A Theoretical Analysis." *Inquiry* 19(1): 68–78.

Durham, G., and B. Kill B. 1999. "Public Health Funding Mechanisms in New Zealand." *Australian Health Review* 22(4): 100–112.

Eichler, R., P. Auxila, and J. Pollock. 2002. "Promoting Preventive Health Care: Paying for Performance in Haiti." In P. J. Brook and S. M. Smith, eds., *Contracting for Public Health Services: Output-Based Aid and Its Application.* Washington, D.C.: World Bank.

Faulkner, L., and H. Schauffler. 1997. "The Effect of Health Insurance Coverage on the Appropriate Use of Recommended Clinical Preventive Services." *American Journal of Preventative Medicine* 13(6): 453–58.

Flessa, S. 2000. "Where Efficiency Saves Lives: A Linear Program for the Optimal Allocation of Health Care Resources in Developing Countries." *Health Care Management Science* 3(3): 249–67.

Frossard, M. 1990 "Hospital Strategy and Regional Planning in France." *International Journal of Health and Management* 5: 59–63.

Fry, J., and W. J. Stephen. 1986. "Primary Health Care in the United Kingdom." *International Journal of Health Services* 16(4): 485–95.

Gertler, P., L. Locay, and W. Sanderson. 1987. "Are User Fees Regressive?" *Journal of Econometrics* 36: 67–88.

Gordon, R. 1983. "An Operational Classification of Disease Prevention." *Public Health Report* 98: 107–109.

Gosden, T., F. Forland, I. S. Kristiansen, M. Sutton, B. Leese, A. Giuffrida, M. Sergison, and L. Pedersen. 2001. "Impact of Payment Method on Behavior of Primary Care Physicians: A Systematic Review." *Journal of Health Service Research and Policy* 6(1): 44–55.

Gosden, T., L. Pedersen, and D. Torgerson. 1999. "How Should We Pay Doctors? A Systematic Review of Salary Payments and Their Effect on Doctor Behavior." *QJM: An International Journal of Medicine* 92(1): 47–55.

Halfon, N., M. Inkelas, and D. Wood. 1995. "Non-Financial Barriers to Care for Children and Youth." *Annual Review of Public Health* 16: 447–72.

Hill, J. P., and G. Ramachandran. 1992. "A Simple Scheme to Improve Compliance in Patients Taking Tuberculosis Medication." *Tropical Doctor* 22(4): 161–63.

Hirdes, J. P., C. A. Botz, J. Kozak, and V. Lepp. 1996. "Identifying an Appropriate Case Mix Measure for Chronic Care: Evidence from an Ontario Pilot Study." *Healthcare Management Forum* 9(1): 40–46.

Hornbrook, M. 1983. "Allocative Medicine: Efficiency, Disease Severity, and the Payment System." *The Annals of the American Academy* 468: 12–29.

Hsiao, W. C. 1995. "Abnormal Economics in the Health Sector." *Health Policy* 32(1–3): 125–39.

Huber, J. H. 1993. "Ensuring Access to Health Care with the Introduction of User Fees: A Kenyan Example." *Social Science and Medicine* 36(4): 485–94.

Hughes, D. and B. Yule. 1992. "The Effect of Per-Item Fees on the Behaviour of General Practitioners." *Journal of Health Economics* 11(4): 413–37.

Hussein, A. K., and P. G. Mujinja. 1997. "Impact of User Charges on Government Health Facilities in Tanzania." *East Africa Medical Journal* 74(12): 751–57.

Ikegami, N. 1992. "Japan: Maintaining Equity through Regulated Fees." *Journal of Health Politics, Policy and Law* 17(4): 689–713.

Institute of Medicine, Committee for the Study of the Future of Public Health, Division of Health Care Services. 1988. *The Future of Public Health*. Washington, D.C.: National Academy Press.

Jelovac, I. 2001. "Physicians' Payment Contracts, Treatment Decisions and Diagnosis Accuracy." *Health Economics* 10(1): 9–25.

Keane, C., J. Marx, and E. Ricci. 2002. "Public Health Privatization: Proponents, Registers, and Decisionmakers." *Journal of Public Health Policy* 23(2): 133–52.

Kouides, R. W., B. Lewis, N. M. Bennett, K. M. Bell, W. H. Barker, E. R. Black, J. D. Cappuccio, R. F. Raubertas, and F. M. LaForce. 1993. "A Performance-Based Incentive Program for Influenza Immunization in the Elderly." *American Journal of Preventative Medicine* 9(4): 250–55.

Kouides, R. W., N. M. Bennett, B. Lewis, J. D. Cappuccio, W. H. Barker, and F. M. LaForce. 1998. "Performance-Based Physician Reimbursement and Influenza Immunization Rates in the Elderly: The Primary-Care Physicians of Monroe County." *American Journal of Preventative Medicine* 14(2): 89–95.

Kress, D., X. Liu, P. Lydon, and A. Crouch. 2002. "Cost and Financing of Immunization Services in the Lao People's Democratic Republic." Report Submitted to Children's Vaccine Program at PATH.

Kutzin, J. 1998. "The Appropriate Role for Patient Cost Sharing." In R. Saltman, ed. *Critical Challenges for Health Care Reform in Europe*. Buckingham: Open University Press.

Larsson, L. 1997. *Glossary of Health Care and Health Care Management Terms*. University of Washington, School of Public Health and Community Medicine, Seattle, Wash.

Leaf, P. J. 1999. "A System of Care Perspective on Prevention." *Clinical Psychological Review* 19(4): 403–13.

Leese, B., and N. Bosanquet. 1996. "Changes in General Practice Organization: Survey of General Practitioners' Views on the 1990 Contract and Fundholding." *British Journal of General Practitioners* 46(403): 95–99.

Lennon, M. A., and others. 1990. "The Capitation Study Two. Does Capitation Encourage More Prevention?" *British Dental Journal* 168(5): 213–15.

Leodolter, I. 1978. "Short Report: The Mother-Child Health Passport: Austria's Successful Weapon against Infant Mortality." *Preventive Medicine* 7: 561–63.

Lillard, L. A., and others. 1986. *Preventive Medical Care: Standards, Usage and Efficiency.* Publication Number R-3266-HHS. Santa Monica, CA: The RAND Corporation.

Liu, X. 2002. *Policy Tools for Improving Allocative Efficiency of Health Resources.* World Health Organization Publications, Geneva.

Liu X., and A. Mills. 2002. "Financing Reforms of Public Health Services in China: Lessons for Other Nations." *Society, Science, Medicine* 54(11): 1691–698.

Loevinsohn, B. P., and M. E. Loevinsohn. 1987. 'Well Child Clinics and Mass Vaccination Campaigns: An Evaluation of Strategies for Improving the Coverage of Primary Health Care in a Developing Country." *American Journal of Public Health* 77(11): 1407–411.

Lohr, K. N., R. H. Brook, C. J. Kamberg, G. A. Goldberg, A. Leibowitz, J. Keesey, D. Reboussin, and J. P. Newhouse. 1986. "Use of Medical Care in the Rand Health Insurance Experiment. Diagnosis- and Service-Specific Analyses in a Randomized Controlled Trial." *Medical Care* 24(9 suppl): S1–S87.

Lurie, N., W. G. Manning, C. Peterson, G. A. Goldberg, C. A. Phelps, and L. Lillard. 1987. "Preventive Care: Do We Practice What We Preach?" *American Journal of Public Health* 77(7): 801–804.

Lynch, M. L. 1994. "The Uptake of Childhood Immunization and Financial Incentives to General Practitioners." *Health Economics* 3(2): 117–25.

McGinnis, J. M., and W. H. Foege. 1993. "Actual Causes of Death in the United States." *Journal of the American Medical Association* 270(18): 2207–212.

McGinnis, M. J., P. Williams-Russo, and J. R. Knickman. 2002. "The Case for More Active Policy Attention to Health Promotion. To Succeed, We Need Leadership that Informs and Motivates, Economic Incentives that Encourage Change, and Science that Moves the Frontiers." *Health Affairs* (Millwood) 21(2): 78–93.

Mills, A. 1997. "Improving the Efficiency of Public Sector Health Services in Developing Countries: Bureaucratic versus Market Approaches." In C. Colclough, ed., *Marketing Education and Health in Developing Countries: Miracle or Mirage.* Oxford: Clarendon Press.

Moran, W. P., K. Nelson, J. L. Wofford, R. Velez, and L. D. Case. 1996. "Increasing Influenza Immunization among High-Risk Patients: Education or Financial Incentive?" *American Journal of Public Health* 101(6): 612–20.

Morisky, D. E. 1990. "A Patient Education Program to Improve Adherence Rates with Antituberculosis Drug Regimens." *Health Education Quarterly* 17(3): 253–67.

Nettleman, M. D., and R. B. Jones. 1989. "Proportional Payment for Pelvic Inflammatory Disease: Who Should Pay for Chlamydial Screening?" *Sexually Transmitted Diseases* 16(1): 36–40.

Organisation for Economic Co-operation and Development. 1998. Health data. Paris.

Petrou, S., and J. Wolstenholme. 2002. "A Review of Alternative Approaches to Health Care Resource Allocation." *Pharmacoeconomics* 18(1): 33–43.

Pilote, L., and others. 1996. "Tuberculosis Prophylaxis in the Homeless. A Trial to Improve Adherence to Referral." *Archives of Internal Medicine* 156(2): 161–65.

Pontes, M. C. 1995. "Agency Theory: A Framework for Analysing Physician Services." *Health Care Management Review* 20(4): 57–67.

Reddy, S. D. 2000. "Examining Hazard Mitigation within the Context of Public Goods." *Environmental Management* 25(2): 129–41.

Ritchie, L. D., A. F. Bisset, D. Russell, V. Leslie, and I. Thomson. 1992. "Primary and Preschool Immunization in Grampian: Progress and the 1990 Contract." *British Medical Journal* 304(6830): 816–19.

Rubin, R. I., and D. N. Mendelson. 1995. "A Framework for Cost-Sharing Policy Analysis." In N. Mattison, ed., *Sharing the Costs of Health: A Multicountry Perspective*. Basle: Pharmaceutical Partner for Better Health Care.

Rundall, T. G., and H. H. Schauffler. 1997. "Health Promotion and Disease Prevention in Integrated Delivery Systems: The Role of Market Forces." *American Journal of Preventative Medicine* 13(4): 244–50.

Schauffler, H. H. 1993. "Disease Prevention Policy under Medicare: A Historical and Political Analysis." *American Journal of Preventative Medicine* 9(2): 71–77.

Schauffler, H. H., and T. Rodriguez. 1993. "Managed Care for Preventive Services: A Review of Policy Options." *Medical Care Review* 50(2): 153–98.

———. 1996. "Exercising Purchasing Power for Preventive Care." *Health Affairs* (Millwood) 15(1): 73–85.

Schauffler, H. H., C. Brown, and A. Milstein. 1999. "Raising the Bar: The Use of Performance Guarantees by the Pacific Business Group on Health." *Health Affairs* (Millwood) 18(2): 134–42.

Solanki, G., H. H. Schauffler,, and L. S. Miller. 2000. "The Direct and Indirect Effects of Cost-Sharing on the Use of Preventive Services." *Health Services Research* 34(6): 1331–50.

Stiglitz, J. E. 1986. Economics of the Public Sector. New York: W.W. Northon and Company.

Unti, L. M., K. K. Coyle, B. A. Woodruff, and L. Boyer-Chuanroong. 1997. "Incentives and Motivators in School-Based Hepatitis B Vaccination Program." *Journal of School Health* 67(7): 265–68.

U.S. Preventive Services Task Force. 1989. *Guidelines to Clinical Preventive Services: An Assessment of the Effectiveness of 169 Interventions*. Baltimore, MD: Williams & Wilkins.

Vladescu, C., and S. Radulescu. 1999. "Improving Primary Health Care: Output-Based Contracting in Romania." World Bank document (http://rru.worldbank.org/Documents/).

Waddington, C. J., and K. A. Enyimayew. 1989. "A Price to Pay: The Impact of User Changes in Ashanti-Akim District, Ghana." *International Journal of Health Planning and Management* 4: 17–74.

Wall, S. 1998. "Transformations in Public Health Systems." *Health Affairs* (Millwood) 17(3): 64–80.

World Bank. 1993. *World Development Report 1993: Investing in Health.* Washington, D.C.

GAVI (Global Alliance for Vaccines and Immunization). 2002. *Immunization Financing Options: A Resource for Policymakers.* Geneva: GAVI Secretariat.

World Health Organization. 2000. *The World Health Report 2000: Health Systems: Improving Performance.* Geneva.

Yoder, R. 1989. "Are People Willing and Able to Pay for Health Services?" *Social Science and Medicine* 29: 35–42.

Yokley, J. M., and D. S. Glenwick. 1984. "Increasing the Immunization of Preschool Children: An Evaluation of Applied Community Interventions." *Journal of Applied Behavior Analysis* 17(3): 313–25.

CHAPTER 11

Buying Results: Contracting for Private Health Care Delivery

Benjamin Loevinsohn and April Harding

To achieve the health-related Millennium Development Goals (MDGs) in developing countries, health services delivery, particularly for poor people, will have to be improved. Nearly 6 of 10 child deaths in developing countries could be prevented through the full implementation of a few effective and low-cost interventions (Bryce and others 2003). Additional resources for the public sector will not be enough, especially as most curative services in developing countries are provided by the private sector (World Bank 2004). Contracting with nongovernmental organizations (NGOs) or other nonpublic entities to manage or deliver health services has been proposed as one approach to improve both coverage and quality of care.

WHY CONTRACT—IDEOLOGY OR PRAGMATISM?

Serious government capacity constraints throughout the developing world have undermined attempts to improve the delivery of health care and other services (Mills, Bennett, and Russell 2001). The evidence base for most service delivery reforms in developing countries is weak, however, and the debate related to contracting is heated. Contracting with nonstate providers is often seen as arising out of an ideological desire to "privatize" publicly financed health services and ultimately to limit or end government involvement in health care (Pfeiffer 2003; Turshen 1999). Another view is that purchaser-provider splits such as contracting are technocratic, neoliberal solutions (driven by the "new public sector management" model), focused excessively on efficiency and giving too little attention to equity.

Discussions with people involved in contracting in developing countries suggest that they are motivated by practical concerns, not ideology. Most contracting initiatives arise either from an absence of government services or from frustration with the poor quality and coverage of government services, especially for poor people. Most advocates of contracting express a desire for increased government financing so that services in the community can be expanded and improved. They also want to see governments engage with private providers, which already deliver the bulk of curative services in developing countries, in order to improve quality of care, access, and coordination.

Potential Advantages of Contracting

Contracting for health service delivery is attractive because it has the potential (Loevinsohn 2000) to:

- Ensure a greater focus on the achievement of measurable results, particularly if contracts define objectively verifiable outputs and outcomes.

- Overcome "absorptive capacity" constraints that often plague government health care systems and prevent them from effectively utilizing the resources made available to them.

- Tap the private sector's greater flexibility and generally better morale to improve services.

- Broaden managerial autonomy and decentralize decisionmaking to managers on the ground.

- Use competition to increase effectiveness and efficiency.

- Allow governments to focus on other roles they are uniquely placed to carry out such as planning, standard setting, financing, and regulation.

Potential Difficulties of Contracting

A number of potential problems have been raised in connection with contracting (Abramson 1999; England 1997; Frick-Cardelle 2003; Mills 1998; Palmer 2000; Slack and Savedoff 2001; Soderlund, Mendoza-Arana, and Goudge 2003). They include concerns that

- Contracts will not be feasible at a sufficiently large scale to make a difference at the country level.

- Contracts will be more expensive than government provision of the same services, partly reflecting greater transaction costs.

- The higher levels of financing usually associated with contracts explain their success, and providing the same resources to public institutions would accomplish the same or better results.

- NGOs and other nongovernmental entities will not want to work in remote or difficult areas and are less capable of providing services to the very poor, thus increasing inequities in health service delivery.

- Governments will have limited capacity to manage contracts effectively.

- Tenders and contract management will create additional opportunities for fraud and corruption.

- NGOs and governments are so weary of each other that they will not be able to work together effectively.

- Even if successful, contracting will not be sustainable.

This review of contracting experience examines the effectiveness of contracting for health service delivery, taking into account the methodological rigor of the evaluations, to find out the extent to which the potential difficulties posited actually occur during implementation. Recommendations are also made for future contracting efforts.

APPROACHES TO CONTRACTING

Contracting for health service delivery can be approached in several different ways. For example, under a *management contract* (table 11.1, arrangement 3), a government contracts with a nonstate entity or an individual to manage existing government services in a specified area. Under a *service delivery contract* (table 11.1, arrangement 4), the contract specifies that a provider will both manage and supply the production infrastructure such as personnel, equipment, and drugs. The arrangements described in table 11.1 are not exhaustive, and there are clearly hybrids. For example, the line between a management contract and a service delivery contract blurs when the contractor uses government health workers but pays them much more than their civil service salaries.

This chapter generally deals with examples of these two types of contracts, management and service delivery contracts, sometimes in comparison with government services. Some experience has been acquired with contracts between national governments and local governments to achieve certain goals (table 11.1, arrangement 2). Though interesting, this arrangement rarely involves a true contract into which the parties enter voluntarily and the contractor can be fired for nonperformance (although other rewards and sanctions may be available). In a few evaluated instances of this approach, a government, a donor, or both commonly make a grant to NGOs (arrangement 5), which define where and what services are delivered. However, these are generally not true contracts, partly because the government has little say in what services are delivered and where. Also, few of these grants have been rigorously evaluated (Connor 2000). Contracts between different levels of government and grants to NGOs are not examined in this review.

STUDY METHODOLOGY

This review focuses on evaluated instances, in developing countries, of contracts between governments, or their agents, with identifiable nonstate providers for delivery of primary health care services including nutrition (but excluding referral hospital care or ancillary services such as food provision in hospitals).

Inclusion Criteria

To be included in the review, the evaluation had to measure quality of care, outputs such as increase in the volume of services provided, or impact on health status. The

TABLE 11.1 Some Service Delivery Arrangements

Arrangement	Initiator (defines services)	Approver	Manager	Production infrastructure	Financing	Example
1. Government services	Govt.	Govt.	Govt.	Govt.	Govt.[b]	Govt. primary health care centers
2. Intergovernmental agreements	Govt.-1[a]	Govt.-1	Govt.-2[a]	Govt.-2	Govt.-1[b]	Transfer of funds from federal to provincial governments
3. Management contracts	Govt.	Govt.	Private sector	Govt.	Govt.[b]	Govt. hires a private sector manager to manage existing govt. health services
4. Service delivery contracts	Govt.	Govt.	Private sector	Private sector	Govt.[b]	Govt. hires NGO to provide services where none currently exist
5. Government grants to private sector	Private sector (most often)	Govt. or donor	Private sector	Private sector	Govt. (+/− NGO or community contribution)	NGOs submit proposals to govt. for needs identified by community or NGO
6. Vouchers	Private sector or govt.	Consumer	Private sector	Private sector	Govt. and/or donor	Female sex workers are provided vouchers for curative care, which they can redeem at practitioners of their choice
7. Franchising	Private sector	Consumer	Private sector	Private sector	Consumer (+/− subsidy from govt. or donor)	Private practitioners join franchise network providing reproductive health services
8. Private sector services	Private sector	Private sector and consumer	Private sector	Private sector	Consumer or NGO/donor	1) NGO establishes health services in slum areas using its own funds 2) For-profit providers establish private clinic

Govt., government; +/−, with or without; NGO, nongovernmental organization.

[a] Govt.-1 and govt.-2 refer to different levels of government.

[b] This may be supplemented by formal or informal user charges.

Source: Authors.

evaluations also had to, at a minimum, involve before-and-after or controlled designs. Hence, evaluations were excluded that described the contracting process but that did not measure some tangible outputs. Also excluded were studies that just provided "after" evaluations with no "before" data or without contemporaneous controls. Although instances of contracts with for-profit entities were not excluded, all the contracting initiatives reviewed involved nonprofit organizations.

Search and Review Methodology

To find as many examples of contracting as possible, experts from a variety of institutions were asked about examples of contracting of which they were aware. Previous reviews of contracting in developing countries were also examined (Abramson 1999; Mills 1998; Palmer 2000; Slack and Savedoff 2001). A computerized search of the published literature was also carried out using ECO (Electronic Collections On-Line, a broad database covering scholarly journals in a wide variety of fields); Periodical Abstracts (covering general and academic journals in business and economics, including transcripts of television and radio news programs); EconLit (covers journals, books, working papers, and dissertations in economics); WorldCat (a database covering books and other resources in a large number of libraries); PAIS (Public Affairs Information Service, which provides selective subjects and bibliographic access to periodicals, books, hearings, reports, gray literature, government publications, Internet resources, and other publications from 120 countries); and PubMed (the U.S. National Library of Medicine's search service for access to Medline and other related databases).

The electronic search was supplemented by a manual review of journals that often publish articles related to health systems in developing countries (*Health Policy and Planning* and *Social Science and Medicine*). Written reports or presentations of the evaluated examples were reviewed and summarized, and considerable attention was given to the evaluation methodology employed. Then an attempt was made to conduct structured interviews with people who had intimate knowledge of the particular example. The summaries were modified accordingly, and the same people were asked to review the summaries before they were finalized.

In the instances where before-and-after data were available from experimental and control groups, the "double differences" were calculated. The *double difference* is the difference between follow-up and baseline results in the experimental group minus the difference between follow-up and baseline results in the control group. Wherever possible, differences are expressed as percentage points.

RESULTS: CONTRACTING CAN QUICKLY IMPROVE SERVICE DELIVERY

From the 10 studies summarized in table 11.2, contracting with NGOs appears to deliver effective primary health or nutrition services, and impressive improvements can be achieved rapidly. Good results have been achieved in a variety of settings and for a variety of different services. All the studies found that contracting

TABLE 11.2. Summary of Contracting Experiences

Location and service type	Contract and intervention type	Scale	Contracting arrangement	Evaluation methodology	Main results	Subsequent history	Comments
Cambodia Rural PHC and district hospital services	SDC compared with MC and CC, that is, government provision of services.	1.5 million population	Competitively bid, formal contract, managed by special unit of MOH. Some problems ensuring good relations with provincial officials. NGOs were paid on time.	Randomized controlled study with 12 districts as experimental units. Household and health facility surveys conducted before and after 2.5 years of implementation.	SDC and MC much better than CC. Median double difference[a] on 7 indicators for SDC vs. CC was 21.3%p[b], for MC vs. CC double difference was 9.3%p.	Expanded to twice as many districts.	Impressive results in contracted districts achieved quickly. SDC performed better than MC but both outperformed government provision. Rigorous methodology. SDC more expensive but reduced out-of-pocket expenditure by community.
Bangladesh Rural community nutrition services	SDC with NGOs compared with control areas with no organized nutrition services (that is, normal government health services with no nutritional component).	15 million population	Fixed-price MOU. Initially sole source selection of NGOs, then competitive. Serious problems with payment and other aspects of contract management.	Controlled, before and after study with 6 experimental and 2 control upazillas. Household surveys conducted by third party.	Malnutrition rates declined 18% in SDC upazillas compared with 13%p in controls (double difference = 5%p; double difference for vitamin A was 27%p.)	Expanded to more than 30 million population.	NGOs were able to successfully implement nutrition interventions on very large scale. Modest difference in change in nutrition status, but larger in coverage of related services. No indication of how government would have done implementing nutrition services.
Bangladesh Urban PHC	SDC with NGOs compared with government provision of services, that is, CCC.	4 million population	Competitively bid formal contracts, managed by special unit of government division. Difficulties encountered paying contractors on time and monitoring adequately.	Controlled before-and-after study with 15 contracts compared with one large area implemented by CCC. Household and health facility survey by third party.	Coverage data not yet published. Double difference for availability of specific services (immunization, family planning) was very large, 57% to 92%.	Contracts not yet completed. Planning for expansion of contracts far advanced and funding secured.	NGOs performed better in ensuring availability of services in spite of having same amount of resources. CCC unable to provide broad package of services in newly built facilities. Coverage data not yet available.
Bolivia Urban PHC	Limited MC in phase 2. MC with expanded authority in phase 3. Control area had continued public sector management.	250,000 population	Single source contract with NGO. Contract management by committee including community representatives.	Controlled, before and after design, but data from routine reporting system; only a few indicators examined.	Double difference for deliveries between MC and control was 21%p, and 1%p for bed occupancy.	Unknown	Relatively small-scale study showed large changes in MC district. Methodological issues. Contract giving greater autonomy to NGO resulted in larger changes.
Guatemala Rural PHC in mountainous areas	MC in selected municipalities and SDC in more remote areas, compared with government provision (control).	3.4 million	Competitively bid contracts with NGOs. Difficulties with financial management and supervision of contracts.	Controlled design based on household survey conducted by third party 3 years after contracting began.	Median difference between MC and control on 5 indicators was 11% (range 5–16%p).	Started as small pilot but expanded rapidly. Now covers 27% of country.	MC appeared to make modest difference in service delivery. Difficult to assess SDC because of remoteness. No baseline data available.

			Input/contract	Design/method	Results	Scale-up	Comments
Haiti Bonuses for NGOs delivering PHC in rural areas	NGOs with SDCs offered performance bonuses based on agreed targets.	534,000 population	Input type of contract changed to one focused on outputs.	Before-and-after (7 months later) design based on household surveys carried out by third party.	Average of follow-up minus baseline ranged from −3%p (prenatal care) to +32%p (vaccination coverage).	Expanded to cover 1.5 million people, 19% of Haitian population.	Rapid and large change in some easy-to-change indicators. No control group.
India Urban TB control services in Hyderabad	NGO under SDC delivered TB control services in defined population and worked with private providers. Compared with publicly managed area of similar size.	500,000 population	Informal contract with existing NGO changed to formal MOU. Government provided drugs and other inputs; NGO paid for staff.	Controlled design with after-only data from recording system verified by national TB program officials. Cost data collected by third party.	NGO found 21% more TB cases and had 14% better treatment success rate. Cost per successful treatment $118 for NGO vs. $138.	Being scaled up in various parts of India with ongoing evaluation.	NGO achieved better results at lower cost than public sector. No baseline data available; relied on recorded but audited data.
Madagascar and Senegal Community nutrition services	Madagascar: SDCs with 50 NGOs. Senegal: SDCs with NGOs that worked through small groups of unemployed youth.	460,000 in Madagascar; 490,000 in Senegal	Madagascar: contract management done by unit in office of the president; in Senegal by parastatal. No serious problems encountered.	Before-and-after (17 months) household survey of nutrition status in Senegal. Third party survey of participation in project and control areas.	Severe and moderate malnutrition declined 6%p and 4%p, respectively. Participation was 72% in project and 35% in control areas.	Continued with NGOs in both countries, but in different format.	Modest effect on malnutrition but effect size uncertain because of absence of control group. NGO successfully used unemployed youths to deliver services.
Pakistan Rural PHC	MC for the 104 basic health units in 1 district.	3.3 million population	Sole source contract with NGO by local government. Received monthly tranche of funds regularly.	Interrupted time-series design based on routine recording and reporting system.	Nearly fourfold increase in number of outpatient visits.	Only started in May 2003.	Dramatic increase in outpatient visits achieved with same budget. Data only from recording system, data on other indicators not available.
India Improving quality of care by private practitioners	SDC for NGO working with private providers to improve MCH services.	54,000 population	NGOs applied for grant from U.S. Agency for International Development and then informally contracted with private providers.	Before-and-after (6 months later) design based on household surveys by community health workers.	Rapid improvement in provider skills ranging from 25%p to 57%p compared with baseline.	Unknown	Small-scale, uncontrolled study, but large and rapid improvement achieved in quality of care.

PHC, primary health care; MC, management contract; SDC, service delivery contract; CC, control contract; NGO, nongovernmental organization; MOH, Ministry of Health; CCC, Chittagong City Corporation; MOU, memorandum of understanding; TB, tuberculosis; MCH, maternal and child health.

a. *Double difference* = difference between follow-up and baseline results in the experimental group minus the difference between follow-up and baseline results in the control group.

b. %p = percentage points.

Source: Authors based on interviews and cited references.

yielded positive results. The most rigorously evaluated cases demonstrated the largest impact. In the four studies where it was possible to calculate it, the median double differences ranged from 9 to 26 percentage points (figure 11.1). All the double differences were positive. Larger double differences were observed for the parameters that are easier to change, such as immunization, vitamin A, and antenatal care coverage. Smaller changes were observed in parameters that require important behavioral changes, such as family planning and institutional delivery.

Contractor vs. Government Performance

Of the 10 studies, 6 compared contractor performance with government provision of the same services. All 6 found that the contractors were consistently

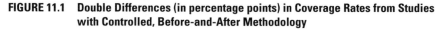

FIGURE 11.1   Double Differences (in percentage points) in Coverage Rates from Studies with Controlled, Before-and-After Methodology

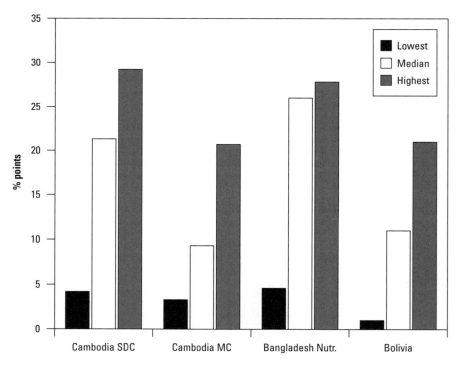

SDC, service delivery contract; MC, management contract.

Note: As an example of the way the double differences were calculated, in Cambodia baseline full immunization coverage was 25.5 percent in SDC districts, 29.9 percent in MC districts, and 34.0 percent in the control districts. The coverage rates found at the follow-up survey were 65.8 percent, 54.4 percent, and 53.0 percent, respectively. This yields a double difference (follow-up minus baseline in the experimental group minus follow-up minus baseline in the control) for SDC versus control of 21.3 percentage points and of 5.5 percentage points for MC versus control. The range and median double differences for the seven indicators included in the contracts are described in figure 11.1 for the Cambodia study.]

**BOX 11.1   CONTRACTOR VERSUS GOVERNMENT PERFORMANCE IN INDUSTRIAL
AND MIDDLE-INCOME COUNTRIES**

There are few examples of contracts initiated for primary health care services in industrial countries. Most countries that contract have always done so. In countries where both contracted and public (salaried) physicians deliver primary health care services, the distinct reimbursement schemes make it virtually impossible to assess the impact of contracting alone (as distinct from that of the payment basis). Hence, opportunities to compare performance are rare. Nevertheless, a few scholars have attempted to assess the difference.

Several Central European countries have initiated contracting for packages of primary health care services. Where contracted services have been compared with those still provided by salaried physicians, results have generally been favorable. In Croatia, evidence of higher productivity was found in contracted practices, including indicators of patient accessibility (Hebrang and others 2003).

In Estonia, where salaried physicians converted to contracted status, a "before-and-after" analysis found improvements in allocative efficiency indicators, technical efficiency indicators (for example, annual number of visits per doctor, number of visits per inhabitant), and immunization rates (from 74 percent to 88 percent). (Koppel and others 2003).

---

more effective than the government, based on a variety of parameters related to both quality of care and coverage of services. The few such studies done in industrial or middle-income countries reported similar results. In the studies reviewed here, the differences between contractor and government performance also tended to be large.

Autonomy

A number of approaches to contracting appear to work quite well, but maximizing the amount of autonomy given to contractors is likely to enhance success. This comes out clearly in the studies from Bolivia and particularly Cambodia, where service delivery contracts were superior to management contracts. This finding is consistent with the experience with hospital autonomy reforms. In conjunction with these reforms, in instances where the hospital management has been given only limited autonomy, performance has improved little (Harding and Preker 2003).

Scale of Contracted Services

A number of possible difficulties have been posited about contracting, some of which can be addressed by the examples reviewed. The concern that contracts are unlikely to provide services on the large scale needed to make a difference at the country level appears to be unwarranted. Half of the examples studied involved populations of millions of beneficiaries, and in one example, contracts now cover a third of rural Bangladesh, more than 30 million people. Furthermore, it appears that there are economies of scale and that larger contracts may be less expensive on a per capita basis than smaller ones.

Cost of Contracting

Contracting is not necessarily more expensive than government provision of the same services, as the studies from Pakistan, urban Bangladesh, Hyderabad in India, and the management contracts in Cambodia suggest. Nongovernmental entities performed better, even when public institutions were provided with similar amounts of resources. Some of the contracts studied were more expensive than government delivery of the same services, although the contractors invariably performed better, and they also appeared to save people in the community money by reducing other out-of-pocket health expenditures. Although the services provided under the different contracts are not strictly comparable, a basic package of primary health services ranged from US$0.65 per capita per year in urban Bangladesh to US$6.25 per capita per year in rural Guatemala. The low price in Bangladesh likely reflects the fact that the better-off urban residents received their care from for-profit providers. Nonetheless, large examples from low-income countries demonstrate that basic primary health care services, including first-level referral hospital care, can be delivered for US$3 to US$6 per person per year.

Equity

The concern that nongovernmental entities will not want to work in remote or difficult areas and are less capable of providing services to the very poor also appears to be unwarranted from the experiences examined. Given the resources and the explicit responsibility, many contractors were willing to work in difficult, previously underserved areas. However, only the evaluation in Cambodia explicitly addressed the issue of whether contracting could improve equity. It found that, when contracts included explicit targets for reaching the poor, contractors were able to significantly improve health services for them. This study also showed that contractors were much better than the government in reducing inequities.

Contract Management

Considerable concern has been expressed that governments will not have the capacity to manage contracts effectively. The experience thus far is that contract management has sometimes been an issue and will require further attention. However, it has not prevented contracting efforts from being successful. Even in rural and urban Bangladesh and Guatemala, where observers believed contract management was not done well, contractors still successfully implemented large programs. The fact that in some situations, as in Cambodia and Senegal, for example, contract management was not an issue, suggests that the problem is tractable. The cases with successful contract management appear to have benefited from either external management support or a limited number of contracts to be administered.

Government–Contractor Relations and Corruption

In most of the situations studied, contracts appeared to have made it easier for governments and NGOs to have a productive relationship. Because of its sensitive nature, it is difficult to know whether corruption was an important issue. However, those with intimate knowledge of the contracting experiences generally believed that it was not a significant issue. In one example, it was only through the presence of an NGO contractor that the central government and the donor discovered the extent and scale of local government corruption.

Sustainability

Given its apparent success, the sustainability of contracting is a genuine concern. Nine of the examples of contracting reviewed had sufficient elapsed experience to judge whether they were sustainable or not. Seven of the nine have been continued and expanded, often dramatically. (Information on the two exceptions is not available.) In Cambodia, Guatemala, rural Bangladesh, Haiti, and India, the scope of contracting has more than doubled from what it was initially, demonstrating that contracting in those countries has been sustainable.

METHODOLOGICAL LIMITATIONS OF THIS REVIEW

This review was based primarily on papers in the gray literature, some of which had not undergone peer review. The review included 10 contracting examples, not a large number from which to draw definitive conclusions. It is almost certain that there are other examples of contracting that we were unable to identify. Other experiences may not have been written up because the results were poor, which would lead this review to more positive conclusions than are warranted. This type of positive results bias is usually more profound when only published articles are used.

Applicability of Findings

All the cases summarized in table 11.2 focused on primary care and nutrition services, where outputs are relatively easy to measure. Other health services, such as specialist inpatient care, present much larger measurement challenges related to quality of care. Also, the providers in these cases were nonprofit organizations. Contracting with for-profit entities, especially self-employed physicians, is common in industrial and middle-income health systems, but not in low-income countries.

Possible Study Biases

Of the 10 examples of contracting that met the inclusion criteria (that is, had at least before-and-after data or data from contemporaneous controls), 4 had before-and-after controlled designs, 3 had controlled designs with a single measure in time, and the remaining 3 were before-and-after evaluations. There was only one randomized trial. Three of the studies also relied on routinely collected data from health information systems of unknown accuracy. In addition, there could have been a pilot-test bias in the examples considered. Because contracting is new and different, it may have received extra attention from managers, donors, and the NGOs, thereby limiting the external validity of the studies. It is difficult to know how serious this problem is. There is some comfort in the fact that many of the contracting examples were done on a very large scale and provided services to many millions of beneficiaries. The history of contracting for social service delivery in the United States and Australia suggests that the initial experiences were problematic and that results improved as governments and contractors ironed out the difficulties they encountered (Domberger 1999; Savas 2000).

In light of the methodological concerns about the cases studied, there is still a need for future contracting efforts to include rigorous evaluations. However, the current weight of evidence suggests that contracting with nongovernmental entities will provide better results than government delivery of the same services. No longer should contracting be considered an untested intervention or a "leap of faith."

IS CONTRACTING A SUSTAINABLE APPROACH?

Almost all the contracting efforts studied have been sustained and substantially expanded. Nonetheless, four major questions have been raised about sustainability:

- Will contracting be financially sustainable, given that sometimes contracts have been more expensive than government delivery?

- Will reliance on international NGOs or expatriate individuals impede development of local capacity?

- What is the long-term role of the government?

- How might contracting affect NGOs and other parts of civil society?

Financial Sustainability

Contracting appears to be an effective means of improving service delivery, and, in some instances, these results have been achieved at the same cost or lower than government delivery of the same services. For these cases, financial sustainability is not an issue. In other cases reviewed, particularly the service delivery contracts in Cambodia, contracting was more expensive for the government, although it reduced out-of-pocket expenditures by the community, particularly the poor, by a larger amount than the contract cost. In this case, sustainability is an issue of whether there is sufficient political will to improve services and efficiently subsidize the poor. The contracts reviewed delivered a basic package of primary health care services for between US$3 and US$6 per capita per year in low-income countries. At these low costs, financial sustainability is a question of the global determination to meet the health MDGs and provide all people with access to basic health services.

Capacity Development

In countries with many indigenous NGOs such as Bangladesh, competitive bids were almost always won by local NGOs. Bidding procedures that are at least partly based on price will, in the long run, select for local NGOs, because expatriates are much more expensive than local professionals. In addition, even "international" NGOs are staffed almost entirely by local health workers. The extent to which contracting efforts encouraged the growth of local NGOs is not yet clear, although access to predictable funding flows is a key determinant of NGO sustainability in virtually all settings (Green 1987).

Long-Term Role of Government

Under contracting, the government's role becomes more strategic and less directly involved in service delivery. Governments will still need to finance health services and carry out essential public health functions such as setting policy and technical standards, collecting information, monitoring and evaluating performance, responding in emergencies, and coordinating all its partners. Because actual service delivery takes up so much time and attention, contracting may well make governments better able to carry out their other, unique roles. If governments want to be stewards of the health sector, they will have to find creative ways of working with the private sector.

Governments already play only a minor role in delivering curative services in many developing countries. Although some people argue that the long-term involvement of governments in delivery of primary care is essential, it would, in fact, be unusual. In most of continental Europe, for example, social health insurance funds contract with independent providers. In Canada, the United Kingdom, and New Zealand, tax-based funding bodies similarly contract with independent providers (or groups) for virtually all primary health care services. Even in Scandinavia, where the government role in service provision is the greatest among the industrial countries, private providers deliver substantial amounts of primary care. In Norway in 2001, 66 percent of primary care services were delivered by private, contracted physicians and only 19 percent by salaried physicians (Sorenson and Grytten 2002).

None of this discussion is meant to diminish the challenges associated with contracting in low-income countries. The intent is merely to underscore that contracting for primary health care services is a widely practiced and accepted means of ensuring delivery of primary care. In other sectors, too, governments have become accustomed to working through contractors. Few countries still have public works departments, but roads continue to be built and maintained.

Effect on NGOs

Concern has been expressed that contracting will result in the "capture" of NGOs by governments so that they will not be able to criticize governments or play an effective advocacy role. The extent to which this problem has actually occurred is not clear. Conversations with NGOs involved in contracts with governments indicate that they themselves do not feel constrained to criticize government policies or actions. In one instance, an NGO went public with accusations of corruption by local officials. Hence, it seems that much depends on the NGO and individuals involved. Contracting also gives NGOs some advantages, through their provision of services on a large scale: increases in their legitimacy, overall size, and presence in communities. Nonetheless, protecting the independence of civil society is important, so there should be space for NGOs to decline to participate in contracts, if they believe it would compromise their other roles. (A contract, by its nature, involves the voluntary participation of two parties for mutual gain.)

RECOMMENDATIONS

Based on the successes thus far, there should be a significant increase in the amount of contracting undertaken in developing countries as a means of rapidly improving service delivery and achieving MDGs. This process will require close monitoring, constant evaluation and reevaluation, and improvements in contract administration.

• Increase the Amount of Contracting

The challenge will be twofold: contracting for services not currently provided by government ("green site" contracting); and—the more challenging task—contracting for services already provided by government but where effectiveness and efficiency could be improved. In both types of contracting, the challenge is to ensure that governments get value for money spent, so that services are improved for the community.

• Continue Evaluation

Future contracting efforts should continue to include rigorous monitoring and evaluation to better determine its effectiveness, obtain robust estimates of the effect size, test it under various conditions, and address remaining issues such as its effects on equity, the utility of performance-based bonuses, and different approaches to bidding. Ultimately, any debate about the effectiveness of contracting should be settled by evidence collected systematically, not by theoretical arguments or ideology.

• Improve Monitoring

One of the big advantages of contracting is that it allows governments to focus on outputs and outcomes, rather than inputs. To do this effectively, monitoring of contracts will need to improve. This will require greater use of health facility and household surveys rather than just data from routine reporting systems; collection of baseline data against which to measure progress; and use of third parties to work with purchasers in establishing monitoring tools and to help with data collection. Third parties have the advantage of being neutral and providing specialized expertise in monitoring and evaluation.

• Ensure Autonomy

According to experience thus far, allowing contractors autonomy yields greater effectiveness and efficiency. Contracts should specify outputs and outcomes but allow the contractor's managers to decide the best way of achieving them. For example, it makes sense to specify that immunization coverage should increase to 80 percent, but it is counterproductive to specify that this must be done by immunizing children on street corners. Process issues must be addressed when it comes to quality (for example, that immunizations are given according to the national technical guidelines), but the bias should be toward "letting managers manage." Obstacles to managerial autonomy include line item budgets; imposition of strategies or approaches that do not have a strong scientific basis; requisite government preapproval of innovations suggested by contractors; and the introduction of new programs or activities into the contract without extensive discussion with contractors.

• Scale

The cases examined in this review suggest that each contract should be fairly large, on the order of 500,000 beneficiaries, to obtain economies of scale and allow proper monitoring and evaluation.

- **Pay Attention to Contract Management**

Although inadequate contract management did not prevent contracting from being successful, improvements in this area could increase its effectiveness. Approaches that may improve contract management include use of management support (consultants or third parties) to help the government with contract management, including monitoring; limiting the number of contracts and the number of payments per contract; and involving civil society and international or multilateral agencies during the contractor-selection process to ensure transparency.

NOTE

The authors gratefully acknowledge the kind assistance and insights of Gerard La Forgia, Tonia Marek, Rena Eichler, Anita Johnson, Nurul Islam, Ashraf Uddin, Brad Schwartz, Indu Bhushan, Ritva Reinikka, Sarbani Chakraborty, Diana Weil, Knut Lonnroth, Silvia Albert, K. J. R. Murthy, Jacques Baudouy, Chiaki Yamamoto, and Shanta Devarajan.

REFERENCES

Abramson, W. 1999. *Partnerships between the Public Sector and Non-governmental Organizations: Contracting for Primary Health Care Services.* Latin America and Caribbean Health Sector Reform Initiative (LACHSR), Pan American Health Organization, Washington, D.C.

Bhushan, I., S. Keller, and B. Schwartz. 2002. "Achieving the Twin Objectives of Efficiency and Equity: Contracting Health Services in Cambodia." ERD Policy Brief Series Number 6. Manila, Philippines: Asian Development Bank, Economic and Research Department.

Bryce, J., S. Arifeen, G. Pariyo, C. Lanata, D. Gwatkin, and J. P. Habicht. 2003. "Reducing Child Mortality: Can Public Health Deliver?" *Lancet* 62: 159–64.

Connor, C. 2000. "Contracting Non-Governmental Organizations for HIV/AIDS: Brazil Case Study." Special Initiative Report No. 30. Abt Associates, Washington, D.C.

Domberger, S. 1999. *The Contracting Organization: A Strategic Guide to Outsourcing.* Oxford: Oxford University Press.

England, R. 1997. *Contracting in the Health Sector: A Guide to the Use of Contracting in Developing Countries.* London: Institute for Health Sector Development.

Frick-Cardelle, A. J. 2003. *Health Care Reform in Central America: NGO-Government Collaboration in Guatemala and El Salvador.* Miami: University of Miami, North-South Center Press. ISBN 1-57454-122-6.

Green, A. T. 1987. "The Role of Non-Governmental Organizations and the Private Sector in the Provision of Health Care in Developing Countries." *International Journal of Health Planning and Management* 2: 40.

Harding, A. L., and A. S. Preker. 2003. *Innovations in Health Services Delivery: Corporatization of Public Hospitals.* World Bank, Washington, D.C.

Hebrang, A., N. Henigsberg, V. Erdeljic, S. Foro, V. Vidjak, A. Grga, and T. Macek. 2003. "Privatization in the Health Care System of Croatia: Effects on General Practice Accessibility." *Health Policy and Planning* 18(4): 421–28.

Koppel, A., K. Meiesaar, H. Valtonen, A. Metsa, and M. Lember. 2003. "Evaluation of Primary Health Care Reform in Estonia." *Social Science and Medicine* 56(12): 2461–66.

Loevinsohn, B. 2000. "Contracting for the Delivery of Primary Health Care in Cambodia: Design and Initial Experience of a Large Pilot-Test." World Bank, Washington, D.C.

Mills, A. 1998. "To Contract or not to Contract? Issues for Low and Middle Income Countries." *Health Policy and Planning* 13(1): 32–40.

Mills, A. S. Bennett, and S. Russell. 2001. "Taking Account of Capacity." In Mills, Bennett, and Russell, eds., *The Challenge of Health Sector Reform.* Hampshire, United Kingdom: Palgrave.

Palmer, N. 2000. "The Use of Private Sector Contracts for Primary Health Care: Theory, Evidence, and Lessons for Low Income and Middle Income Countries." *Bulletin of the World Health Organization* 78(6): 821–29.

Pfeiffer, J. 2003. "International NGOs and Primary Health Care in Mozambique: The Need for a New Model of Collaboration." *Social Science and Medicine* 56(4): 725–38.

Savas, E. 2000. *Privatization and Public Private Partnerships.* Washington, D.C.: CQ Press.

Slack, K., and W. D. Savedoff. 2001. "Public Purchaser – Private Provider Contracting for Health Services: Examples from Latin America and the Caribbean." Publication No. SOC-111. Inter-American Development Bank, Washington, D.C.

Soderlund, N., P. Mendoza-Arana, and J. Goudge, eds. *The New Public/Private Mix in Health: Exploring the Changing Landscape.* Geneva: The Global Forum for Health Research. ISBN 2-940286-13-2.

Sorenson, R., and J. Grytten. 2002. "Service Production and Contract Choice of Primary Physician." *Health Policy* 66: 73–93.

Turshen, M. 1999. *Privatizing Health Services in Africa.* New York: Rutgers University Press. ISBN 0-8135-2581-0.

World Bank. 2004. *World Development Report 2004: Making Services Work for Poor People.* Washington, D.C.: International Bank for Reconstruction and Development. ISBN 0-8213-5468-X.

CHAPTER 12

Purchasing Hospital Services: Key Questions for Policymakers

Eric de Roodenbeke

F inding the best way to buy hospital services is a critical issue for policymakers. Providing a set of questions within a framework can help them choose the most appropriate options for their specific country context. We list these major questions and the issues they raise. To use such a framework in making purchasing decisions, however, some major criteria have to be met in the areas of financing, autonomy, and stewardship.

KEY CRITERIA FOR EFFECTIVE PURCHASING DECISIONS

Purchasing hospital services can act as a major trigger for improvements in hospital efficiency and equity in delivering care if the hospital fulfills some basic financing, autonomy, and stewardship criteria.

Financing

Health care *financing* must rely on third-party payment mechanisms either through insurance or public funds. Both can be funded through premiums and taxes. Third-party payers will buy services for the population it covers. Therefore, up to a point, the purchaser

- Decides on the type of coverage provided within any national framework on mandatory coverage.

- Negotiates with providers to buy what the purchaser considers best for the groups for which it is accountable.

- Makes its own choices within corporate priorities, the market environment, and social pressure.

Autonomy

Hospitals must have *autonomy*. Ownership can be public or private, for profit or not for profit. This autonomy does not have to be total—in many countries, public hospital management of human resources is subject to civil service regulations.

Although a limitation on autonomy may reduce their impact, purchasing mechanisms will still trigger major benefits as long as hospitals have some freedom to

- Change the scope of services in order to adapt to shifting demand (qualitative, in the nature of care or service, as well as quantitative).

- Discuss prices and resource flow with the payer (for example, payment scheme, prices within the scheme, billing system).

- Decide on priorities for resource utilization (operation expenditures, including costs related to human resources but also investments in plant and equipment).

Stewardship

National or local governments are responsible for *stewardship* and regulating the health care system. Allowing third-party payers to buy services does not mean that health care delivery will operate in a free market; both buyers and providers have to comply with certain rules. Nonetheless, market mechanisms give better results than other allocation mechanisms. To be effective, purchasing mechanisms will benefit from government oversight in

- Defining the level of equity, solidarity, and social balance to be achieved in the health care system.

- Setting priorities for hospital services in relation to public health priorities and goals to be reached within a specified time.

- Financing public health services in accordance with social and health priorities.

Under this set of hypotheses, an analytical framework can be devised for addressing the key considerations when attempting to buy the best hospital services for the money. This analytical framework can help guide decisionmakers contemplating major changes in a national health financing scheme. It will reveal the range of factors that hospitals and funding organizations should discuss before plunging into a new health financing scheme.

However, when using this framework, reader should keep in mind that in most analyses of efficiency or equity in health care delivery, hospitals are usually examined as a whole and compared with primary health care (PHC) facilities. Such broad brush strokes hide the details of a complex picture (Liu and Mills 2003) that must be studied, looking for mechanisms to improve hospital efficiency and equity in delivering care. In line with this consideration, it is important to be mindful of this diversity when addressing the question of how to buy hospital services more effectively.

FOR WHOM TO BUY?

Once coverage of every individual's basic health needs has been made a national priority (that is, providing everyone with adequate services for their specific needs), a baseline must be established for what is currently being delivered. This is the springboard for answering the first question: Who should benefit the most from hospital care financing? The two major dimensions of access are geographic and economic (Fournier and Haddad 1995); a third is sociocultural access. Anthropological studies in West Africa have shown the importance of cultural beliefs in an individual's health care decisions, but also the major role of health care staff behavior (Jaffré and Olivier de Sardan 2003).

Utilization of Hospital Services

Utilization data, based on consumption, not need, are a rough proxy for estimating demand. The major limitation of such an estimate is also related to diversity of care responding to diversity of clinical need. Because many different services are bundled together to obtain an overall utilization rate, it may hide overutilization of certain services and underutilization of others. Nevertheless, an attempt at an overview of the present provision of hospital care can be made through major indicators covering the two key functions of the hospital: inpatient and outpatient services. Hospitals undertake almost every diagnostic and treatment activity for either inpatients or outpatients, but a weak information system will not be able to capture all the details.

Service utilization is usually monitored, and overall population data can be used for differential utilization analysis. However, such data cannot be analytically extended beyond a region. District hospitals are not evenly distributed over a country, and data at the district level will not match a facility's actual catchment area, thereby skewing results. Although referral hospitals are supposed to have a national clientele, most of their patients come from the town or region where the hospital is located. Services delivered at the referral hospital can therefore be added to the regional total. For a better understanding of utilization patterns at the district level, specific analysis should be undertaken at the regional level with a focus on spatial distribution and patient orientation. This requires a specific prospective survey of a patient sample over a defined time. In countries where such surveys have been undertaken (for example, Burkina Faso, de Roodenbeke 1995; Côte d'Ivoire, Vilayleck 1999; Cameroon, Blatt 1996), most hospital outpatients came from the immediate area, and less 15 percent of the inpatients came from outside the district.

WHAT DO WE KNOW ABOUT INPATIENT SERVICES?

Data on all hospitals, public, and private (including for-profit) facilities should be filled into table 12.1. What is considered a hospital should be precisely defined so that the same measure will be applied throughout the country. Table 12.1 highlights differences between regions regarding bed coverage and facility utilization. Special attention should be paid to occupancy rates and length of stay to see whether productivity gains make extra capacity available. When hospitals have high occupancy rates and short stays, provision of care has to be investigated in detail to see whether admissions can be reduced by promoting other types of care (for example, day care, home supervision). Increasing the

TABLE 12.1   Hospital Inpatient Utilization within Regional Facilities

Region	Number of hospitals	Population	Beds	Admissions	Admissions per population	Population	Beds per deaths	Deaths per admission
X	5	2,909,645	1,919	78,258	2.69%	0.066%	4,957	6.33%
Y	11	1,580,052	1,268	50,497	3.20%	0.080%	2,822	5.59%
....								
National	131	18,077,883	15,288	650,981	3.60%	0.085%	32,812	5.04%

Source: National information system.

number of beds should always be the last resort after every other option has been ruled out. Purchasing mechanisms can be used to promote alternative treatments to reduce inpatient care. Budget funding, in contrast, might promote adding capacity.

For inpatient services, efforts to compensate for regionally unequal access might take into consideration any national commitment to poverty reduction. In relation to the Millennium Development Goals (MDGs), a special emphasis can be put on use of services for communicable diseases and for maternal and infant care. In most low-income countries, those services represent between one-half and two-thirds of inpatient services utilization.

WHAT DO WE KNOW ABOUT OUTPATIENT SERVICES?

Analyzing gross hospital outpatient services data will not reveal the diversity of services between hospitals and within a hospital. In many hospitals, although there is a formal referral care pattern, outpatient clinics offer a mix of PHC and district hospital-level care. Not infrequently, as in Ghana (Ghana Ministry of Health 2004), basic care represents more than 50 percent of the total outpatient day (OPD) hospital attendance. It is difficult to collect data to show how much of hospital outpatient care should have been provided in a subreferral facility. Similarly, there are practically no systematic regional data to show how activity at a referral hospital comes from actual referrals.

Fee-for-service policy has favored the extension of outpatient services to meet popular demand. Outpatient services are a significant source of income for hospitals. Moreover, outpatient services generate a good bit of inpatient and diagnostic business.

National information systems cover all OPD activities (public and private). Filling out table 12.2 will reveal the overall contribution of hospitals in OPD activity and differences between regions. Data will also indicate whether, at the regional level, there is any specific connection between overall outpatient utilization and hospitals' share of this activity. Hospital outpatient care can be efficient, if right-sized and highly qualified staff resources are not squandered on scraped knees. Hospitals play a major role in providing outpatient care to

TABLE 12.2   Regional Outpatient Activity

Region	Population	Total outpatients	Outpatients/ population	Number of hospital outpatients	Outpatients/ hospital activity
X	2,887,596	2,226,059	0.77%	1,125,247	0.50%
Y	917,250	604,645	0.66%	252,473	0.42%
....					
National	18,077,883	9,340,180	0.52%	2,181,462	0.40%

Source: National information system.

address the health care priorities. This role might expand, if the economic barrier posed by fee policy is significantly diminished. Special attention should therefore be paid to gatekeeping mechanisms to avoid misuse of specialized care. When analyzing outpatient activity, it is always difficult to estimate the role of traditional medicine, an important alternative to western medicine in many countries (Senah, Adusei, and Akor 2001). Some regional differences in access may reflect different cultural approaches to health care.

Outpatient care should not compete with PHC or traditional medicine but should complete it, especially in urban areas where both demand and access to hospital outpatient care are high. Purchasing arrangements can help reduce demand on hospital outpatient services by supporting hospitals giving assistance to PHC facilities, for example, consulting physicians who monitor their activities. This is an interesting, systematic way of responding to an urban population's demand for health care.

Understanding the Patient Profile

The second major influence on hospital utilization is related to patient health and socioeconomic status.

Information on health status on admission to a hospital can indicate how referral care is handled and how much referral care hospitals actually deliver. Patient health status can be tracked only when an information system is reliable and critical information is systematically entered. These data will be significant if a district health information system can provide a population health index. Because such data are unavailable in most countries, the best way to obtain a proxy of hospital patient health status is by doing a survey of medical records (if accurate) through a section analysis or through a retrospective analysis.

Studies demonstrate that a patient's socioeconomic status influences access to hospital inpatient care and raise issues of equity even in countries with extensive insurance coverage (Aligon and Grandfils 1997). A household's lack of resources is a major reason for delaying access to hospital care. Cultural factors and perceived quality of care are also important (Jaffré and Olivier de Sardan 2003).

Often, data from broad surveys (such as demographic and health surveys) are not specific enough to identify hospital clients (type of services used and health status per patient). In nationwide studies, there is always a structural bias: Average revenues per capita are always higher in towns than in the countryside, and hospital catchment areas are mostly urban. Outpatient services represent the bulk of hospital utilization, when it is measured only through the overall figures. Wealthier patients usually overuse outpatient services, but outpatient services overall make up a minor part of hospital costs.

Further sociodemographic studies are needed to see whether critical care is provided equitably across all population groups within a catchment area. Without such a baseline study, equity improvements will be difficult to promote through purchasing hospital care.

Setting Priorities

In conjunction with national health policy priorities, the purchasing mechanism can promote different components of hospital care related to equity and public health priorities.

Equity considerations can focus on

- *Geographical differences*. An effort can be made to include people living in remote areas or having poor access to hospital facilities.

- *Socioeconomic differences*. Specific groups can be targeted to promote appropriate use of hospital care.

- *Sociodemographic differences*. An effort can be made to reach age and gender groups (for example, for maternal and infant care).

Public health considerations can focus on

- *Disease type*. Major communicable diseases are an example—making immunizations and other needed services readily available.

- *Care type*. Services can be organized in a way that differentiates between acute and chronic care.

The type of care and the response will depend on priorities. Purchasing will be an effective policy tool only if it is *situation and goal connected*. That is why a baseline study of actual hospital use and a clear view of priorities are indispensable when using purchasing mechanisms to enhance hospital performance.

WHAT TO BUY?

When deciding what to buy, different, competing alternatives at different levels must be considered. The final mix will draw on different sources of financing to cover the health care expenditures. In few developing countries is the hospital network up to meeting the growing demand for quality care. The national authorities will have to upgrade some facilities with the available resources, which means setting priorities for both capital investments and the development of human resources. But before deciding how to allocate their resources, these purchasers must know what they want to buy.

Public Health Priorities and Hospital Care

For low-income countries, public health priorities can be read through their commitment to the MDGs. Reducing maternal and infant mortality means that all pregnant women have pre- and postnatal care and assisted deliveries. The PHC centers are the cornerstone of these activities, but the judicious use of referral hospital care is critical to reduce mortality rates. Combining assisted deliveries and access to district hospitals for referrals (cesarean sections) is a priority to reach the maternal and child health MDGs.

Hospital outpatient services play a major role in treating children under five years of age (under-5) and fighting major diseases. In low-income countries such as Ghana, under-5 and obstetrics make up about half of all hospital admissions (World Bank 2004: 150).

Take, for example, communicable diseases in Sub-Saharan Africa. Malaria is always among the first reasons reported for attending outpatient care and is also significant for inpatient services. Human immunodeficiency virus (HIV) treatment is the upcoming challenge. Hospitals have to play a major role in launching and monitoring antiretroviral treatment, which will take a huge part of their resources. Financing will largely determine what hospitals can do about this new challenge.

Efficiency of Hospital Care

When resources are scarce, ever-closer attention should be paid to efficiency. Cost-effectiveness assessment is important so that funding can be channeled to the facilities that are best at delivering health care at least cost.

Previous works on this subject have shown how cost-effective African district hospitals were when responding to medical need for common pathologies (World Bank 1994).

For inpatient services, cost-effectiveness analysis has to consider the respective roles of district, regional, and teaching hospitals. Outpatient services will be cost-effective when adequate technical skills are mobilized to deal with the complexity of pathologies presented.

To fulfill their referral missions, hospitals have to bear important structural costs. Promoting better utilization is important to increase hospital productivity—and sometimes more relevant than creating a new first-line response with lower unit costs but higher marginal cost. Analysis of overall cost to the population should lead the decision on what to buy. The cost-effectiveness of health care delivery is specific to each district and region: a local purchasing scheme should be the most effective at figuring out the best mix for the locality. Nationwide rules might be inefficient because theoretical low unit costs do not necessary result in actual low overall costs.

Major Hazards and Hospital Response

How will major health hazards be taken into consideration? For the population at large, major hazards are not a priority because they affect a small number of individuals. For those individuals, major health hazard is indeed a major concern, because they will probably not have enough resources to pay for treatment. Covering major hazard lowers the risk of overutilization, but risk management is difficult when the population covered is small. Extensive basic care coverage dramatically increases the risk of overutilization. Purchasing mechanisms can help draw a line between these two concerns.

When dealing with major health hazard, there is a difference between acute illness and chronic disease. Most acute illness can be related to emergencies and considered a priority even though the treatment cost might be high. Excluding such an event from coverage becomes an ethical concern, when the chance of saving a life is good and medical resources are available. For example, if the available neurosurgery can save a life after a traffic accident, should only rich people be saved because the actual cost is too expensive for the poor?

Decisionmaking for chronic diseases is less obvious. In this case, the cost of care is high and demand is growing with epidemiological transition. Low-income countries cannot afford to treat every chronic disease by the latest medical standard. Making choices will exclude all or part of treatment for some chronic diseases from collective purchasing arrangement, although they are a major health hazard. A line has to be drawn between affordable treatments and highly costly treatments. A national authority should review annually a list of priority treatments that could be covered by collective purchasing arrangement. Such a list will depend on how much a country is willing to spend for health.

If insurance is intended to provide protection, not only basic care coverage, but also major acute hazard should be covered. This option may necessitate a reinsurance scheme, if resource pooling at the district level may not suffice to cover expenses. Collective purchasing arrangements can dramatically improve referrals from inner country to regional and national hospitals, but limits will have to be set by contract or regulation.

Hospital Care as an Essential Public Health Service

Hospitals provide private individuals with services that are also a public health service for the community. A hospital is like a fire department in that people hope not to use it but know it is there if needed. The best example of this function is the emergency department. Although the hospital as an institution can be considered a public good, part of its services are private. Therefore, the overall cost of hospitals should be shared between individual and solidarity-related mechanisms.

If a collective purchasing arrangement recognizes hospital production of public health services, and not just delivery of private individual services, financial arrangements should reflect this recognition. Some hospitals receive budget subsidies to finance this dimension of public good, but rules should be set to ensure that most of those funds go into priority services, the ones of critical importance to saving patients' lives. In that case, collective purchasing arrangements can finance individual risk at its real cost. Considering the public health functions of hospitals, public financing could cover the fixed costs, while insurance covers the variable costs of individual treatment. No rules can be set defining a better mix to address this issue. The important point is that it be taken into consideration when a collective purchasing arrangement does not cover all hospital expenditures.

In-Hospital Training

Costs and constraints related to training health care professionals are often included as part of a hospital's operation costs. Training is a major specific service offered by hospitals and, potentially, not just university hospitals. Should purchasing mechanisms share in the cost of training? There are no consistent data on cost of training in hospitals in low-income countries. Most hospital training costs are incurred in the human resource time spent in on-site training of future professionals. In-hospital training also raises treatment costs, because trainees tend to order more exams and larger prescriptions than seasoned health care professionals. If this production of service is not rewarded, hospitals may try to use interns as low-cost labor, while full-time staff spend minimal time teaching. The result will be low-quality care and badly trained future health workers and physicians.

This extra cost has to be financed, but it should be paid under public financing schemes, if education is considered part of public service. When education is considered a personal investment, hospitals should estimate the cost of training and bill the student or supporting organization. There is no reason a patient should pay for training when seeking care.

A selection of providers based on better prices can be a shortsighted strategy, when the price is lower because a hospital does no in-house training and therefore has a lower overhead.

Transportation

The cost of transportation often precludes access to referral care, if transportation is not considered part of the health services package. Even if care is free, access to health services will remain a major problem in remote areas, because most people living below the poverty line cannot afford transportation. If transportation is not supported by specific financing, however, it will not expand to respond to population health needs. In rural areas where population is scattered, synchronizing transportation to available outreach services might make more sense than building a hospital. In some urban areas, a good transportation network can also be a means of improving delivery of primary care services.

If a collective purchasing arrangement covers transportation fees (under certain rules), hospitals will have to decide whether it is worth competing with private companies in this market. Public health authorities will have to take responsibility for regulating health transportation.

FROM WHOM TO BUY

Level of Care

Most health systems in low-income countries are designed—on paper—with three levels of hospital referral. Actually, the referral system works on two consistent operational levels:

- *Referral hospitals for PHC*. Level 1 referral for PHC is part of the district health care organization. The district hospital is the referral for all the primary health care facilities. Its role and functions are well documented through many guidelines and case studies (World Health Organization [WHO] 1992). Its major contribution to the district health care system as a backup to primary health care is well documented (WHO 1987: 88, WHO 1992; World Bank 1994).

- *Referral hospitals for district hospitals*. Level 2 referrals can be either regional or teaching/national hospitals. In practice, geographical access and transportation costs limit most people's access to teaching hospitals outside the region in which they reside. Although teaching/national hospitals may have more specialized services and sophisticated equipment, these elements can be considered specific features of an organization of the same type. Teaching hospitals are different from regional hospitals mainly in their responsibilities for training health workers, although this mission can (and should) be shared with the regional hospitals. Responding to major public health needs is not the sole objective of second-level referral hospitals; training is (or should be) part of their mission.

Purchasers will have to adopt strategies for each level of hospital after analyzing their current context and addressing key issues within that framework. In some areas, however, there might not be much difference between level 1 and level 2 hospitals or between poorly functioning level 1 hospitals and upgraded PHC facilities.

This first breakdown of the hospital entity is insufficient to cover the story of purchasing hospital services. Hospitals produce health care around some major

TABLE 12.3   Care Delivery Matrix

Level of service	First-line care	First-referral hospitals	Second-referral hospitals
Health care type	Outpatient	Inpatient	Inpatient
Health care nature	Minor cuts	General surgery	Orthopedic surgery

Source: Author.

product line: outpatient, inpatient, diagnosis and treatment technical units, or emergency care.[1] Some of these functions may offer services close to the ones delivered on the primary level (outpatient, diagnosis), while others are specific to hospitals (inpatient and emergency care). Whatever level the hospital belongs to, purchasing will have to take into account the difference between hospital-specific and nonspecific services (nature of service). A third dimension related to specialty type should be added to this matrix because many outpatient and diagnostic services should not be available at the PHC level (type of service). Table 12.3 is an example of a care delivery matrix where the highest level of service can also provide services offered at the lower levels. Collective purchasing arrangements will influence the evolution of hospital product line.

To maintain a referral system, purchasing strategies will have to be combined. As long as subsidies cover a significant part of the budget and most of the employees are paid directly from the national budget, purchasing policies in relation to care level can be efficient if there is an overall approach combining collective purchasing arrangements with subsidies-allocation mechanisms. If the arrangements do not allow referral care to be bought, referral hospitals will compete with PHC and district hospitals to keep a share of the market. There is some evidence that regional and national referral hospitals derive a significant part of their revenue from profitable basic outpatient activities. Loss of these revenues would lower the quality of care even for referral services that benefit from cross-subsidization within the hospital.

To buy wisely, collective purchasing arrangements should promote a policy of selecting providers at different levels to deliver the same types of care. There should also be gatekeeping mechanisms. Copayment, for example, can be very efficient.[2]

What Place for the Private Sector?

Depending on the country, the private sector delivers more or less of the hospital care, mostly at the district level and in major urban areas.

Some countries (Ghana, Cameroon) have a network of mission hospitals, whose reputation is good overall. Their fees are usually higher than in the public sector, however, not because their operating costs are higher but mainly because they are less subsidized than the public hospitals. In some areas where the private sector is the sole provider, a collective purchasing arrangement has no choice but to buy. In areas where facilities may compete, private providers' higher fees may put them at a disadvantage. Collective purchasing arrangements might then have to take into consideration quality for price. A look at productivity might change purchasing perspectives.

A human resource assessment can evaluate a hospital's labor productivity. Detailed analyses—facility by facility (rather than by sector, public versus private)—might reveal significant contrasts. Both high inpatient bed occupancy and bed turnover are indicative of the overall productivity of inpatient care assets. This is another measure of a facility's productivity.

When competition is possible, a collective purchasing arrangement will have to analyze hospital performance on the use of capital as well as labor to favor the most efficient facilities, and not just buy on the cheap. When competition is not possible, purchasing policy will have to be designed in a way that motivates hospitals to improve productivity.

Collective purchasing arrangements should take a long-term view of efficiency. It would be disastrous if purchasing mechanisms put most productive hospitals out of business, simply because lack of subsidies forced them to charge higher fees than subsidized competitors.

Collective purchasing arrangements may be an opportunity for private for-profit business in the wealthier urban areas. If equity is a national priority, pricing and supervision of services can forestall profiteering from money raised under collective purchasing arrangements intended to be propoor and prosolidarity. Collective purchasing arrangements will not answer the question of ownership performance. Many researchers have concluded that public and private facilities are extremely hard to compare and that assessments can vary widely, depending on the criteria used to evaluate the delivery system (Raisa 2002).

Service Provision by Collective Purchasing Organizations

No evidence supports the theory that integrated systems (health maintenance organization-type) are always more efficient than purchasing systems (different provider and insurer). Nevertheless, poor quality care limits the lessons that can be learned from the experience of mutual insurance in West Africa (Audibert, Mathonnat, and de Roodenbeke 2003). So, where facilities are scarce or of poor quality, collective purchasing organizations may want to become providers. It can also be an alternative when care providers are too dominant.

For hospital care, assets are an important barrier to getting into business; investment returns will take a long time to materialize. Delivering outpatient services might be an interesting option—no major asset investments and immediate returns for high-productivity facilities.

Insurers may be tempted to get into this business, but implementation of collective purchasing arrangements requires a major mobilization of resources to finance the organization's administrative and transaction costs. It is important that most of the resources collected pay for care instead of covering mostly administrative and investments costs. A collective purchasing arrangement should be able to conduct medical assessments to challenge dominant positions through negotiations with providers. This might be an alternative to health maintenance organizations and a priority in a purchasing scheme.

HOW TO PAY?

Fee for Service

From country to country, there are many fee-for-service formulas with more or less comprehensive packages covered by various premiums. Most often, drugs are sold separately with a positive margin policy that may vary from hospital to hospital. Fees for service are a major incentive, even at subsidized public hospitals where they may be a minor part of overall revenue. These resources bring in the additional funds hospitals need to buy goods and services to ensure smoother operations. From the provider's perspective, these resources must be kept and expanded. Fee for service is a good purchasing instrument when a collective purchasing arrangement can

- Negotiate the lowest possible fees to maintain a specified quality standard.

- Pay only for service received.

- Pay for the poor when they need care.

In a mixed financing scheme, hospitals will favor revenue-generating activities. A decade of experience has shown that services under subsidies (usually not covering full cost) cannot compete with those getting fee for service.

Limiting overhead expenses by constraining prices and volume is important. For providers, it is an incentive for higher productivity: the more it produces, the more it is paid. It can also be a good incentive for quality, if high quality is rewarded with bonuses.

Fee for service rather than a fee per episode makes sense. Few hospitals in low-income countries have the information system needed to run a fee-per-episode billing system. Management capacity is often too weak to set up and operate such a system.

A national price list allowing fee adjustment by regional economic status is consistent with a policy of subsidizing care in the poorest regions more liberally than in better-off areas. For effective purchasing, bonuses and penalties related to the quality of care can be added or subtracted from the price on the national list. Quality of care can be measured against a health outcome index and patient satisfaction. A collective purchasing arrangement must also track volume to avoid being cheated by hospitals or patients.

Fee for service makes it easier for hospital management to track resource flow, activities, and input utilization. The billing system is easy to run under fee-for-service schemes. Hospitals can estimate service costs and compare them with revenues, seeking to raise productivity and raise prices. But fee for service cannot cover all the hospital production costs described here.

Capitation Payment

Capitation payment can be partially combined with fee for services. Capitation payment favors enrollment—hospitals have to enroll as many individuals as possible to get revenues. It is an incentive for hospitals to be more demand responsive when patients have alternative choices. Where hospital utilization is low, this option is worth considering to make hospital demand proactive.

Capitation favors activities where patient follow-up is recommended and cost of service is fairly flat. Maternal care, for example, is a good prospect for capitation payment—the number of visits and list of exams pre- and postdelivery can be set. Capitation payment can be combined with fee for service if extra activities are requested.

Where competition is weak, capitation payment does not favor quality of care. Hospitals may give capitation patients less attention than they give their fee-for-service patients. In that case, a collective purchasing arrangement has to protect clients' rights and threaten providers: no service equals no payment.

Capitation payment must be supported by a detailed contract and a monitoring process to enforce it. Each party must know exactly what is included and what is not.

How to Maintain Cash Flow for Hospitals with a Billing System

When there is no third-party payment, fee for service brings an immediate cash inflow. Under a collective purchasing arrangement, financial barriers to access are reduced, offering hospitals the prospect of additional revenues. Asking patients to pay up front and seek reimbursement from the insurer is one way hospitals could maintain their cash revenue. This system has major drawbacks in terms of patient access (most people cannot pay cash in advance) and supervision (hospitals have no incentives to provide information to insurers). Billing insurers for services is the only realistic option in most low-income countries. Hospitals will have to verify patients' entitlement to services and send the bill to the insurer.

To put together a billing system, most hospitals will have to upgrade their administration departments. Ideally, all activities will be tracked, and the patient will be billed by the end of the next month. When switching from a patient-payer to a collective purchasing system, the latter should make advance payments to the hospital. At first, it will be difficult for hospitals to bill in less than 60 days. Routinely, the rule should be payment upon presentation of the bill covering the most recent month's activity, minus adjustments from the previous month after checking the bills against the services actually delivered.

Billing will cost, so hospitals must track those costs and figure out how to recover them. There are several recovery options. The collective purchasing arrangement will have to pay (for example, average billing charge added to fee, lump sum), or the billing cost will be covered by subsidies in cash or nature (by civil servant salaries). If billing costs are recovered through a subsidy, every hospital should be entitled to it.

The imperative of reorganizing accounting services for billing in most hospitals also opens an interesting opportunity to introduce new managerial approaches to other aspects of contracting. Monitoring the accounting function can trigger productivity-enhancing changes in other hospital management practices.

AT WHAT PRICE?

What price to pay for service is a major concern for both collective purchasing arrangements, looking for the "right price," and hospitals, trying to avoid delivering underpaid services. Estimating service cost and deciding between pricing per service or per episode are prerequisites to negotiations on a payment mechanism. Per episode pricing looks like a nearly impossible option, however, considering that most hospitals contemplating collective purchasing arrangements have to quickly organize accounting departments and customer services and build capacity to assemble reliable, basic information needed for sound management in general and pricing in particular. Most countries lack the capacity to conduct cost analysis on the economic price of services or to run price simulation models. Even if these analyses are done, capacity will still have to be built to develop an information system that will eventually allow correct costing of services.

Estimating Cost of Services

Hospitals should estimate service costs, but with an awareness that a correct cost estimate of each activity or episode is elusive (Shepard, Hodgkin, and Anthony 2000). Tracking systems for such information are costly and not fully reliable. Proposals to introduce sophisticated information systems—where not even basic information is available today—should be eyed skeptically. No information system can be a substitute for missing managerial skills, nor can it be operated without them. Comprehensive information systems also need a strong technical infrastructure, also missing in most low-income countries. Most service costing within a hospital is a management tool used, for example in Eritrea, for targeting performance incentives (Nusau 2003) but not to estimate fees for collective purchasing arrangements in a national framework.

Thus, although service cost estimates may look like an obvious point of departure for any collective purchasing arrangement, hospitals in most low-income countries will have to struggle to develop the capacity to make reasonably close estimates. In any case, the theoretical economic cost might be far different from the effective cost, and major differences in costs affect pricing sustainability. In addition, hospital fee regulations contain a long list of exemptions, and donors now support capital investment. Baseline fair prices are all the more difficult to estimate or compare because service quality also influences costs.

Nonetheless, even if a country is not yet able to estimate the cost of hospital services, this should not prevent it from getting into a collective purchasing arrangement. The insurer can start buying hospital services at the historical price (actual prices under fee for service) and monitor, together with the hospitals, trends in expenditures (by type and by major activity) and in the volume and quality of services. The minimum requirement is an accounting and activity reporting system to implement financial controls.

Marking Prices Up and Down to Better Cover Risks

One of the major roles of hospitals is to provide care for the small number of individuals who face major health risks. If this coverage is not mandatory, most people will not want to pay a high premium for a low-probability risk. In most low-income countries, if this kind of care is priced at its real cost, practically no one will have access to it, even with complementary insurance coverage.

Collective purchasing arrangements play a major role in pooling risks (healthy people pay for sick people) but hospitals can also pool risk by under-pricing major health risks and marking up minor health care (minor care pays for major care). The volume of minor activities is usually so high that cross-subsidizing can greatly reduce the price charged for major health risks to make it affordable. Such an approach can help attenuate adverse risk selection in a collective purchasing arrangement where stakeholders may be reluctant to pay for costly care. The impact of such a pricing policy will be limited on minor risk and affordable for most people. Overall, it will make no difference in expenses for care, but the approach has a strong psychological impact: insurance subscribers feel they are getting their money's worth.

Whether prices can be marked up or down depends on the nature of the overall financing scheme and coverage of all hospital expenditures. Compensatory pricing will be possible if it is consistent throughout a country. If it is not, pressure to buy at the lowest price may force hospitals to limit their major risk services in order to remain competitive with other providers. Whether this second-level pooling is needed depends on the design of the benefit package: If major health risk coverage is mandatory and hospitals receive enough income to undertake major risk activities, pooling at the hospital level becomes less relevant. Government will be responsible for deciding to what extent people should have access to major risk treatment. For nonpriority risks, marking down prices would subsidize the richest of the population segment. The poor would be unable to pay, even when subsidized. For better social justice, these services could therefore be priced at cost.

How to Deal with Subsidies?

Subsidies play a major role in pricing in countries where fees for service are derived from the residual cost of inputs. The whole subsidy policy should be revisited, including direct payment of health workers, if a country wants enough transparency in the delivery system to make it more efficient. At the same time, subsidy policy should be clarified for capital investment and operating costs, which may not answer to the same rules.

One way of revising operating cost subsidies is to shift from budget subsidies to outcome-related subsidies, so that the government purchases services. This can be a way of addressing the question on sharing health risk. The ministry of health (MOH) could subsidize major health risks, leaving coverage of minor risks and first-level care to health insurance. In theory, such an approach is feasible and has a major advantage: all facilities (public and private) will have the same subsidy for the same service. A purchasing mechanism could also replace a budget allocation system for services provided under an exemption policy.

Changes in subsidization, because of their complexity, have to be phased in during a transition period. For the MOH, tracking resource use within hospitals will be difficult. For hospitals, multiple sources of financing are hard to manage, and the borderline between insurance financing and MOH financing will never be clear-cut. Within three to five years, when the insurance scheme should be well organized, it should finance all operating costs.

In low-income countries, capital investment financing is monitored by the MOH in conjunction with donors, if there is a common funding basket, for example, under a Sector Wide Approach Program. To promote hospital efficiency, capital investment plans should be tied to effective access to good quality care. Judicious use of capital investment is a strong incentive for major improvements in general and medical management. Capital investment should be considered a specific component of a purchasing scheme. Including depreciation and interest costs (when borrowing), however, makes no sense when estimating the operation cost component of service prices. Subsidies should be maintained for capital investment, but they can be allocated in a competitive process that awards them only to hospitals that can estimate all costs and their impact on services.

Copayments

If care becomes free for patients, overutilization is a risk, especially for first-line outpatient care in urban areas. Copayment can reduce this risk. To be effective, the copayment does not have to be high. It can also be wholly or partly reimbursed by insurance (if this can be done without a large transaction cost).

If copayment is chosen, it should be simple, or hospitals will have to pick up most of the administrative burden. To make it simple, there are two major choices: either lump-sum or percentage-of-price payment. Lump sum will limit minor, inexpensive care, because the copayment can be a major share of the price. For expensive care, this lump sum will not reduce access to care. Lump sum is easy to manage for hospitals: everybody pays the same amount. These arguments should make lump sum the option of choice. If lump-sum payment does not curtail overutilization, the percentage-of-price option can be considered.

For major expenditures related to inpatient services where overutilization is not a risk, because patients are always referred by health workers, there is no need for copayment. Copayment may put an additional burden on patients, although the risk is unrelated to patient demand. To reduce risk of hospital-driven overhospitalization so as to maximize revenues under a fee-for-service system, medical supervision—and penalties for proven, systematic overhospitalization—should be written into any collective purchasing arrangement.

Opportunity Cost

Opportunity-cost analysis explains why, when cost is low or service free, people might not use health services. Opportunity cost (for example, time lost from productive activities) plays a major role in minor care and a minor role in critical care. It has a large impact when consumers perceive no immediate benefit, as in preventive care. The opportunity cost adds to the paid cost: waiving fees for service is good for individuals who can afford to absorb the opportunity cost. Because the poor, especially those in rural areas, are usually very sensitive to opportunity costs, the insurer should endeavor to reduce those costs. Monitoring health service utilization is the first step to identify areas where opportunity cost plays a significant role. Then the insurer can conduct surveys to find out why certain services in some areas are underutilized. These surveys are neither expensive nor technically difficult to monitor and will provide the necessary information to reach people who underutilize health services because of the opportunity cost.

MOVING FORWARD

Most documents and working papers report hospitals' weak management capacity in low-income countries (de Roodenbeke 2003). The current situation varies—from hospitals with skilled management teams to district hospitals staffed by unskilled clerks. In Ghana and most other developing countries, hospitals are involved mostly in routine, repetitive activities performed according to established procedures, systems, and regulations. They devote little time or energy to strategic planning and efficient use of resources (Ghana Ministry of Health 2003).

Accountability is low and human resource management almost nonexistent. Accountability has to become a major driver for management progress in the hospital sector. As long as hospital managers do not have to bear the consequences of their own poor management, the chance of progress is slim. Accountability can be demanded only when managers are appointed because of their capability and skills. Corruption and under-the-table payments should be prosecuted. A purchasing mechanism will not work without governance.

To introduce accountability as part of good governance, trained staff and incentives for a managerial approach are needed throughout an organization (de Roodenbeke 2001). Results-based incentives are a good trigger for replacing bureaucracy by management. Introducing performance indicators to boost hospital performance is likely to succeed only if incentives are significant, and rewards are based on effective, reliable performance indicators. In most Sub-Saharan African countries, the MOH has not effectively exercised its stewardship function to lead hospitals toward efficiency improvements. Most reforms have been supply oriented, with multiple prerequisites related to guidelines, processes, and provision of resources. This approach has failed, because these inputs do not invite the significant behavioral change that is key to successful reform. Better organization will come not from inputs but from an output-driven process. Instead of building norms and guidelines, the MOH should provide guidance and training to help facilities reach objectives corresponding to public health needs and community demand. Introducing a purchasing mechanism through collective purchasing arrangements can be an additional trigger to drag public hospitals upward (Preker and Harding 2003). The challenge will be to combine several triggers, because none will by itself promote a well-managed organization.

Accreditation deserves special mention. Most purchasing systems include accreditation as a major instrument for quality enhancement. Although accreditation is a regulatory instrument, it was developed after the advent of collective purchasing arrangements. Before accreditation, collective purchasing arrangements relied on other regulatory instruments such as contracting and medical supervision.

- *Contracting.* Contracting offers the advantage of being much less normative than accreditation and more results oriented. Contracting leaves room for sound dialogue between hospitals and insurers. Regulations can draw guidelines for contracting, but purchasing arrangements should be negotiated at the local level. Accreditation and contracting are not mutually exclusive, however, but can be mutually reinforcing.

- *Medical supervision.* Medical supervision can be used to prevent health care abuse and to guarantee good medical practice. The insurer's own physicians should provide the supervision and should be given free access to all medical records and patients within a hospital. For effective medical supervision, hospital records must be complete and accurate, so implementation of a medical records policy is important.

Collective purchasing arrangements can promote or ignore disease prevention and the choice of the best treatment in times of illness. Purchasing has to

FIGURE 12.1   Where Best to Buy What?

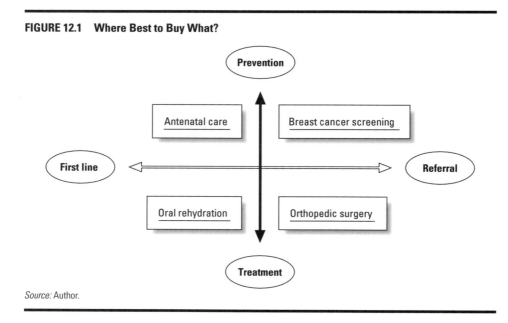

Source: Author.

deal with more than just efficient use of hospitals when care is needed. It has to address the overall efficiency of the health care system by trying to buy, considering price and quality, what is most relevant for public health priorities.

This perspective can be of particular importance in the context of poverty reduction strategy where the MDGs in health are mostly in a prevention-treatment mix within a first line-referral mix.

NOTES

1. Emergency care refers to a 24-hour facility open all year equipped to address major vital medical or surgical distress with access to diagnostic exams and technical equipment. Referral will become part of emergency care. Obstetrical care, which also has to be accessible 24 hours a day all year, is a specific part of emergency care.

2. A copayment might be 100 percent of a fee when there is direct access to referral care, while it would be 50 percent when a patient is referred from a PHC facility.

REFERENCES

Aligon, A., and N. Grandfils. 1997. "Analyse socio-économique des dépenses d'hospitalisation en 1992." No. 1157. Paris, CREDES, p. 94.

Audibert, M., J. Mathonnat, and E. de Roodenbeke. 2003. *Le financement de la santé dans les pays d'Afrique et d'Asie à faible revenu.* Paris: Karthala.

Blatt, A. 1996. "Évaluation des facteurs influençant le recrutement des patients de l'hôpital central de YAOUNDE." Technical document. Yaoundé, OCEAC, p. 37.

de Roodenbeke, E. 1995. "L'hôpital Africain, bilan et perspectives." M. d. l. Coopération, Paris, p. 313.

———. 2001. "La dynamique du projet d'établissement." Paris, La documentation francaise.

———. 2003. "Privatisation des hôpitaux dans les pays en développement." - http://www.univ-lille1.fr/bustl-grisemine/pdf/colloque/G2003-9.pdf.

Fournier, P., and S. Haddad. 1995. "Facteurs associés a l'utilisation des services de santé dans les pays en développement." Montreal, PUM/AUPELF-UREF.

Ghana Ministry of Health. 2003. "Hospital Strategy: A Document for Hospital Reforms in Health Sector." Accra, p. 115.

———. 2004. "Ghana Clinical Services Review. Vol. 1 - main report, p. 59.

Jaffré, Y., and J. Olivier de Sardan. 2003. *Une médecine inhospitalière : les difficiles relations entre soignants et soignés dans cinq capitales d'Afrique de l'Ouest*. Paris: Karthala.

Liu, X., and A. Mills. 2003. *Economic Models of Hospital Behavior and Their Application to Provider Payments Systems*. Washington, D.C.: World Bank.

Nusau, S. 2003. "Improving Hospital Management Skills in Eritrea: Costing Hospital Services." Partners for Health Reform Plus Project. Abt Associates Inc. Bethesda, Md., p. 31.

Preker, A. S., and A. Harding. 2003. *Innovations in Health Service Delivery: The Corporatization of Public Hospitals*. Washington, D.C.: World Bank.

Raisa, B. 2002. "Delivering Health Care Services: Public, Not for Profit or Private." Discussion Paper No. 17. Toronto, Commission on the Future of Health Care in Canada, p. 52.

Senah, K., J. Adusei, and S. Akor. 2001. "A Baseline Study into Traditional Medicine in Ghana." MOH/DANIDA Project, p. 80.

Shepard, D., D. Hodgkin, and Y. Anthony. 2000. *Analysis of Hospital Costs, a Manual for Managers*. Geneva: World Health Organization.

Vilayleck, M. 1999. *Rapport stage EDH 98-99*. Rennes: ENSP, p. 51.

WHO (World Health Organization). 1987. "Hôpitaux et santé pour tous. série de rapports techniques." No. 744. Geneva.

———. 1992. "Hospitals in Rural and Urban Districts." Geneva.

World Bank. 1994. *Better Health in Africa: Experiences and Lessons Learned*. Washington, D.C.

———. 2004. "Mutual Health Insurance in Ghana: Fiscal Sustainability and Strategic Purchasing of Priority Health Services." Washington, D.C.

PART IV

Purchasing Inputs

CHAPTER 13

Paying for Health Care Labor

Pascal Zurn and Orvill Adams

Human resources for health care are central to managing and delivering health services (Murray and Dimick 1978; World Health Organization [WHO] 2002a). People—the various clinical personnel, managers, auxiliary staff, and others—are needed to perform each health intervention. It is also they who diagnose problems and determine which services will be provided, when, where, and how. The performance of any organization depends on the availability, effort, and skill mix of its workforce.

Because recruitment and retention policies are key issues for purchasers, gaining insights into labor-purchasing mechanisms may permit them to be addressed more effectively. This chapter is intended to provide a brief introduction to health labor purchasing and to discuss the mechanisms through which it can have an impact on the delivery of health services and on health system performance.

PURCHASING HEALTH CARE LABOR

We shall define *health care labor purchasing* as an employment relationship whereby health workers are directly or indirectly hired to perform specific work under given conditions. In other words, health labor purchasing reflects either a direct hiring of health workers—as when a hospital contracts directly with individuals—or indirect hiring, through the purchase of health services—as when a hospital contracts with an outside entity to obtain nursing services.

Directly or indirectly, purchasing health labor aims at delivering health services. The provision of health services refers to the combination of inputs into a production process taking place in a particular organizational setting and leading to the delivery of a series of interventions (Murray and Frenk 2000).

Purchasing can be viewed from different perspectives: those of government, hospital director, or health insurance supplier. For instance, a government perspective would be broad, covering the needs of the population, the priorities of the system, and the behavior of the providers.

FRAMEWORK FOR PURCHASING HEALTH LABOR

In this section, a framework is developed to foster understanding of health labor purchasing mechanisms (figure 13.1). It shows how labor purchasing affects the

FIGURE 13.1   Framework for Purchasing Health Care Labor

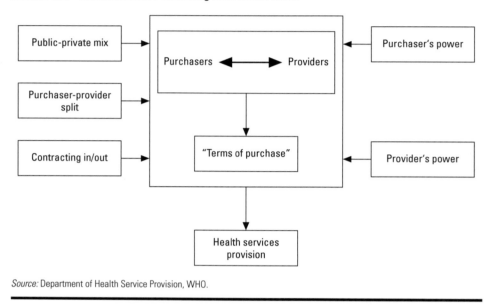

Source: Department of Health Service Provision, WHO.

provision of health services. Insight into this relationship is crucial, since the provision of health services is one of the key determinants of health.

We shall first consider purchasers and providers. Thereafter, the "terms of purchase"—that is, health labor working conditions, remuneration, and benefits—are presented and their impact on health services discussed. Finally, contextual and policy factors related to the health care system and labor market, such as public–private mix and purchasing power, are discussed in light of their impact on labor purchasing and health system performance.

Purchasers

The different characteristics and perspectives of purchasers have consequences for labor purchasing. Many authors discuss the wide range of institutional stakeholders involved in shaping human resources in health (Brito 2000; Egger, Lipson, and Adams 2000; Martineau and Martinez 1997). In the context of labor purchasing, we differentiate among categories (table 13.1).

TABLE 13.1   Types of Purchasers

State (central and local government)

Private, for-profit organizations (self-employed, private, semiprivate)

Private, not-for-profit organizations (nongovernmental organizations, religious institutions)

Source: Martineau and Martinez 1997.

THE STATE

The state, through its various ministries, is a major employer for health sector workers in many developing countries (Martineau and Martinez 1997). The mechanism through which public health workers are employed is a system of civil service or its facsimile.

PRIVATE, FOR-PROFIT ORGANIZATIONS

Private, for-profit organizations include self-employed individuals (for example, self-employed doctors providing primary care) and individuals employed by private organizations (for example, health workers in a private hospital). One key feature in private, for-profit organizations is the nature of ownership, which affects the incentives for purchasing and managing services (Milgrom and Roberts 1992).

PRIVATE, NOT-FOR-PROFIT ORGANIZATIONS

Private, not-for-profit organization such as nongovernmental organizations or religious institutions play an important role in some developing countries, particularly in Africa. In Chad, for example, an estimated 20 percent of the health institutions are private, not-for-profit organizations (Diallo and Gupta, in press). In terms of recruitment, wage, and work motivation, personnel in this sector are likely to differ from those in the two other categories of institutions. The specificities of the not-for-profit sector are well reviewed by Salamon and Anheier (1996).

Providers

In the context of labor purchasing, we shall consider human resources for health as providers. In the *World Health Report 2000*, *human resources for health care* are defined as "the different kinds of clinical and non-clinical staff who make each individual and public health intervention happen (WHO 2000, p. 77). This includes individuals in both private and public sectors and different domains of health systems such as personal curative and preventive care, nonpersonal public health interventions, disease prevention, health promotion services, research, management, and support services.

Terms of Labor Purchasing

Purchasers hire health labor or services to obtain a set of health interventions. The transactions for labor are mediated by contracts. In contracting, one major issue is motivating one person or organization (agent) to act on behalf of another (principal) in a situation of asymmetric information. This problem is known as the principal–agent problem (Hölmstrom and Tirole 1989). Monitoring, use of competing sources of information, and explicit incentive contracts are some of the means of controlling for this asymmetry of information. Accordingly, the degree of specification of the work to be performed is likely to differ from one contract to another, but typically contracts are imprecise. Among the factors preventing complete contracting are the difficulties of foreseeing all events that might arise over time (Milgrom and Roberts 1992).

By "terms of labor purchasing," we mean elements such as working conditions (career development, contract duration, working time and shift work, work autonomy, and separation), remuneration, and benefits. These elements determine, to a large extent, workers' behavioral responses such as willingness to apply for and accept employment and job satisfaction. In turn, these behavioral responses are likely to affect performance through the volume, quality, and distribution of health services (figure 13.2).

In the following, the terms of labor purchasing are examined and discussed in the light of workers' behavioral responses and impact on health services.

WORKING CONDITIONS

Under working conditions, we consider career development, contract duration, working time and shift work, work autonomy, and separation.

Career development. Career development is most commonly defined as a process in which goals are set and specific talents, capabilities, and interests are identified. The possibility of career development for the health workforce is crucial, especially in an environment characterized by a phenomenal growth in knowledge related to health sciences, coupled with technological advances. In such an environment, continuing education is a vital prerequisite for safe practice and for improving the quality of health services.

Contract duration. Purchasers may hire labor for different lengths of time. It is common to differentiate among short-term contracts, fixed-term contracts, and

FIGURE 13.2   Terms of Purchasing and Health Services

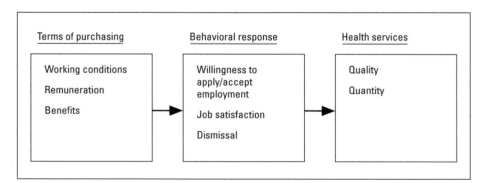

Source: Department of Health Service Provision, WHO.

permanent employment. The designation and duration of each contract varies according to the national labor market legislation. In general, there are two principal differences between temporary and permanent employment. Permanent employees enjoy job security, while temporary employees have renewable contracts. Temporary personnel are often not entitled to benefits enjoyed by permanent staff. Furthermore, the use of short-term staff is a way to avoid the requirements and procedures applied to the recruitment or dismissal of fixed-term or permanent employees. These differences in job security have important implications for health workers' performance (Alcazar and Andrade 2001). However, the excessive use of temporary workers may compromise quality of care, owing to the absence of "team spirit" or lack of familiarity with the patients (Arrowsmith and Mossé 2000).

Working time and shift work. Limitations on working hours and the provision of rest periods are of particular importance to health care workers because they have a direct impact on the quality of services (International Labour Organisation 1998). In terms of job satisfaction, the increased use of overtime is frequently cited as a key area of job dissatisfaction among nurses (Federation of Nurses and Health Professionals 2001). Accordingly, part-time working is often considered a means of improving recruitment and retention, and hence improving the delivery of health services. Although problems of recruitment and retention of nurses in Britain and France persist, there are some quantitative indications of a growth in part-time work (Arrowsmith and Sisson 1999).

Work autonomy (professional autonomy). Work autonomy, defined as control over one's own work, is among the key variables explaining job satisfaction. Autonomy was reported among the most significant variables explaining nurses' job satisfaction in a study reviewing the characteristics of "magnet hospitals" (Gleason-Scott, Sochalski, and Aiken 1999). *Magnet hospitals* are defined as hospitals successful in recruiting and retaining professional nurses. Recent investigations within magnet hospitals document a significant relationship between nursing and quality of care, as well as patient satisfaction (Aiken, Smith, and Lake 1994; Kramer 1990).

Separation. Rules on separation affect purchasers' and providers' behavior. For instance, in their hiring decisions, employers take into account the cost of firing or laying off employees (Milgrom and Roberts 1992). Similarly, a guarantee of long-term employment is attractive to risk-averse workers. Rules on separation are likely to vary from one country to another, from the public to the private sector, and possibly from one profession to another.

REMUNERATION

Providing adequate and timely remuneration is important to guarantee the recruitment of motivated and qualified staff (Martineau and Martinez 1997). Furthermore, the way in which providers are paid also influences service quality

(WHO 1999). Wage costs account for between 65 and 80 percent of the recurrent health system expenditure (Kolehamainen-Aiken 1997; Saltman and von Otter 1995). Accordingly, the payment of health care workers is a major concern for health policymakers. Moreover, in public health systems, wage changes (both increases and decreases) regarding health personnel are a particularly complex and sensitive issue, because these personnel are civil servants and any changes regarding their status is likely to give rise to a reaction by all civil servants.

Countries have tried different ways of funding health care labor—physicians in particular—with different impacts on health services. Fee for service, capitation, and salary are the usual modes of payment.

Fee for service. Under fee for service, providers are funded retrospectively. Doctor itemize their services on a bill, and the sickness fund pays the doctor or reimburses the patient. The usual approach is that the medical association and health insurance negotiate the fee schedule, and the government provides guidelines to limit costs (Ensor, Witter, and Sheiman 1997).

Remunerating doctors by fees for each item of service rewards doctors according to the amount of work performed (Donaldson and Gerard 1993). This method of payment allows doctors a large degree of autonomy.

However, one concern associated with this payment method is its potential to increase health care costs. Because doctors derive their income from the number of medical acts prescribed, they may induce patients' demand to reach "an income target" (Evans 1974).

This method of paying doctors is found in industrial countries such as Australia, Belgium, Canada, France, Germany, Japan, the Republic of Korea, New Zealand, Norway, Switzerland, and the United States (Abel-Smith 1994; Boerma and Flemming 1998). It is also found in developing countries such as China, India, and Nigeria, where private health expenditures make up more than 50 percent of total health expenditures (WHO 2002b).

Salary. Under this system, the doctor is paid a fixed salary per unit of time, regardless of the amount of work done. One advantage of this system is that it makes health care planning easier, as doctors' salaries are known in advance (Maynard, Marinker, and Gray 1986). However, doctors may not be motivated to provide the best quality of care, as they may want to minimize time spent with patients. Low salaries are likely to favor absenteeism and development of a second occupation in the private sector. For instance, a survey in public hospitals in Costa Rica showed that 3 of 10 doctors attributed work absenteeism to low salaries (Cercone, Duran-Valverde, and Munoz-Vargas 2000).

Capitation. Under a capitation system, the doctor is paid a negotiated amount for each patient registered with her, regardless of how much treatment they require during a year (Ensor, Witter, and Sheiman 1997). This is a prospective payment method, which transfers financial risk for delivering services from budget or fund-holding institutions (for example, village or community prepayment schemes or commercial health insurance) to health care providers (WHO 1999). This system encourages doctors to compete for registered patients, but, once patients are registered, to deliver as little care to them as possible. This might be countered by the competitive process itself, which should lead patients to choose a general practitioner who provides good service. If a doctor fails to provide good treatment, then the patient has the option of registering with another doctor. Similarly, there is also a potential for *cream skimming*—that is, doctors may be inclined to prevent high-need patients from registering on their list.

In actuality, these methods of payment are seldom observed in pure form, and most health care systems combine the different payment methods. For instance, general practitioners in the United Kingdom receive, in addition to their salary, financial incentives linked to health outcomes (for example, the vaccination rate). To balance the potential of fee for service to increase health care costs, different approaches have been developed. For instance, the unit value of each service provided is decreased after a certain volume of care (Grignon, Paris, and Polton 2002). Nonfinancial measures such as the diffusion of best-practices protocols or peer-reviewed individual practices are also used.

BENEFITS

In addition to wages, a variety of benefits might also be offered by employers as strategies to recruit new staff. A survey of hospitals in the United States shows that richer benefits such as health insurance and vacation time are the most commonly used incentives (American Hospital Association 2001). Hospitals may offer other recruitment and retention benefits such as tuition reimbursement, contract-signing bonuses based on experience or length of commitment, or advantageous pension plans.

Special benefits are often used to attract health care workers into outlying areas to improve the distribution of health services. For instance, a study in Indonesia found that to attract medical graduates from Jakarta to the outer islands, a bonus of as much as 100 percent of the normal salary would be necessary (Chomitz and others 1998).

CONTEXTUAL AND POLICY FACTORS

Contextual and policy factors related to the health care system and the labor market also affect labor purchasing, health services delivery, and health system performance. Under this category, we review the public–private mix, the purchaser–provider split, contracting in and out, purchaser power, and provider power.

PUBLIC–PRIVATE MIX IN HEALTH CARE

The issue of public–private mix can be examined from different perspectives: financing (how are services paid for?) or delivery (how are health services provided to recipients of care?) (Deber and others 1995).

In many countries, the public health care sector has been dominant. For instance, general government expenditure on health as a percentage of total expenditure on health is above 60 percent in countries such as Australia, Canada, Chad, Costa Rica, Germany, Madagascar, Papua New Guinea, and Zambia (WHO 2002b).

However, debate has been growing on the issue of expanding the private health care sector. Arguments developed by proponents of expanding private care emphasize the value of competition and the strengthened incentives for efficient performance associated with private institutions. In particular, the introduction of private insurance is said to encourage innovation and efficiency because of its flexibility, the profit motive, and the increase in choice for the consumer (Chollet and Lewis 1997). Proponents of expanding public systems stress the issue of market failures implicit in health markets (Maynard and Dixon 2002).

The public–private mix in health care is likely to have an impact on labor purchasing. Competitive markets are expected to increase the flexibility of health care systems and hence of the labor-purchasing process. In effect, purchasers should be able to choose from among different providers. Moreover, the public sector may be perceived as less flexible, due to political and budget constraints. For instance, because health personnel are often civil servants, the government may be reluctant to make any major changes such as increasing remuneration of health personnel, for fear that other civil servants would make similar demands.

Differentiating between the public and private health labor force is often complex, however, as health workers may work in both sectors. For instance, in Angola nearly 8 of 10 doctors who work for the Ministry of Health also work in the private sector, but only 1 in 5 of them with official authorization (Fresta, Jorge, and Ferrinho 2000).

PURCHASER–PROVIDER SPLIT

Over the past years, health care reforms to separate public purchasing from public provision have been introduced in several countries. The purchaser–provider split is a term that usually refers to government legislation reshaping public authorities into bodies for purchasing health services, rather than organizations for managing and employing health service providers (Ovretreit 1995). The extent of the purchaser–provider split varies. Some public providers are managed entirely by another public body while others may be totally privatized (a *total split*). In other cases, a public authority may retain management of some services *(partial split)*.

A well-defined separation of functions between purchasers and providers of health services has existed in some European countries for a long time; others have recently introduced it (Savas 2000). Purchasers may be a public agency, as in Sweden and in the United Kingdom; a health insurer, as in Germany; or primary health care physicians, as with general practitioner fundholders in the United Kingdom.

The main reason for splitting purchasers and providers is to create markets or quasi-markets for health services delivery (Le Grand and Bartlett 1993). Some observers argue that purchasers may be able to use their purchasing power to induce providers to offer better value for money. Stronger provider account-ability and empowerment of citizens are also emphasized as advantages of the purchaser–provider split. Observers on the other side argue that transaction costs and purchasers' opportunistic behavior have been identified as potential problems associated with the purchaser–provider split.

CONTRACTING IN AND OUT

In contrast to a wholesale adoption of a contracting framework at the system level (purchaser–provider split), we shall now consider contracting at lower lev-els and differentiate between "contracting in" and "contracting out." *Contracting in* can be defined as an employer–employee contract. For instance, an employer such as a hospital contracts with an individual employee to perform specific tasks. *Contracting out* refers to the purchase of services provided by a company or self-employed individuals to resolve some subsector problems.

An organization may contract out to provide a service directly to the public or to provide a public hospital with "support" service such as catering or laundry services. For instance, large-scale government contracting of nongovernmental organizations to extend basic health services to the poor has developed in Guatemala (Nieves, Forgia, and Ribera 2000). India and Sri Lanka also contract out many support services such as catering and cleaning, especially in large cities (Bhatia and Mills 1997; Russel and Attanayake 1997).

Efficiency incentives, lower costs, and flexibility of work arrangements are among the arguments in favor of contracting out. In effect, the replacement of direct, hierarchical management structures by contractual relationships between purchasers and providers is said to promote increased transparency of prices, volumes, and quality in trading, as well as managerial decentralization, both of which should enhance efficiency (Mills and Broomberg 1998). Moreover, such a process is expected to increase competition among providers, in the further expectation that lively competition will enhance supply-side efficiency.

Opponents of contracting out claim that its overall benefits may be out-weighed by the potentially substantial costs involved in its creation and mainte-nance (transaction costs), as well as lower wages for employees (Ovretreit 1995).

PURCHASER POWER

A single entity that is the sole purchaser of labor is a *monopsony*. One example is the potential monopsony power of hospitals in hiring nurses or the ministry of health in hiring the health workforce. The amount of labor demanded will influence the price the monopsonist must pay for it. In contrast to the situation in a competitive market, the monopsony is a price maker, not a price taker. Monopsony results in lower wages and employment of nurses compared with a competitive market. For monopsony to occur, nurses must also have limited mobility (Feldstein 1999).

A number of studies have tested whether or not hospitals possess monopsony power with respect to nurses, and the results are contradictory. Sullivan (1989) and Staiger, Spetz, and Phibbs (1999) conclude that hospitals have a substantial monopsony power. In contrast, Hirsch and Schumacher (1995) find no empirical support for the monopsony model.

PROVIDER POWER

Unions and professional associations seek to increase their members' market power, employment, and income (Maceira and Murillo 2001). Labor-purchasing conditions will therefore be influenced by their power.

Seldon, Jung, and Cavazos (1998) suggest that physicians in the United States have market power through such avenues as restricting supply and price fixing. In France, trade unions are granted an institutional role at establishment level (Mossé and Tschobanian 1999). In India and Sri Lanka, a clear constraint to support services contracting was the inability to counter the power of the public service unions in dictating employment terms and conditions (McPake and Mills 2000).

The varying degree of homogeneity of the different professional groups may also explain their relative success in maintaining a monopoly of practice. In Iceland, one of the factors that contributed to breaking the professional monopoly of pharmacists was division within the profession (Morgall and Almarsdottir 1999).

CONCLUSIONS

The framework presented in this paper encompasses a wide diversity of elements, but the role of yet more factors should also be investigated. For instance, the role of cultural or political factors is likely to affect labor purchasing. The effects of migration on labor purchasing should also be considered.

A better understanding of the interaction between the elements of the framework would reinforce the analysis. For instance, the type of interaction between government and unions may vary greatly from place to place. Sometimes grouping of many health personnel in public service creates a condition of bilateral monopoly between large unions and the government (Tirole 1988). The structure of a bilateral monopoly gives both the government and the unions an incentive to be confrontational, because each side knows the other can accept a broad range of conditions.

The central role of human resources in the health system shows that labor-purchasing issues have to be understood. In an attempt to improve understanding of such issues, this chapter has presented a framework and reviewed its main elements to show how labor purchasing may affect health services delivery and health system performance.

NOTE

Many thanks are due to William Savedoff, Health Financing and Stewardship, for his useful comments and suggestions, and to Janet Clevenstine, Department of Health Service Provision, both of the World Health Organization.

REFERENCES

Abel-Smith, B. 1994. *An Introduction to Health, Policy, Planning and Financing.* New York, N.Y.: Longman Group Limited.

Aiken, L., H. Smith, and E. Lake. 1994. "Lower Medicare Mortality among a Set of Hospitals Known for Good Nursing Care. *Medical Care* 32(5): 771–87.

Alcazar, L., and R. Andrade. 2001. "Induced Demand and Absenteeism in Peruvian Hospitals." In R. Di Tella and W. Savedoff, eds., *Diagnosis Corruption: Fraud in Latin America's Public Hospitals.* Washington, D.C.: Inter-American Development Bank.

American Hospital Association. 2001. "The Hospital Workforce Shortage: Immediate and Future." *Trend Watch* 3(2): 1–8.

Arrowsmith, J., and P. Mossé. 2000. "Health Care Reform and the Working Time of Hospital Nurses in England and France." *European Journal of Industrial Relations* 6(3): 283–306.

Arrowsmith, J., and K. Sisson. 1999. "Pay and Working Time: Towards Organization-Based Systems?" *British Journal of Industrial Relations* 37(1): 51–75.

Bhatia, M., and A. Mills. 1997. "The Contracting for Dietary Services by Public Hospitals in Bombay." In S. Bennett, B. McPake, and A. Mills, eds., *Private Health Providers in Developing Countries: Serving the Public Interest?* London: Zed Books.

Brito, P. 2000. "Health Sector Reform and Its Impact on Human Resources and Employment Management within the Health Sector." *Revista Panamericana de Salud Publica* 8(1-2): 43–54.

Boerma, W., and D. Flemming. 1998. *The Role of General Practice in Primary Health Care.* London: The Stationary Office.

Cercone, J., F. Duran-Valverde, and E. Munoz-Vargas. 2000. "Compromiso de gesión, rendición de cuentas y corrupción en los hospitales de la Caja Costarricense de Seguro Social." Latin America Research Network Working Paper R-418. Inter-American Development Bank, Washington, D.C.

Chollet, D., and M. Lewis. 1997. "Private Insurance: Principles and Practice." In G. Schieber, ed., *Innovations in Health Care Financing: Proceedings of a World Bank Conference*, March 10–11, 1997. Washington, D.C.: World Bank.

Chomitz, K., G. Setiadi, A. Azwar, N. Ismail, and P. Widiyarti. 1998. "What Do Doctors Want? Developing Incentives for Doctors to Serve in Indonesia's Rural and Remote Areas." Policy Research Working Paper 1888. World Bank, Washington, D.C.

Deber, R., L. Narine, P. Baranek, N. Sharpe, K. Duvalko, R. Zlotnik, P. Coyte, G. Pink, and P. Williams. 1995. "The Public/Private Mix in Health Care." Canadian National Forum on Health. Internet communication of December 8, 2002 at http://wwwnfh.hc-sc.gc.ca/publicat/public/idxpuble.htm.

Diallo, K., and N. Gupta. In press. *Assessment of human resources in Chad*. Geneva: World Health Organization.

Donaldson, C., and K. Gerard. 1993. *Economics of Health Care Financing: The Visible Hand*. London: Macmillan.

Egger, D., D. Lipson, and O. Adams. 2000. "Achieving the Right Balance: The Role of Policymaking Processes in Managing Human Resources for Health." Issues in Health Services Delivery, Discussion Paper 2, Evidence and Information for Policy. World Health Organization, Department of Organization of Health Services Delivery, Geneva.

Ensor, T., S. Witter, and I. Sheiman. 1997. "Methods of Payment to Medical Care Providers." In S. Witter and T. Ensor, eds., *Introduction to Health Economics for Eastern Europe and the Former Soviet Union*. New York, N.Y.: John Wiley and Son Ltd.

Evans, D. 1974. "Supplier-Induced Demand: Empirical Evidence and Implications." In M. Perlman, ed., *The Economics of Health and Medical Care*. New York, N.Y.: John Wiley and Sons.

Federation of Nurses and Health Professionals. 2001. *The Nurse Shortage: Perspective from Current Direct Care Nurse and Former Direct Care Nurses*. Washington, D.C.

Feldstein, P. 1999. *Health Care Economics*. 5th ed. New York, N.Y.: Delmar Publishers.

Fresta, E., M. Jorge, and P. Ferrinho. 2000. "The Internal Brain-Drain in the Angolan Health Sector." In P. Ferrinho and W. Van Lerberghe, eds., *Health Personnel Performance and Providing Health Care under Adverse Conditions*. Studies in Health Services Organization and Policy 16. Antwerp, Belgium: ITG Press.

Gleason-Scott, J., J. Sochalski, and L. Aiken. 1999. "Review of Magnet Hospital Research: Established Findings and Implications for Professional Nursing Practice." *Journal of Nursing Administration* 29(1): 9–19.

Grignon, M., V. Paris, and D. Polton. 2002. "Influence of Physician Payment Methods on the Efficiency of the Health Care System." Discussion Paper 35. Commission on the Future of Health Care in Canada, Ottawa.

Hirsch, B., and E. Schumacher. 1995. "Monopsony Power and Relative Wages in the Labor Market for Nurses." *Journal of Health Economics* 14: 443–76.

Hölmstrom, B., and J. Tirole. 1989. "The Theory of the Firm." In R. Schmalensee and R. Willig, eds., *Handbook of Industrial Organization*, Vol. 1. Amsterdam: North Holland.

International Labour Organisation. 1998. "Terms of Employment and Working Conditions in Health Sector Reforms." Report for discussion at the Joint Meeting on Terms of Employment and Working Conditions in Health Sector Reforms. Geneva.

Kolehamainen-Aiken, R. L. 1997. "Decentralisation and Human Resources: Implications and Impact. *Human Resources for Health Development Journal* 2(1): 1–14. http://www.moph.go.th/ops/hrdj/Hrdj_no3/table_contents.html.

Kramer, M. 1990. "The Magnet Hospitals: Excellence Revisited." *Journal of Nursing Administration* 20(9): 35–44.

Le Grand, J., and W. Bartlett. 1993. *Quasi-Markets and Social Policy*. Basingstoke: Macmillan.

Maceira, D., and V. Murillo. 2001. "Social Sector Reform in Latin America and the Role of Unions." Working Paper 456. Inter-American Development Bank, Research Department, Washington, D.C.

Martineau, T., and J. Martinez. 1997. "Human Resources in Health Sector: Guidelines for Appraisal and Strategic Development." Health and Development Series, Working Paper 1. European Commission, Social and Development Unit, Brussels.

Maynard, A., and A. Dixon. 2002. "Private Health Insurance and Medical Savings Accounts: Theory and Experience." In E. Mossialos, A. Dixon, J. Figueras, and J. Kutzin, eds., *Funding Health Care: Options for Europe, European Observatory on Health Care Systems Series*. Buckingham, United Kingdom: Open University Press.

Maynard, A., M. Marinker, and D. Gray. 1986. "The Doctor, the Patient and Their Contract: Alternative Contracts: Are They Viable?" *British Medical Journal* 242: 1438–40.

McPake, B., and A. Mills. 2000. "What Can We Learn from International Comparisons of Health Systems and Health System Reforms. *Bulletin of the World Health Organization* 78(6): 811–20.

Milgrom, P., and J. Roberts. 1992. *Economics, Organization, and Management*. Englewood Cliffs, N.J.: Prentice-Hall.

Mills, A., and J. Broomberg. 1998. "Experiences of Contracting: An Overview of the Literature." Macroeconomics, Health and Development Series, Technical Paper 33. World Health Organization, Geneva.

Morgall, J., and A. Almarsdottir. 1999. "No Struggle, No Strength: How Pharmacists Lost Their Monopoly." *Social Science and Medicine* 48: 1247–58.

Mossé, P., and R. Tschobanian. 1999. "France: The Restructuring of Employment Relations in the Public Services." In S. Bach, L. Bordogna, F. Della Rocca, and D. Winchester, eds., *Public Service Employment Relations in Europe: Transformation, Modernization or Inertia?* London: Routledge.

Murray, V., and D. Dimick. 1978. "Contextual Influences on Personnel Policies and Programs: An Explanatory Model." *Academy of Management Review* October: 750–61.

Murray, C., and J. Frenk. 2000. "A Framework for Assessing the Performance of Health Systems." *Bulletin of the World Health Organization* 78(6): 717–31.

Nieves, I., G. La Forgia, and J. Ribera. 2000. "Large-Scale Government Contracting of NGOs to Extend Basic Health Services to Poor Populations in Guatemala." Case presented at the international conference on "The Challenge of Health Reform: Reaching the Poor," San José, Costa Rica, May 2000, under the auspices of the World Bank, the Inter-American Development Bank, and la Caja Costarricense de Seguro Social.

Ovretreit, J. 1995. *Purchasing for Health: A Multidisciplinary Introduction to the Theory and Practice of Health Purchasing*. Health Services Management Series. Buckingham, U.K.: Open University Press.

Russel, S., and N. Attanayake. 1997. "Reforming the Health Sector in Sri Lanka: Does Government Have the Capacity?" The Role of Government in Adjusting Economies, Paper 14. Development Administration Group, University of Birmingham, United Kingdom.

Salamon, L., and K. Anheier. 1996. *The Emerging Nonprofit Sector: An Overview*. John Hopkins Nonprofit Sector Series 1. Manchester, United Kingdom: Manchester University Press.

Saltman, R. B., and C. von Otter. 1995. *Implementing Planned Markets in Health Care: Balancing Social and Economic Responsibility*. Buckingham, United Kingdom: Open University Press.

Savas, S. 2000. *A Methodology for Analysing Contracting in Health Care.* Copenhagen: World Health Organization, Regional Office for Europe.

Seldon, B., C. Jung, and R. Cavazos. 1998. "Market Power among Physicians in the U.S. 1983–1991." *The Quarterly Review of Economics and Finance* 38(4): 799–824.

Staiger, D., J. Spetz, and C. Phibbs. 1999. "Is There a Monopsony in the Labor Market? Evidence from a Natural Experiment." Working Paper 7258. National Bureau of Economic Research, Cambridge, Mass.

Sullivan, D. 1989. "Monopsony Power in the Market for Nurses." *Journal of Law and Economics* 32: S135–78.

Tirole, J. 1988. *The Theory of Industrial Organization.* Cambridge, Mass.: MIT Press.

WHO (World Health Organization). 1999. *The World Health Report 1999: Making a Difference.* Geneva.

———. 2000. *The World Health Report 2000: Health Systems: Improving Performance.* Geneva.

———. 2002a. "Human Resources for Health: Developing Policy Options for Change." Background paper prepared for the WHO workshop on Human Resources and National Health Systems, Geneva, December 2–4, 2002.

———. 2002b. *The World Health Report 2002: Reducing Risks, Promoting Healthy Life.* Geneva.

CHAPTER 14

Purchasing Pharmaceuticals

Ulrika Enemark, Anita Alban, Enrique C. Seoane-Vazquez,
Andreas Seiter

Pharmaceuticals are a critical input to the proper functioning of the health services. Most curative and many preventive health services depend on pharmaceuticals. Patients perceive availability of pharmaceuticals in a facility as an indicator of the quality of health services, and drug availability helps explain overall utilization of health services. Despite significant progress in increasing the number of people with access to essential medicine over the past decades, a substantial share of the world's population (more than a third worldwide and more than half in the poorest parts of Africa and Asia) still lack access to reliable supplies of essential medicines (World Health Organization [WHO] 2000).

Many factors influence whether poor people can obtain affordable essential drugs of standard quality. Increased access to drugs depends on an efficient resource allocation and purchasing (RAP) system including rational selection and use of medicines, adequate and sustainable financing, affordable prices, and reliable health care and drug supply systems.

This chapter is based on literature found by systematic search of published literature, particularly in Africa and Asia. Search criteria included pharmaceuticals/drugs and developing countries combined with key parameters regarding RAP (Enemark, Alban, and Seoane-Vazquez 2004).

PHARMACEUTICAL RAP IN DEVELOPING COUNTRIES

The importance of pharmaceuticals for patients is illustrated by the fact that drug expenditures constitute a greater share of total health expenditures in developing countries than in industrial countries (figure 14.1). Drug expenditures in developing countries represented, for example, 24 percent of the health care expenditures in South Africa and 66 percent in Mali in the 1990s (WHO 2000).

Most spending on pharmaceuticals in developing countries is privately financed—between 45 and 90 percent of all drug expenditures (WHO 2000). Private drug expenditures represent a higher percentage of total expenditures than in the case of health care expenditures. Correspondingly, the larger part of household health care expenditures is spent on pharmaceuticals (WHO 2002).

FIGURE 14.1   Pharmaceutical Spending

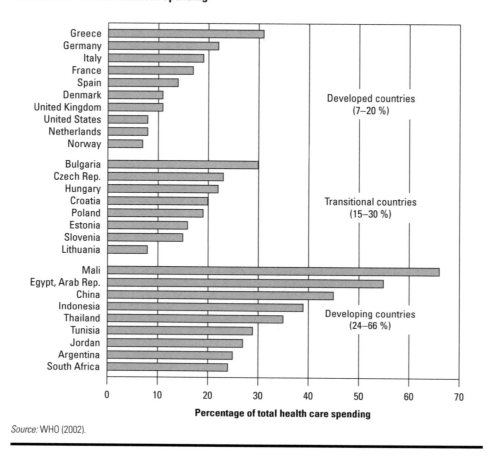

Source: WHO (2002).

The high level of private financing suggests that individual market transactions are highly prevalent, and pooled purchasing is less common. Private and social insurance cover an insignificant share of total health sector spending in most developing countries, although social security coverage is fairly common in Latin America and some Asian countries. Private drug insurance is only in its beginnings in developing countries because of the complex challenges involved. Ghana is currently introducing such insurance, and it will be interesting to see how successful this model will be.

The private sector is the main player in the pharmaceutical sector of developing countries. The private sector has the largest number of manufacturers, wholesalers, and community pharmacies, and the value of private drug sales is larger than the public (Velasquez, Madrid, and Quick 1998). But the public sector is a main source of health care and medicines for the poorest part of the population of those countries. Self-medication and use of drugs following advice by unskilled pharmacy personnel is common in developing countries (Ensor and San 1996; Paphassarang and others 2002). For example, 60 percent of pharmacy clients in Accra, Ghana, are estimated to have no prescription (Mayhew and others 2001).

RAP Arrangements

In most developing countries, the individual patient buys drugs for cash from a pharmacy, a physician, a private drug seller, or a shop. Revenues from selling drugs are used to purchase new supplies either on the private market or through a dedicated supply chain with pooled purchasing. Public or donor subsidies exist in varying degrees, filling gaps if revenues from drug sales fall short of what is needed to restock the supply chain.

Agents that allocate resources and purchase pharmaceuticals include central government agencies, local government agencies, social health insurance schemes, private drug insurance plans, community drug-financing schemes, employer-provided health services, and nongovernmental organizations. Often, several RAP arrangements coexist in a country. For example, decentralization may take place for RAP of some pharmaceuticals but not for others used in vertical programs (for example, in Argentina, health is a responsibility of the states, but the central government established Programa Remediar in 2002 to provide essential drugs to the poor), and nongovernmental schemes often operate alongside a tax-funded public system.

CORE POLICY RAP STRATEGIES TO INCREASE ACCESS TO DRUGS

The strategic options to improve drug access entail measures to stimulate optimal functioning of the market through incentives, regulation, and information. These strategies may largely be classified into demand-side interventions, supply-side interventions, and pricing and incentives.

Demand-Side Interventions (For Whom to Buy?)

All RAP arrangements attempt to ensure availability of a set of defined drugs to potential users covered by the arrangement. The problem is that in many countries too little funding is available to purchase enough medicines to satisfy demand and that poor people, in particular, are not reached by the existing arrangements. Poor people have to navigate several access hurdles: price of drugs, knowledge about availability of treatment, trust in the system that delivers the treatment, distance and transportation costs, and discrimination based on gender, religion or ethnicity.

Agreement is widespread that available subsidies should be used to improve access to essential drugs for the poor and use of pharmaceuticals for high-priority services (maternal and child health, family planning) and for diseases of public health importance such as tuberculosis (Bitran and Giedion 2003).

SUBSIDIZING DRUGS FOR TARGET POPULATION GROUPS

Government or donor agencies provide subsidies for health services, including pharmaceuticals. Drugs often have high copayments, but exemptions and waivers are given to certain target groups (Gilson, Russell, and Buse 1995). These groups are often broad and, in practice, patients rather than services are exempt, causing problems of sustainability. A pregnant mother, for example, may receive free medicines and redistribute them to other family members. Community financing schemes (concerned about moral hazard) limit subsidies for poor people (Atim 1999; Bennett, Creese, and Monasch 1998; Gilson and others 2001; Musau 1999). The general experience is that the success of an exemption program depends to a large extent on the existence of a functioning financing mechanism to compensate for lost revenue from drug subsidies (Bitran and Giedion 2003). Waivers for the poor appear to be most successful under card systems involving local authorities in the identification of eligible persons (Gilson and others 1998; Gilson, Russell, and Buse 1995). However, in many cases exemption-based systems fail to deliver the expected results. This is one reason Ghana, for example, is replacing exemptions with a health insurance model that offers subsidized membership for the poor.

Another way of targeting pharmaceuticals to the poor is to ensure that populations in deprived areas get an allocation of funding for drugs reflecting their needs. While needs-based geographical resource allocation criteria are proposed for funding certain recurrent expenditures (Ghana, Tanzania), these criteria do not often apply to drug budgets.

PROMOTING RATIONAL DRUG USE

To ensure optimal utilization of limited resources, any RAP arrangement has to address the widespread problem of irrational use of drugs such as overprescription, polypharmacy, overuse of antibiotics, abuse of injections, underuse of effective products such as oral rehydration salts, and use of dangerous drugs (for example, Al Serouri, Balabanova, and Al Hibshi 2002). These problems arise under the influence of economic pressures, lack of information, inadequately trained health workers, lack of supervision and accountability, perceived patient expectations, drug company promotions, and financial gains from prescribing and dispensing.

Most interventions to improve rational prescription include training or other educational activities of prescribers and drug dispensers (Laing, Hogerzeil, and Ross-Degnan 2001; Oliveira-Cruz, Hanson, and Mills 2001). Other interventions include the development and implementation of standard treatment guidelines, drug utilization review, and encouragement of the use of generic drugs, including generic substitution. The outcomes of these interventions are mixed, but overall results are positive in terms of decreased average number of drugs prescribed and correct selection and dosage of drugs (Oliveira-Cruz, Hanson, and Mills 2001). Ghana has had good results by combining education and monitoring of prescribers.[1]

Adequate patient use of pharmaceuticals also demands attention. Poor people turn to self-medication more often than rich people (Ching 1995; Gilson and others 2001; Mbugua, Bloom, and Segall 1995). Inappropriate use of self-medicated drugs or lack of compliance compromise the potential gains related to drug utilization. Health education and building of trust between patients and prescribers appear to be successful interventions for addressing these problems (Oliveira-Cruz, Hanson, and Mills 2001). Additionally, compliance can be addressed by improving the affordability of medicine. This was demonstrated in the case of tuberculosis (Homedes and Ugalde 2000).

Supply-Side Interventions

The selection of drugs and providers is a key issue for RAP agents managing a limited resource pool. Supply-side interventions may be targeted at production, wholesale and retail. Most RAP arrangements would not, however, involve interventions regarding production.

STRATEGIC SELECTION OF PHARMACEUTICALS TO BENEFIT THE POOR (WHAT TO BUY?)

One tool for controlling costs and making drugs more accessible is an essential drugs list, coupled with a rational procurement policy (for example, Laing, Hogerzeil, and Ross-Degnan 2001). Worldwide, 156 countries have adopted an essential drugs list (figure 14.2). Most drugs in the WHO model Essential Drugs List (EDL) are out of patent, allowing procurement agencies to compare prices and conditions from various companies and select the best provider in terms of quality, reliability, and price (WHO 2002).

The EDL needs to be updated (ideally every year) to account for changes in medical practice, availability of newer drugs that have reached the end of their patent life and are now available as generics, and changes in the country's economic situation if these affect the budget available for pharmaceuticals.

The EDL may or may not include drugs used in secondary or tertiary care levels depending on the main sources of financing for drugs on these levels. It usually does not restrict the private market for pharmaceuticals, which is limited only by the general regulatory framework that defines which drugs can be registered and who can import, manufacture, and sell these drugs.

Few insurance schemes have a pharmaceutical policy that is consistently practiced (Atim 1998, 1999; Bennett, Creese, and Monasch 1998; Musau 1999). The successful ones engage in selective contracting. For example, one scheme in Tanzania (UMASIDA) contracts care from providers who agree to restrict drug use to

FIGURE 14.2   Countries with a National Essential Drugs List, December 1999

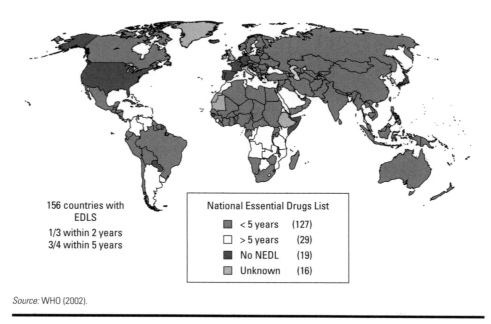

156 countries with
EDLS

1/3 within 2 years
3/4 within 5 years

National Essential Drugs List

■	< 5 years	(127)
□	> 5 years	(29)
■	No NEDL	(19)
▨	Unknown	(16)

Source: WHO (2002).

the WHO EDL and to prescribe only by generic name. The prescribing habits of providers are monitored. A provider who violates the agreement on essential drugs will not be reimbursed (Bennett, Creese, and Monasch 1998).

A serious constraint to the implementation of an essential drugs and generics policy is the widespread preference among patients and doctors for brand drugs and the perceived linkage between brand and quality. In the Republic of Yemen, cost-sharing schemes using the EDL guidelines have reduced the use of injections, intravenous drips, and syrups (Al Serouri, Balabanova, and Al Hibshi 2002). However, patients perceive the limited drug lists and the amounts provided as deterioration of services. There was also dissatisfaction with the use of drugs from India (generic) rather than from the United Arab Emirates (brand names). The same was reported from Ghana, where the new health insurance schemes will have to address this issue if they want to avoid "negative selection" based on the perception of poor quality: People who are better off can join a private insurance plan that can offer more choices of drugs outside the EDL. The recommendation for Ghana is to introduce a visible, decentralized quality assurance system that helps to build trust in the public procurement and supply policy and the drugs offered under the new insurance plans. Such a system exists already within the Catholic Health Service in Ghana, where pooled purchasing is combined with decentralized delivery to regional centers, which have the capacity to monitor drug quality on a regular basis.[2]

SELECTING SUPPLIERS (FROM WHOM TO BUY?)

The process of selecting from whom to buy drugs is important. Active competition between the public and private sector on price, quality, and volume of drugs at the stage of selecting the providers is likely to reduce prices and increase value for money. The various suppliers of drugs include:

- *Public supply agency*. Until recently the standard approach in many developing countries has been to have a centralized public system such as government central medical stores, essentially a monopoly, supply drugs to government health facilities. Some countries started a process of transforming the central supply agency into a parastatal or autonomous agency to stimulate accountability and more businesslike operations (Tanzania).

- *Producers*. Drugs can be purchased directly from domestic or international drug producers. It may be government policy to restrict purchases from international producers for reasons including constraints on use of foreign exchange (for example, Mauritania [Audibert and Mathonnat 2000]) or a policy to protect home industry (for example, before the World Trade Organization's Agreement on Trade-Related Aspects of Intellectual Property Rights, most developing countries—including India and Argentina—had a policy requiring local manufacture of drugs).

- *Private supply agency*. This can be either a private for-profit supply agency that specializes in procurement and distribution of drugs (for example, Crown Agents—based in the United Kingdom, but operating worldwide, or a non-profit organization such as mission-based MEDS in Kenya).

- *Private retailers*. The RAP agent may choose to allow patients to buy from any retailer, from retailers licensed by the public authorities (SEWA in India), or from licensed retailers abiding by additional criteria set by the RAP arrangement (UMASIDA in Tanzania) (Bennett, Creese, and Monasch 1998).

An important issue is to ensure the quality of supplies. Regulation to ensure quality and access may take the form of registration and licensing arrangements and monitoring by regulatory bodies. Reimbursement may be restricted to drugs prescribed and dispensed by licenseholders from an agreed list of drugs.

Pricing and Incentive Regimes

The nature of the market for pharmaceuticals—with its information asymmetries and combination of a relatively competitive retail market and a less competitive production and wholesale level—poses a substantial risk of supplier-induced demand, irrational prescription, overpricing, and unequal distribution. Behavioral changes may be stimulated through the use of financial incentives, penalties, or other regulatory measures. The main intervention areas include the design of payment mechanisms and control of prices.

INCENTIVE REGIMES (HOW TO PAY?)

The payment system for physician visits will influence prescribing patterns and drug use. An additional factor influencing drug overuse is when physicians combine the prescribing and dispensing roles (Guyana or the Republic of Korea).

There are three general types of provider payment, which have different incentives for prescription of drugs:

- *Budgetary transfer.* Budgets may be allocated in the form of an earmarked, line-item budget for medicine and supplies (conditional grant). Global budgets, however, encourage efficiency because they allow the reallocation of funds across budget lines.

- *Capitation.* Capitation is not a common payment method in developing countries. Preliminary findings for a prepayment scheme in Rwanda suggest that members seek care earlier, and therefore need fewer drugs and recover faster (Schneider, Diop, and Bucyana 2000).

- *Fee for service.* This is the most common payment mechanism for private insurance as well as for individual purchases. It provides incentives for increasing the number of services and drug utilization.

Financial incentives may be used to stimulate rational prescription. In Nepal, the establishment of a user charge per prescription rather than per drug item prescribed showed improved efficiency, with fewer drugs prescribed per patient, lower costs per prescription, lower wastage due to inappropriate prescribing, and a larger share of prescriptions adhering to standard treatment guidelines (Holloway and others 2002; Holloway, Gautam, and Reeves 2001).

In addition to the modality of payment, the flow of funds also affects drug prescribing. In some RAP arrangements, patients make the payment to the pharmacy and later seek full or partial reimbursement from the RAP agent *(indemnity cover;* SEWA in India). In others, the payment is made directly by the RAP agent to the provider (UMASIDA in Tanzania [Bennett, Creese, and Monasch 1998]).

The structure of *dispensing margins* (allowed markups on cost) and *dispensing fees* affects the use of drugs. A fixed-percentage markup encourages dispensing of the most expensive drugs. A declining markup percentage with increasing price reduces this incentive. A markup with a fixed dispensing fee is neutral, unless a higher rate applies for generic dispensing, thus encouraging the dispensing of low-cost drugs. Experience with applying dispensing margins and fees in developing countries is limited, but the economic incentives behind the failure to adhere to regulation are strong (Kumaranayake and others 2003).

CONTROLLING PRICES (AT WHAT PRICE?)

Increasing the affordability of drugs requires that purchases be made at the lowest prices for the same standard quality.

RAP arrangements may harvest the benefits from *competition,* as the example of antiretrovirals illustrates (figure 14.3), by buying generic rather than branded

FIGURE 14.3   Competition as a Price Inhibitor: The Example of Antiretrovirals

Cost per capsule or tablet (in U.S. dollars)

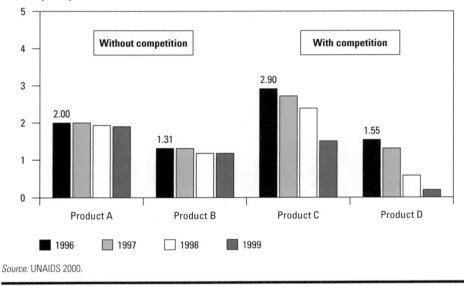

Source: UNAIDS 2000.

drugs and by broadening the pool of potential providers to include both public and private sector providers. Also, a choice has to be made whether to engage in price negotiations to make a drug price agreement part of a service contract. The ability of RAP agents to influence the price is likely to vary with their size and scope, with larger RAP agents such as government agencies and social insurance schemes having more bargaining power.

Governments can *regulate* manufacturer, wholesale, and retail drug prices. Prices may be set locally or centrally. Typically, governments set the initial price of a drug—and authorize future changes in this price—using a process that combines negotiation with the companies and the application of a set of economic and clinical criteria. In price regulation, there is a danger of corruption, which may lead to higher prices in some regulated markets than those that can be achieved by rational procurement and market forces in countries without price regulation. An effective price control mechanism requires a monitoring and enforcement capacity unusual in developing countries owing to limitations in staff, funding, and delegation of authority. An alternative approach might be to make import prices public and encourage competition between private wholesalers and retail pharmacists, or to regulate only a certain category of drugs: in India, for example, the strictest price control is on the essential drugs, requiring clear specification of the retail price on the drug containers for easy reference by consumers (Berman 1997).

There is little systematic research on the enforcement of pharmaceutical markups. In practice, pharmaceutical markups seem to vary greatly between facilities and to be higher than the markups officially established (in Nepal [Levison 2003], Ghana [Nyanator, Asare, and Tayvia 2002], and Costa Rica [WHO 1995]).

Although purchasing agencies have a potential role in controlling strict adherence to price control regulations and in *bargaining* for low prices, they rarely exercise it (Atim 1999; Bennett, Creese, and Monasch 1998; Musau 1999). Exceptions include a scheme in the Philippines that negotiates favorable prices for essential drugs from local suppliers (Bennett, Creese, and Monasch 1998) and another in Tanzania where the dispensing unit can bill only according to a price list (based on generic drug prices) attached to the contract (Musau 1999).

ORGANIZATIONAL AND INSTITUTIONAL ARRANGEMENTS

Organizational and institutional arrangements set the framework within which RAP of pharmaceuticals works. The efficiency of RAP depends on the characteristics and responsibilities of the decisionmakers and the level of resources pooling. The drug policy and regulation set out the framework of the pharmaceutical sector.

Organizational Issues

The private retail drug market in developing countries is highly dispersed, relying largely on individual transactions in an open market. Establishment of community financing and other insurance schemes represents an increasing concentration on the demand side, although these schemes still function effectively as active purchasing agents, bargaining for drug price and quality and setting restrictions on drug use. Most countries also have some sort of third-party payment system, which often includes drug benefits but requires a copayment and limits drug use to a defined list of drugs. In some countries, separate drug benefit schemes exist. This separation provides cost-shifting incentives that may not be optimal from a societal point of view, as cost-minimizing health plans may urge providers to prescribe drug-intensive strategies, financed under the separate drug plan rather than alternatives.

Health care providers and pharmacies may be licensed to undertake different activities. In Zimbabwe, for example, private practitioners are allowed to dispense drugs only under certain circumstances (long distance to nearest outlet) (Bennett and Ngalande-Banda 1994). In other places, such as Ghana and India, private clinics are allowed to offer integrated services including dispensing of pharmaceuticals. The lack of separation between prescribing and dispensing roles, particularly in Asia, gives practitioners an incentive to overprescribe, because the prescription is directly linked to financial gains. In fact, the number of prescriptions written is higher when prescribing and dispensing functions are combined (Govindaraj and Chellara 2002; Trap, Hansen, and Hogerzeil 2002; Witter 1996).

While government RAP agencies are often tied to purchasing from the public sector supply agency, this is not the case for many community financing and insurance schemes. Public sector RAP agencies at the decentralized level are also increasingly free to use other sources for procurement. However, key questions are: How is the quality of drugs ensured? and Do the benefits of purchasing from smaller supply agents in a competitive environment exceed the benefits of large-scale procurement through centralized procurement agents with the inherent inefficiencies of monopoly public sector institutions?

The most common practice for government RAP arrangements is to have budgets earmarked for drugs and medical supplies, often tied to spending with a particular statal or parastatal supply agency. Drug revolving funds, often used by the public sector, have limited accountability to users. The separation of demand-side activities (the financing arrangement) from supply-side activities might encourage active purchasing, but the capacity to do so is low in many developing countries.

The health sector reform process in developing countries often entails a combination of measures such as strengthening the district health services and giving autonomous status to major hospitals and public central supply agencies (Ghana, Guyana, Mozambique, Tanzania, Uganda). The process has often been slow, however, and competition has not been introduced, because many districts, regions, and hospitals are still compelled to acquire the drugs from the public central supply agency.

Fragmentation of purchasing functions is often problematic. Good experience has been gained from pooled purchasing arrangements at the country level, for example, by allowing private nonprofit facilities to buy drugs from government stores in several countries (Bennett and Ngalande-Banda 1994); by pooling donor funds for purchase of pharmaceuticals in Mozambique (Pavignani and Durão 1999); and, at the multinational level, by negotiating the price of antiretroviral drugs in Latin America and the Caribbean, as a result of which antiretroviral drug prices dropped significantly (Pan American Health Organization 2002).

With increasing decentralization, competitive procurement may also be introduced by local RAP arrangements, either by selection between procurement agents or by own-procurement (local tendering). Increasing the number of smaller procurement units, however, could reduce drug procurement efficiency.

Institutional Arrangements

Many governments in developing countries have established national drug policies and regulations to ensure efficacy, safety, and rational drug use, mainly in a comprehensive approach that includes the use of competitive bidding, management control, distribution strategy, educational activities in the rational use of drugs, premarket registration, licensing, and other regulatory requirements. Few community financing and insurance schemes have their own drug policy and regulation, although district health management boards are sometimes allowed to make local adjustments to the EDL (Kenya).

Evidence of the impacts of national drug policies on actual use of medicine is limited, but approaches combining several strategies seem to have advantages (Gilson and others 2001; Ratanawijitrasin, Soumerai, and Weerasuriya 2001).

The implementation of a national drug policy is often a slow process, and the lack of monitoring and information dissemination constrains the stewardship function of the public sector.

The combination of high prices transferred from the concentrated wholesale drug market to the retail level and the pressure put by the competitive environment of the retail market on quality and information asymmetries generates a challenge for the regulatory environment and quality assurance system to ensure affordable prices and standard drug quality. For a successful generic drug policy, continued trust in the quality of drugs is essential. Bhutan is an example of a country that buys generic drugs through international competitive bidding and uses part of the savings to pay for drug-quality testing in high-standard laboratories in Bangkok.

Health services in developing countries are increasingly decentralized, thereby separating stewardship and governance. Decentralization of control over drug budgets, however, has been particularly slow. Drug budgets in government facilities are often given as conditional grants tied to purchases from one supply agent, the public central supply agency. Although theoretically a pooled procurement system, if run effectively, is likely to be more efficient, the district medical services may find that a large private sector supply agent (for example, MEDS, the supply agent for the mission sector in Kenya) can provide supplies at competitive prices and quality, and faster than a public central supply agency.

In some developing countries, decentralization has resulted in a weakening of the regional health service (Tanzania), jeopardizing the already weak monitoring and supervisory functions over rational prescription and drug store management. It may also decrease the opportunities for monitoring and enforcing adherence to regulations.

Regulation is a key instrument employed by governments to align the behavior of the players in the pharmaceutical sector with their public policy objectives. The effects of regulatory measures regarding pharmaceuticals in developing countries are poorly documented. Most countries have established a basic legal regulatory framework (Kumaranayake and others 2000), but enforcement in both the public and the private sector is the key problem. Regulatory control is reported to be ineffective or at best weak owing to insufficient information collection, lack of sound rules for monitoring, and lack of capacity to enforce compliance (Berman 1997; Kumaranayake and others 2000). Additionally, drug manufacturing standards are difficult to enforce, and counterfeit drugs are widely available (Berman 1997). Weak enforcement of regulation results from lack of human resources, inadequate financing, outdated systems, and from the lack of commitment in an environment too focused on direct service delivery (India [Berman 1997] and Ghana [Asibuo and Ampofo 2001]). In the absence of effective enforcement, some major providers have developed a capacity for decentralized monitoring, using, for example, the German Pharma Health Fund Minilab. Empowering the consumer side of the supply chain and creating a transparent quality control system appears to be a good way to discourage trade in substandard or counterfeit drugs. Simplifying the supply chain, for example, by asking licensed suppliers to deliver directly to regional distribution hubs instead of a big central warehouse is another element of an anticounterfeiting strategy. Both are applied by the Catholic Health Service in Ghana.[3]

When health facilities receive drugs only through a kit[4] (push) system, accountability is likely to be lower than in a demand-driven (pull) system in which health facilities order and buy drugs using funds held either locally (cost-sharing funds, decentralized budgets) or in central accounts earmarked for drugs by health facility or by district health services.

FROM PASSIVE TO ACTIVE PURCHASING OF PHARMACEUTICALS

In many developing countries, the health care insurance and provision functions continue to be integrated, although Ghana and some other countries have worked with soft performance contracts within the government and mission sector. A community drug scheme may both collect premiums and supply the drugs (RDF Nyamira, Kenya), and facility-based schemes have no separation between the supply and demand sides. Few insurance schemes for the informal sector act as active purchasers (Bennett, Creese, and Monasch 1998).

Theoretically, active purchasing should be easier to introduce in the area of pharmaceuticals, because drugs are actually purchased outside the health facilities. In principle, larger RAP agents should be better able than small buyers to exert collective consumer influence over large providers, thereby making more effective purchases ensuring high-quality services and drugs at affordable prices. One way forward could be to encourage networking and associations of small schemes to strengthen their bargaining positions.

To separate the health financing and provision functions, the separation of ownership and governance can take place through decentralization of ownership, decentralization of the budget process (to regional or district health authorities), and creation of semiautonomous agencies. Decentralization and the establishment of agencies is the current trend in many developing countries, but the process has proved slow (Kenya, Ghana). Several countries are undergoing a process of recentralization in the national government of pharmaceutical-related functions that were previously decentralized in local institutions. This recentralization responds to health care crisis (Argentina) and particularly to the human immunodeficiency virus crisis that generated the establishment of vertical programs at the national level, instead of local programs using decentralized institutions (Guyana).

There is insufficient evidence on the effects of pharmaceutical interventions focused on the poor and disadvantaged. More research is needed to find out which interventions most effectively reach these groups. Evidence from developing countries is also limited regarding the implementation and enforcement of regulations and particularly regarding their effectiveness. Was the impact achieved the one intended? Information is also scant on the functions of community financing schemes and drug revolving funds with regard to resource allocation and purchasing of drugs and ensuring access to drugs for poor people.

NOTES

1. Personal communication, Rebecca Nordor, director of pharmacy, Korle-Bu Teaching Hospital, February 26, 2004.

2. Personal communication, Charles Kofi Allotey, chief pharmacist, Catholic Drug Center, Ghana, March 2, 2004.

3. Personal communication, Charles Kofi Allotey, chief pharmacist, Catholic Drug Center, Ghana, March 2, 2004.

4. A standard package of drugs (in terms of contents and quantities) used for all health facilities and distributed on a regular basis irrespective of stock situation at individual facilities.

REFERENCES

Al Serouri, A. W., D. Balabanova, and S. Al Hibshi. 2002. "Cost Sharing for Primary Health Care: Lessons from Yemen." Oxfam Working Papers. Oxfam, Oxford, United Kingdom.

Asibuo, S. K., and K. K. K. Ampofo. 2001. "Review Study of Health Sector Regulation in Ghana." Ministry of Health, Accra. Unpublished.

Atim, C. 1998. "Contribution of Mutual Health Organizations to Financing, Delivery, and Access to Health Care: Synthesis of Research in Nine West African Countries." Technical Report No. 18. Partnerships for Health Reform, Abt Associates, Bethesda, Md.

———. 1999. "Social Movements and Health Insurance: A Critical Evaluation of Voluntary, Nonprofit Insurance Schemes with Case Studies from Ghana and Cameroon." *Social Science & Medicine* 48(7): 881–96.

Audibert, M., and J. Mathonnat. 2000. "Cost-Recovery in Mauritania: Initial Lessons." *Health Policy and Planning* 15(1): 66–75.

Bennett, S., and E. Ngalande-Banda. 1994. "Public and Private Roles in Health: A Review and Analysis of Experience in Sub-Saharan Africa—Current Concerns," SHS Paper 6. World Health Organization, Geneva.

Bennett, S., A. Creese, and R. Monasch. 1998. "Health Insurance Schemes for People Outside Formal Sector Employment: Current Concerns." ARA Paper 16. World Health Organization, Geneva.

Berman, P. 1997. "Supply-Side Approaches to Optimizing Private Health Sector Growth." In W. Newbrander, ed., *Private Health Sector Growth in Asia. Issues and Implications.* Chichester, U.K.: Wiley & Sons.

Bitran, R., and U. Giedion. 2003. "Waivers and Exemptions for Health Services in Developing Countries." Social Protection Discussion Paper No. 0308. Social Protection Unit, Human Development Network, World Bank, Washington, D.C. Available at www.worldbank.org/sp.

Ching, P. 1995. "User Fees, Demand for Children's Health Care and Access across Income Groups: The Philippine Case." *Social Science and Medicine* 41(1): 37–46.

Enemark, U., A. Alban, and E. C. Seoane-Vazquez. 2004. "Resource Allocation and Pur-chasing of Pharmaceuticals in Developing Countries." HNP Discussion Paper. World Bank, Washington, D.C. Forthcoming.

Ensor, T., and P. B. San. 1996. "Access and Payment for Health Care: The Poor of Northern Vietnam." *International Journal of Health Planning and Management* 11(1): 69–83.

Gilson, L., S. Russell, and K. Buse. 1995. "The Political Economy of User Fees with Target-ing: Developing Equitable Health Financing Policy." *Journal of International Develop-ment Special Issue* 7(3): 369–402.

Gilson, L., D. Kalyalya, F. Kuchler, S. Lake, H. Oranga, and M. Ouendo. 2001. "Strategies for Promoting Equity: Experience with Community Financing in Three African Coun-tries." *Health Policy* 58(1): 37–67.

Gilson, L., S. Russell, O. Rauyajin, T. Boonchote, V. Pasandhanathorn, P. Chaisenee, A. Supachutikul, and N. Tantigate. 1998. "Exempting the Poor: A Review and Evalua-tion of the Low Income Card Scheme in Thailand." PHP Departmental Publication 30. London School of Hygiene and Tropical Medicine, London.

Govindaraj, R., and G. Chellara. 2002. "The India Pharmaceutical Sector. Issues and Options for Health Sector Reform." World Bank Discussion Paper 437. World Bank, Washington, D.C.

Holloway, K. A., B. R. Gautam, T. Harpham, and A. Taket. 2002. "The Influence of User Fees and Patient Demand on Prescribers in Rural Nepal." *Social Science and Medicine* 54(6): 905–18.

Holloway, K. A., B. R. Gautam, and B. C. Reeves. 2001. "The Effects of Different Kinds of User Fees on Prescribing Quality in Rural Nepal." *Journal of Clinical Epidemiology* 54(10): 1065–71.

Homedes, N., and A. Ugalde. 2000. "Improving the Use of Pharmaceuticals through Patient and Community Level Interventions." *Social Science and Medicine* 52: 99–134.

Kumaranayake, L., C. Hongoro, S. Lake, P. Mujinja, and R. Mpembeni. 2003. "Coping with Private Health Markets: Regulatory (In)effectiveness in Sub-Saharan Africa." In N. Soderlund and P. Mendoza-Arana, eds., *The New Public-Private Mix in Health: Exploring the Changing Landscape.* Geneva: Alliance for Health Policy and System Research/EHO.

Kumaranayake, L., S. Lake, P. Mujinja, C. Hongoro, and R. Mpembeni. 2000. "How Do Countries Regulate the Health Sector? Evidence from Tanzania and Zimbabwe." *Health Policy and Planning* 15(4): 357–67.

Laing, R., H. Hogerzeil, and D. Ross-Degnan. 2001. "Ten Recommendations to Improve Use of Medicines in Developing Countries." *Health Policy and Planning* 16(1): 13–20.

Levison, L. 2003. "Policy and Programming Options for Reducing the Procurement Costs of Essential Medicines in Developing Countries." Concentration Paper. Boston Univer-sity School of Public Health, Department of International Health. Unpublished.

Mayhew, S., K. Nzambi, J. Pepin, and S. Adjei. 2001. "Pharmacists' Role in Managing Sex-ually Transmitted Infections: Policy Issues and Options for Ghana." *Health Policy and Planning* 16(2): 152–60.

Mbugua, J. K., G. H. Bloom, and M. M. Segall. 1995. "Impact of User Charges on Vulnera-ble Groups: The Case of Kibwezi in Rural Kenya." *Social Science and Medicine* 41(6): 829–35.

Musau, S. N. 1999. "Community-Based Health Insurance: Experiences and Lessons Learned from East and Southern Africa." Technical Report No. 34. Partnership for Health Reform, Abt Associates, Bethesda, Md.

Nyanator, F., F. B. A. Asare, and H. Tayvia. 2002. "From the Central Medical Store to the Patient—A Situation Analysis of Mark-ups on Drugs in the Volta Region." *Bulletin of Health Information* 1(2&3): 32–36.

Oliveira-Cruz, V., K. Hanson, and A. Mills. 2001. "Approaches to Overcoming Health Systems Constraints at the Peripheral Level: A Review of the Evidence." CMH Working Paper Series. Paper WG5: 15, 1–121. Commission on Macroeconomics and Health, Geneva.

Pan American Health Organization. 2002. "AIDS Drug Prices Drop 54 Percent in Latin America, Caribbean." July 18. http://www.paho.org/English/DPI/pr020718.htm. Accessed June 28, 2003.

Paphassarang, C., K. Philavong, B. Boupha, and E. Blas. 2002. "Equity, Privatization and Cost Recovery in Urban Health Care: The Case of Lao PDR." *Health Policy and Planning* 17 (Suppl. 1): 72–84.

Pavignani, E., and J. Durão. 1999. "Managing External Resources in Mozambique: Building New Aid Relationships on Shifting Sands?" *Health Policy and Planning* 14:243–53.

Preker, Alexander S. 2004. *Economic Sector Work Ghana*. Washington, D.C.: World Bank.

Ratanawijitrasin, S., S. B. Soumerai, and K. Weerasuriya. 2001. "Do National Medicinal Drug Policies and Essential Drug Programs Improve Drug Use? A Review of Experiences in Developing Countries." *Social Science and Medicine* 53(7): 831–44.

Schneider, P., F. Diop, and S. Bucyana. 2000. "Development and Implementation of Prepayment Schemes in Rwanda." Technical Report 45. Partnership for Health Reform, Abt Associates, Bethesda, Md.

Trap, B., E. H. Hansen, and H. V. Hogerzeil. 2002. "Prescription Habits of Dispensing and Nondispensing Doctors in Zimbabwe." *Health Policy and Planning* 17(3): 288–95.

Velasquez, G., Y. Madrid, and J. D. Quick. 1998. "Health Reform and Drug Financing: Selected Topics." DAP Series No. 6. *Health Economics and Drugs*. World Health Organization, Geneva.

Witter, S. 1996. "'Doi Moi' and Health: The Effect of Economic Reforms on the Health System in Vietnam." *International Journal of Health Planning and Management* 11(2): 159–72.

WHO (World Health Organization). 1995. "Alternative Drug Pricing Policies in the Americas. DAP Series No. 1 (WHO/DAP/95.6). *Health Economics and Drugs,* Geneva.

———. 2000. "Global Comparative Pharmaceutical Expenditures." EDM Series No. 3. *Health Economics and Drugs,* Geneva.

———. 2001. *How to Develop and Implement a National Drug Policy.* 2nd ed. Geneva.

———. 2002. On-line annex tables for *World Health Report 2002.* www.who.int/whr/2002/annex/. Accessed April 2003.

———. n.d. WHO Health System Profiles Database. Accessed April 2003 at www.who.int.

CHAPTER 15

Paying for Capital

Jon Sussex and Sandra Sosa-Rubi

Most health care systems have room for improving efficiency in the use of physical capital—particularly buildings and equipment. Efficiency incentives are often weaker in the processes by which capital is allocated and paid for than in those for use of labor, medicines, and other inputs.

Where assets are effectively donated by governments or aid organizations, health care providers have an incentive to overdemand capital investments initially and then to undermaintain them subsequently. There is also no penalty for underusing assets once procured. Wrongly located or inappropriate facilities, only partially used and poorly maintained, are the result. Such facilities provide a poor standard of care, divert resources away from where they could be used more effectively, and damage staff morale, thus weakening services further.

This chapter summarizes the principles of effective, efficient, and equitable capital financing and capital charging in health care systems and reviews the options for putting these principles into practice. Examples from international practice are provided.

THE COMMERCIAL MODEL

The size of the private sector[1] can vary between countries, from the almost negligibly small to the dominant-ownership pattern, but private hospital providers exist in most. Organizations operating in competitive markets succeed or fail by their ability to earn enough from their investments to pay for the asset base plus interest on debt and returns to equity holders on the capital they have invested. Accounting standards are enforced to ensure that lenders and shareholders are informed about the use and cost of capital. The incentive to stay in business and earn profits provides firms' managers with a strong, direct stimulus to acquire and manage capital assets efficiently. However, many health care systems lack such incentives and need explicit policies on capital investment and capital charging.

The basic commercial model of capital financing and capital charging has the following characteristics:

- Allocation of capital between activities and locations is the outcome of manifold individual business decisions. It is not planned by any central body. Allocative efficiency depends on competitive markets for the goods and services produced and efficient labor and capital markets.

- Finance is provided by private capital markets or from businesses' retained profits. Private capital markets determine the cost of capital for any given investment project according to the risk involved and the balance of capital supply and demand prevailing at the time.

- Capital charging covers both depreciation of assets and payment of a return on investment—interest, dividends, and retained profits.

Health care markets are unlike normal commercial markets, however. Rice (1998) reviews the numerous reasons for "market failure" in health care. Even in the United States, the country that most relies on private businesses operating in competitive markets to purchase and provide health care, about half of all health care expenditure is by the public sector. Governments everywhere plan and fund health care to some degree. In many places, providers of health care are also state owned. Hence, governments are closely involved in the allocation and financing of capital investment in the sector.

CAPITAL FINANCING

Public sector health care providers earn most of their revenues from public sector or "social" payers such as the country's national health service or social insurance funds. Publicly owned health care providers might, in principle, borrow from any or all of: government,[2] international lending organizations, or the private sector, with or without government guarantees that debts will be honored. In addition, capital finance may be provided in the form of grants from governments, aid organizations, and philanthropic private individuals or companies. For example:

- In Italy, public hospitals fund most major investments with grants from the national government, paying no capital charges, although a few schemes are now privately financed in part. In Germany, the regional tier of government makes the grants.

- In Ghana, hospitals receive grants from the national government, a portion of which the government borrows from (and so must repay to) international lending organizations.

- In Bulgarian public hospitals, capital investment is funded by both national and municipal government, and some of the cost of capital charges is recovered in the prices hospitals charge the National Health Insurance Fund.

- In India, private hospitals that provide public health care services borrow capital from private sources but may in addition receive grants from state government.

- Australia and the United Kingdom have mixed systems, with capital funded by both government loans and borrowing from private capital markets. The costs of both types of capital are included in the prices charged by the hospitals.

From the perspective of the health care provider, the most cost-effective source of capital finance is the one that charges the lowest rate of interest. However, this may not be the most socially desirable solution. Interest rates on government borrowing may not accurately reflect the risk involved in public sector investments. If private capital markets are efficient, one line of economic argument goes, whatever rate of interest the private sector would require to lend for a particular investment is the true cost of capital for that investment. If the government lends for the same purpose at a lower interest rate, according to this argument, it is subsidizing the loan, knowing that it can coerce future taxpayers to pay for any adverse risks that might materialize (Klein 1997). But where private capital markets are not perfectly efficient, the cost of a private loan may reflect not just risk but the ability of the lender to extract supernormal profits. Even where private capital markets are efficient, the private cost of capital may exceed the public cost by a small amount, even after proper account is taken of risk (Sussex 2001, chapter 6).

The rate of interest charged by private lenders for a public investment project depends on the extent of any government guarantees that payments to private lenders will be met. If the government guarantees that interest charges will always be paid and the principal duly repaid, there is no more risk to the lender in financing the project in question than in buying government securities, so the interest rate should be correspondingly low. But a government willing to make such a guarantee might as well lend the capital to the health care provider itself, because it gains nothing—transfers no risk—by involving the private sector and will probably have to pay higher transaction costs in doing so. If the government makes no, or only limited, guarantees to private lenders, the rate of interest will be higher, because some risk is being transferred to the private sector.

If capital is available from international lending organizations at a lower interest rate than from either government or private capital markets, then from the national perspective, this will be the most cost-effective source. If there is any implied subsidy in the interest rate being charged, the international lending organizations' funders will eventually have to pay for it.

CAPITAL CHARGING

In nearly all health care systems, the problem is to replicate the incentives and constraints that stimulate efficiency in commercial markets, so that:

- Health care providers invest the right amount of capital in the right mix of buildings and equipment.

- Finance is obtained from the most cost-effective source.

- Assets are procured, used, maintained, replaced, and disposed of efficiently.

Achieving all three objectives depends on managers being given incentives to take account of the costs, as well as the benefits, of capital investment. In many nonmarket-based health care systems that does not happen. Although it may be difficult to obtain permission from health care payers (for example, social insurance funds, local or national government) to purchase assets, permission is commonly accompanied by a grant of capital funds. The buildings and equipment purchased with the grant are effectively a "free good." No depreciation charge has to be included in the income and expenditure account. No interest has to be paid or return on the capital earned.

Once assets have been purchased, the health care provider has to find the funds to operate and maintain them. At that point, the provider may decide that it can afford to run its new facility only at less-than-full capacity, if at all. Although there is no cash or accounting cost to doing so, there is a clear opportunity cost, namely the forgone value of the use to which the resources used to create those under- or unused assets could otherwise have been put. Capital charging would make these costs obvious.

Capital charges comprise two elements, which may either be separated or combined into a single rental charge:

- *Depreciation*—the extent to which the asset is used up during a year. It is conventionally calculated on a "straight line" basis: as one n^{th} of the asset's initial value, where n is the assumed useful life of the asset in years.[3] Alternative depreciation profiles are rarely used and are not discussed here. Broadly speaking, the funds accumulated in a depreciation reserve should be sufficient to replace assets at the end of their lives.

- *The cost of capital*—the opportunity cost of not investing the funds elsewhere in the economy. The cost of capital is the return forgone from the next-best alternative investment. Because the cost of capital is related to the riskiness of the investment undertaken—the higher the risk, the higher is the expected return required by lenders—the relevant cost of capital is the marginal social return expected from investments of similar riskiness.

If health care provider managers have to include depreciation as an expense and must pay for the cost of capital, then unless they enjoy the luxury of unlimited budgets they will have the same incentive to use capital efficiently and not overinvest, as they do to use staff efficiently and not overhire. The objectives of capital charging are thus to:

- Make managers aware of the costs of using capital.

- Provide an incentive to invest in the most efficient mix of capital and labor, to maintain assets efficiently and for as long as it is appropriate to do so, and then to dispose of them in the way that maximizes their disposal value or minimizes the disposal cost.

- Aid performance management by enabling comparison of the costs of different providers.

- Establish a basis for fair competition between public and private providers—the latter cannot avoid the costs of capital and depreciation.

Where the introduction of capital charging into public sector organizations has been evaluated, it has been deemed a success at achieving some or all of the above objectives without excessive implementation and administration costs. Heald has published numerous assessments of the implementation of capital charging in the United Kingdom National Health Service since April 1991 and concludes that: "capital charging is a valuable but flawed tool, which is much better than the asset invisibility it replaced" (Heald 2000: 26). Heald and Scott (1996) quote from assessments by the management consultants Price Waterhouse in 1992 and 1993 of the New Zealand policy since July 1991 of capital charging in the public sector, and report that it had a beneficial influence on the behavior of public sector managers.

Options for the precise type of capital charging to be implemented can be selected along four dimensions. The decision about where to locate capital charging policy on any one dimension can be made independently of decisions about the other three. The following paragraphs look at each of these dimensions in turn.

NEW ASSETS OR ALL?

Capital charging can be readily applied to newly acquired assets. Their prices are known, as are the terms of any loans to finance their procurement. It is straightforward to establish prospectively an asset register and a balance sheet for all new assets acquired after a certain date and their matching debt liabilities, and to enter corresponding depreciation and interest charges in the interest and expenditure accounts. Interest and depreciation would be included in the expenditures to be recovered in the prices charged for the health services provided. The interest charges would be actual cash payments to lenders, whether government, international lending organization, or private sector. Depreciation would not be a cash charge but a cost to the income and expenditure account and would be paid into a depreciation reserve.

As old assets are replaced by new, the proportion of the health care provider's asset base for which it pays capital charges would increase. However, it would be many years before all of its assets were on the balance sheet and being depreciated and paid for out of revenues. Existing buildings can have remaining lives measured in decades. Also, because land is typically not depreciated, the opportunity cost of using land would never be accounted for, unless the health care provider relocated or expanded and had to buy new land. Thus, a (gradually declining) proportion of assets would continue to be a "free good," which managers would have little incentive to use efficiently.

A policy of applying capital charges only to new assets has two other failings. First, the performance of different providers with different mixes of old and new assets could not be compared. A provider that, when capital charging is introduced for new assets, has modern buildings and equipment will, over the coming years, need less new investment than one with older capital stock and so will face lower capital charges. Thus, the first provider will appear to have lower costs even though it uses just as many resources as the second.

Second, if publicly owned providers compete with private providers for any business, whether from public or private sector payers, the private provider will be placed at an unfair competitive disadvantage unless the public provider pays appropriate capital charges on all of its assets. Applying capital charges only to newly purchased assets would progressively reduce this unfair disadvantage but not remove it completely.

To avoid these problems, it is preferable to apply capital charges to both new and existing assets. Indeed, it is the approach adopted in the places where we have found capital charging being employed: Australia, Bulgaria, New Zealand, and the United Kingdom.

The only disadvantage is the administrative cost of the capital charging system, but this is small relative to the potential benefits from more efficient use of capital. Applying capital charging to existing as well as new assets requires all such assets to be identified and assigned a value and estimated remaining useful life over which they should be depreciated. This approach proved feasible in the United Kingdom, though with some teething problems due to software and staff-training problems, and was largely implemented a year after the policy was announced.

There may be a case for restricting capital charging to new investments in the unlikely event that the distribution of existing assets among publicly owned health care providers is equal (in both quantity and quality terms)—perhaps all existing assets are so decrepit as to be nearly worthless—and there is no competition between public and private sector providers. Otherwise it makes more sense to include both existing and new assets.

NOTIONAL VERSUS REAL CAPITAL CHARGES

Notional capital charges would suffice to meet the objective of informing managers of the costs they incur by their acquisition and retention of assets. Management accounts could be created to show the notional balance sheet and include notional depreciation and the cost of capital charges in the income and expenditure account, that is, only as memorandum items. No cash would flow between public sector "lenders" and "borrowers." A notional system would give managers information and permit comparison between providers, but it would not give them incentives to act on that information.

Real capital charges, however, would provide that incentive. They would also mean fairer competition with private providers, because public providers would then have to recover in their prices the full costs of the capital they use.

A notional capital charging system would incur the same administrative costs as a real charging system, where cash changes hands. Assets would have to be identified and valued; accounts would have to be kept. A similar input of time by skilled and senior staff would be required.

Unlike a real charging system, however, a notional system would require no working capital. In a real capital charging system, funds must initially be paid out by government, via whatever agencies it has established for purchasing health care. The element of the prices charged by the public sector providers to cover their capital charges will eventually return to the government as lender but only after a lag. Although there is no net increase in public expenditure (extra money paid out equals extra money paid back), there is a requirement for working capital because of the time lag.

The balance of pros and cons appears to favor the use of real capital charges rather than relying on a purely notional system, unless severe constraints on government finance make it difficult to supply the working capital needed in a real system. Indeed, Australia, Bulgaria,[4] New Zealand, and the United Kingdom all use real capital charges for their public hospitals.

A transition period of a few years is desirable. Time is needed for managers to become familiar with the implications of capital charging, for accounting systems to be tested, and for staff to be trained. Also, managers cannot, even if they wish to, change the mix and scale of their asset base within a year.

In the United Kingdom and New South Wales (Australia), the transition was smoothed by establishing the (real) capital charging system over a few years rather than all at once. The United Kingdom system was set up with real cash flows from day one, in April 1991. But the government managed the transition by initially giving each provider, as part of its revenues, the exact sum that it had to pay back to the government in capital charges. Thus, a provider finding itself relatively overendowed with assets was allowed, in the first year, to charge correspondingly higher prices for its health care services paid for by state-funded agencies. This financial neutrality was then progressively withdrawn until after a few years no further allowance was made for differences between providers in capital charges. The same approach was adopted by New South Wales for the introduction of "capital asset charges" in 2001/02.

TIME PROFILES OF CAPITAL CHARGES

Various depreciation profiles are possible, but health care providers have little reason to depart from the conventional straight line approach.

There are two main options for the profile of the cost of capital element of capital charges:

- An interest/dividend charge equal to a percentage of the average net, depreciated, value of the assets employed during the year. As the net value of an asset declines each year as a result of straight line depreciation, the annual interest charge, and hence the total capital charge (depreciation plus interest) also declines.

- A constant annuity.

If an asset is assumed to deliver broadly the same service throughout its life, a constant annuity is appropriate. The declining capital charge profile resulting from the first method is appropriate only if the value of the annual service provided by the asset is expected to decline, and at that particular rate, year by year. But there is in general no reason to expect this to be the case. Using the declining profile would mean that health care providers with older assets would be able to charge lower prices. When those providers eventually replace their major assets, such as buildings, their capital charges would jump up, even if they continued to produce the same volume and quality of health care services as before.

The declining profile has been used by the United Kingdom National Health Service, but the only apparent rationale for this choice is a mistaken belief that it is administratively simpler than a constant annuity and that it more closely replicates normal commercial practice. However, both options require the same information: asset value, life, and required rate of return. Administrative costs are therefore the same. Furthermore, the constant annuity option is commonly used by commercial businesses to manage their assets (Pratten 1993).

It is therefore recommended that capital charges be levied on each asset at a constant annual rate throughout the asset's life unless there are exceptional reasons to do otherwise.

ASSET VALUATION

Commercial organizations value their assets on a *historic cost* basis. The purchase price of the asset is entered onto the balance sheet. Depreciation is applied to that historic cost value, which remains unchanged whatever happens to the level of prices in the economy generally or to the price of that type of asset. Over time, given positive general price inflation, the historic cost value will increasingly understate the true value of the asset, both because the nominal price of the outputs it helps to produce is rising and because the nominal cost of eventually replacing the asset is also rising. This problem is worst for long-lived assets during periods of rapid inflation. Furthermore, in many places it will be impossible to attribute accurate historic cost values, because records of assets' original acquisition prices will not have been kept.

In Bulgaria, post-1991, asset values have been estimated for the existing assets of public hospitals and depreciation charges levied accordingly. However, the low values attributed to the assets means that the depreciation reserves being accumulated will be too small to fully fund modern replacement assets (Firestine and Tafradjiysky 2002).

It is therefore generally preferable to use some form of current cost (that is, inflation-adjusted) accounting for publicly owned assets. Determining the current values of assets is not, however, entirely straightforward.

Most major health care assets are specialized, with no significant second-hand market, although there will be one for general equipment such as computers and vehicles. Hence, it is practically impossible to determine an *open market value* in their existing use for most major health care assets. An open market value in alternative use might be obtained, for example, as if hospital buildings were to be sold for conversion to commercial or residential use. But this would be unrelated to the value of the hospital's outputs and probably only a fraction of what it would cost to replace the hospital. An open market value in alternative use is relevant only where an asset is no longer required for health care.

It is preferable to value assets at their *depreciated replacement cost*—the cost of replacing the asset, reduced to take account of how much of the asset's expected total life has been used up—unless an asset's depreciated replacement cost exceeds its *value in use*. If the value of the services derived from the asset is less than its depreciated replacement cost, that value in use is what the asset is worth unless the asset could be sold for some other purpose for a higher *net realizable value* (the sales proceeds realizable on the open market, net of selling expenses). But this is unlikely in the case of health service assets. This well-established valuation basis is expressed diagrammatically in figure 15.1.

An asset's replacement cost part way through its life can be estimated either as its initial purchase cost revalued in line with an index of the inflation in prices of such assets over the intervening period or by directly estimating the cost of building that asset today. This approach to valuation may need to be modified, however, if a modern substitute for an asset would be markedly different from the original. In that case it is desirable to use the cost of the *modern equivalent asset* as the starting point for valuation rather than the cost of replacing like with like.

The task of valuing assets may be undertaken by a government agency or by regulated private sector organizations.

FIGURE 15.1 Depreciated Replacement Cost Valuation of Assets

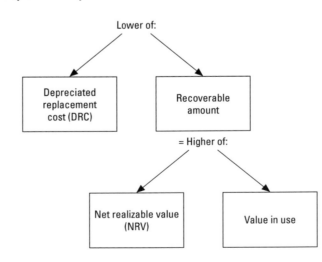

Source: Authors.

CONCLUSIONS

Finance for investment in the physical capital of health care provision may be available from government, international lending organizations, or the private sector. But whatever the source of finance, the application of capital charging for publicly owned health care providers is a practical and worthwhile measure that has the potential benefits of:

- Making managers aware of the costs of capital.
- Improving the efficiency with which capital is used and ensuring an appropriate mix of capital and labor.
- Enabling comparison of costs between providers.
- Establishing a basis for fair competition between public and private sector providers.

A range of options exists for the precise form that capital charging may take. The balance of pros and cons between these options suggests the following approach in most cases:

- Apply to existing as well as new assets.
- Use real, not just notional, capital charges but allow a transitional period.
- Use a constant annuity rather than a declining time profile of charges over an asset's life.
- Value assets on a depreciated replacement cost basis.

Although capital charging is not widespread internationally, a few countries have started to use the approach and with some success. No country has reversed the policy having once introduced it.

NOTES

1. Throughout this chapter, "private" is used to mean both commercial enterprises and voluntary, not-for-profit institutions—anything not owned by local, regional, or national governments.

2. For the purposes of this discussion no distinction is drawn between national and subnational tiers of government. The discussion is phrased in terms of borrowing from national government because subnational tiers are seldom fully self-financing—for example, from local taxes and charges—and so ultimately rely on central government.

3. Land is not usually depreciated in accounts, because in most cases it is not "used up" but should be just as available for further use in 100 years' time as it is today. An exception is where land is contaminated as a result of use, in which case the depreciation of its value should be entered as a cost in accounts.

4. In Bulgaria these are limited to depreciation charges—no other cost of capital is charged.

REFERENCES

Firestine, R., and B. Tafradjiysky. 2002. *Municipalities and Hospital Capital Spending in Bulgaria*. RTI and USAID Bulgaria Health Project. April.

Heald, D. 2000. *Capital Charging in Public Healthcare*. Aberdeen Papers in Accountancy, Finance & Management Working Paper 0016. University of Aberdeen, Department of Accountancy. http://www.abdn.ac.uk/accountancy/web_pgs/public/dept/Wps/Working_Papers.htm.

Heald, D., and D. Scott. 1996. "Assessing Capital Charging in the National Health Service." *Financial Accountability and Management* 12(3): 225–44.

Klein, M. 1997. "The Risk Premium for Evaluating Public Projects." *Oxford Review of Economic Policy* 13(4): 29–42.

Pratten, C. 1993. "Accounting for Property Assets in the Private and Public Sectors." University of Cambridge Department of Applied Economics Working Paper. September.

Rice, T. 1998. *The Economics of Health Reconsidered*. Chicago: Health Administration Press.

Sussex, J. 2001. *The Economics of the Private Finance Initiative in the NHS*. London: Office of Health Economics.

CHAPTER 16

Paying for Knowledge and Research

Dean T. Jamison

The 20th century witnessed a global transformation in human health (Jamison 1999). Chile's experience illustrates the magnitude of this transformation. By the mid-1990s Chile's per capita income had reached about US$4,000 (adjusted for purchasing power), and Chilean women had achieved a life expectancy of 79 years. A century ago, in 1900, today's high-income countries also had income levels around $4,000—and, therefore, had resources sufficient to provide their populations with adequate food, water, shelter, and sanitation. Yet, for them, female life expectancy at the time was perhaps 30 years less than it is in Chile today. Why has health improved so dramatically *after controlling for income and, hence, availability of commodities that, like food, are essential for health?* Although there can be no unambiguous answer to this question, an important factor has been advance in scientific knowledge and its application both in creating powerful interventions and in guiding behavior. Acquisition and utilization of health research and development (R&D) or its products becomes, then, an essential function of a country's health system.

Much knowledge is embodied in global public goods: once a vaccine for hepatitis B has been developed anywhere it becomes, in some sense, available everywhere. Although monopoly pricing made possible by patents may slow the diffusion of some innovations, the temporary nature of patent-induced monopoly pricing limits this effect. But an innovation's being cheap, powerful, and globally available in no way entails its global use. There indeed appears to be enormous variation in the rate at which different countries make use of knowledge and products that are globally available. A recent assessment (Jamison, Sandbu, and Wang 2004) found, for example, that the rate of "technical progress" in reducing infant mortality in 1960–90 ranged from 5 percent a year in some countries down to none at all in others.[1] While infant mortality could certainly decline somewhat from income improvements in the absence of technical progress, a 5 percent rate of technical progress would lead to a halving of the infant mortality rate in 15 years beyond whatever improvements may have resulted from gains in income and education levels. The implication is clear: globally available knowledge and products offer enormous opportunities to countries, but national policies and national health systems determine whether this knowledge is put to local use. Additionally, and importantly, some information for improving outcomes is local and must be locally produced.

This chapter discusses acquisition of knowledge as an important function of national health systems.[2] Hence, in the nomenclature of this volume, resource allocation and purchasing (RAP) for R&D are important policy issues. The chapter will use the term "acquisition" rather than "purchasing" for the most part because of its more general connotation. That said, most of the issues discussed in chapter 1 concerning agency and organization that are important for RAP in general are likewise important with respect to R&D.

This chapter is organized into two main sections. The first discusses main topics that R&D needs to address. The second has sections on the role of the government that deal with areas of knowledge that governments should both pay for and produce; areas that governments should pay for but purchase externally; and, finally, areas that governments should neither pay for nor produce but should encourage, for example, by creating intellectual property or by investing in R&D capacity. The perspective throughout is that RAP policies need to be informed by the particular character of knowledge as a commodity: major fixed production costs leading to a need to focus effort. Nevertheless, although published knowledge can be considered freely available, there are genuine barriers to the diffusion and use of knowledge that RAP policies—institutional designs— need to address.

PRIORITY AREAS FOR R&D

In 1996, the World Health Organization's Ad Hoc Committee on Health Research Relating to Future Intervention Options published the report of its deliberations.[3] The committee proposed creation of a mechanism, now institutionalized as the Global Forum for Health Research, which provides annual updates of the status and directions of health R&D for developing countries. The priority areas identified by the committee (Ad Hoc Committee 1996) have been broadly followed by the forum and may be summarized as observing that four challenges to health systems will remain important for decades to come and, hence, that specific R&D initiatives would contribute significantly to meeting these challenges. These challenges are the unfinished agenda, the continually changing nature of microbial threats, epidemics of noncommunicable diseases and injury, and the efficiency and fairness of health systems themselves.

- *The unfinished agenda.* Despite progress, there remains a huge and unnecessary burden of infectious disease among the poor that can be addressed with available cost-effective interventions. Addressing this unfinished agenda is mostly a matter of political will and (modest) commitment of resources. This unfinished agenda relates closely to the Millennium Development Goals (MDGs) for health and emphasizes the priority needs of those in poverty. R&D can help through operational and behavioral research to facilitate implementation (often by developing and evaluating linked packages of care, such as integrated management of childhood illnesses) and by selective development of new tools, including improvements in vaccines.

- *Continually changing microbial threats.* A more global class of challenges results from the continually changing nature of microbial threats. New pathogens— such as human immunodeficiency virus—and evolution of drug-resistant variants of familiar ones (for example,, ones causing tuberculosis and malaria) create needs for biomedical understanding, for understanding systemic determinants of the spread of drug resistance, and for new drugs and vaccines.

- *Noncommunicable diseases and injury.* Low- and middle-income countries increasingly face major (and hitherto neglected) epidemics of noncommunicable diseases and injury. Selected psychiatric conditions, heart disease, stroke, and road-traffic accidents dominate the disease profile projected for these countries for the year 2020. R&D is required to ascertain ways of preventing and managing these conditions under budgetary constraints far more stringent than in the high-income countries, which have dealt with the problems far longer.

- *Efficiency and fairness of health systems.* Finally, health systems themselves vary greatly in how efficiently and equitably they provide services. Research can assist decisionmakers in solving specific problems, learning from the experience of others, and placing the performance and characteristics of their systems into international and historical context. Such research should pay careful attention to measurement of performance and should include investigation into health systems and their finance, the determinants of the behavior of health care providers and the behavior of individuals and households.

RAP FOR R&D

In some cases, additional resources (probably from lower priority areas within national health budgets or health aid budgets) will be required to meet these R&D needs adequately. In many cases, institutional change will be necessary to create the information and incentives required for efficient RAP. At the international level, resource allocation has often lacked focus (resulting in failure to bring results to the point of application) and has neglected important conditions and issues while providing (relatively) generously for less important ones. Reform is needed. Successful models of competitively driven international funding (and experience-sharing) networks should be applied to currently neglected clusters of conditions.

The conduct of research and development in low- and middle-income countries is commonly hampered by brain drain to the richer nations. For those who remain, there are considerable problems at the operational level that RAP policies must address. We summarize them here.

Just as the quality and productivity of research efforts vary dramatically from one institution to another within the established market economies, they vary in the low- and middle-income countries. Exemplary work is done in a number of institutions and countries; but, in general, the obstacles to high quality are greater when countries' incomes are lower. Inadequate training, insufficient staff motivation, and lack of competition prevent many institutions from attaining their potential. The instability of short-term funding, isolation from peers, and poor access to the research literature all compound the problem and prevent researchers from responding rapidly to ever-changing demands. Salaries are generally poor; rewards to productivity are hampered by nonmerit considerations in the appointment and promotion of senior staff and by restrictive personnel policies. Core support for the maintenance of libraries, databases, equipment, and buildings is inadequate, and communication between scientists at the regional and international levels is difficult. Recent communications improvements resulting from electronic mail and distance learning programs have so far benefited mainly those who are already internationally networked, not those who are most isolated.

The basic cell of research is a laboratory or unit headed by a senior scientist, with each research institute or university employing a number of senior scientists. A department or institute's interests will tend to be multidisciplinary, while each basic cell will focus on one discipline or a small set of closely related ones. Crucial to the success of research is the ability to respond quickly to change—both at the level of the cell and the institute as a whole. The basic cell must respond by acquiring new technologies and skills; the institute must respond by acquiring new or more developed disciplines. In the public sector at least, this ability to respond is continually compromised by the very nature of the mechanisms that fund R&D. Governments usually provide basic core funding for R&D institutes, and their civil service personnel policies tend to push research institutions too heavily toward management structures that lack accountability, thereby creating institutions that become unproductive and unable to respond to new challenges. Over time, salaries often devour core budgets, reducing maneuverability still further. To overcome the structural weaknesses in institutions, network centers of the type described above have evolved in some countries.

Lessons Learned for Institutional Development

Individual teams, institutions, and programs have demonstrated that it is possible to do first-rate research in low- and middle-income countries. Their experience and advice have been well documented elsewhere (see, for example, the interviews with individual leading researchers in TDR 1995). Specific RAP policies seem likely to facilitate the success of institutions and programs, including the following:

- Autonomous management

- Appropriate compensation policies that will attract young and talented scientists

- The capacity to train a large number of individuals from whom subsequent leaders can emerge

- A large enough number to allow for transfer to other sectors and other losses

- Stable core funding

- A significant element of competitive funding that might be allocated to research projects, or to individual development, or to institutional development

- Internationalization and collaboration not only with institutions in the north but also with other institutions in the south

- Increased use of electronic media for peer review and publication as a first step toward reducing the regional bias in established publishing formats.

Investors and institutions could take a number of steps to make these factors more widespread. More institutions in low- and middle-income countries should be freed from civil service management procedures, as is happening already in other government-funded institutions worldwide. This step would enable institutions to offer salary scales that will give them a competitive advantage and begin to combat the brain drain. To secure good staff, institutions should be enabled to recruit by active search and on the basis of peer-reviewed competition. Some—and possibly many—national governments will conclude that the financial, administrative, and even political costs of these steps exceed their benefits. This may be a reasonable choice, but it creates an environment where science is unlikely to flourish and where competition for international support is unlikely to be effective.

Institutions are more likely to succeed if they receive stable core funding, but also if a proportion of their work is funded competitively. They may decide to support some extramural work, set up collaborative networks with an element of competition, or develop internal competition mechanisms. Some institutions such as the Oswaldo Cruz Foundation in Brazil have already moved in these directions with great success, for example, by freeing up intramural resources for competitive allocation between groups and within the institution, with assessments being made by an external review group. There have also been notable successes with the formation of networks such as the International Clinical Epidemiology Network and, more recently, the Global Forum for Health Research.

High-quality research increasingly depends on international collaboration, and almost no institution can now perform effectively without an international element. Institutions should therefore expect that some of their staff will be foreign nationals, although restrictive policies in some countries may, at present, prevent this. Where foreigners may not be employed, it is at least preferable for the scientific advisory board of the institution to contain some international representation. Staff should be enabled to participate in international fellowship schemes, exchanges, and other mechanisms that foster long-term links and enhance the capacity of reciprocating institutions.

Private Sector Involvement

The contribution of the private sector to health research, in the traditional pharmaceuticals (drugs, vaccines, diagnostics, devices) industries, and in a growing list of other health products such as health education materials, has been highly significant in recent decades. Public sector requirements for new product development are dependent on industry for many reasons, including the industry's expertise in development, its efficiency as a manufacturer and distributor, its knowledge and skills in market research and, not least, its financial power. Officials in a number of countries are exploring the ethics and potential of new collaborative ventures between the private and public sectors, and their efforts may bring significant new funding sources to address unmet health needs.[4] For the present, however, both private and public sectors recognize that the health problems of the world's poorest are neglected by industry. The problem is more acute in relation to pharmaceutical products, and we shall focus on them here.

As a result of these limitations on what can be expected from the private sector, national and international research programs in the public sector (with support from the private foundations) have increasingly accepted that they must take some responsibility for researching and developing products themselves, through new mechanisms of collaboration with industry. At the same time, the pharmaceutical industry is itself adapting to recession and other factors to turn itself more into an integrated organizational framework that is comparable to some of the international R&D programs financed by the public sector. This is partly because of the growing interdependence of different types of skill and capacity in the industry, as, for example, in the relationships between the small biotechnology companies and the larger, more stably resourced, pharmaceutical companies. The industry increasingly contracts out its research and manufacturing components, locating each component in the most economically and technically suitable place rather like an assembly industry. The increasing integration has been described as a move toward an "extended family" network and offers major opportunities for developing country participation in private sector R&D.

The failure of current incentive structures to produce health products for the lowest income groups demands remedial action. In essence, the public sector must either harness the skills, energy, and capacity of the private sector to develop and bring promptly to market products for the lowest income groups, or it must take responsibility for doing so itself. In reality, a combination of the two is likely. Public sector RAP policies may engage the private sector in each of the following ways:

- By supporting the costs of the early stages of product development, from compound screening through to phase II trials, if necessary, and offering to support postmarketing surveillance.

- By providing the industry with detailed analyses of the potential market and of the risks and benefits of introducing a product.

- By providing the industry with guaranteed markets for new products such as vaccines. In such schemes, national governments agree to purchase a known quantity of a specified product, raising the financing either from their national budget or through special loans. The up-front investments needed for successful collaborations of this type must be large.

- By streamlining the regulatory controls imposed by the public sector on the industry to the minimum necessary for good standards, in order to cut the industry's costs.

- By carefully designed tax-relief schemes.

- By financial incentives within the patent system. A number of attempts to modify the patent system have been attempted, such as the Orphan Drug Act of 1983 in the United States. This gives companies tax breaks and lengthened exclusivity rights for drugs with small markets, creating strong incentives where there are third-party reimbursement mechanisms that are relatively insensitive to cost. However, the act has not reversed the downward trend in R&D on drugs for diseases that are prevalent in demographically developing countries, and further extension of the period of patent protection—beyond the 20 years recently internationally agreed in the Uruguay Round—is unlikely to substantially affect incentives, pointing to the need for additional mechanisms.

- By making the best use of the extraordinary commitment of individuals and particular companies within the private sector. Some have already demonstrated themselves willing to undertake research and development, production, and supply of drugs on a break-even or defined-profit basis; more may be encouraged to do so. The example of some individuals is clear. For example, Jonas Salk, when asked who owned the patent on his polio vaccine, answered: "Well, the people, I guess. There is no patent. Could you patent the sun?" Salk believed that public goods should be common property for all time. There is certainly a major role for patents among the RAP instruments designed to stimulate innovation. Yet the spirit that Salk conveys—of personal or corporate commitment—represents an important additional resource to draw upon. Likewise, innovation at public expense, even if in the private sector, requires an important reduction in unrestricted patent rights, as, for example, through guaranteeing relatively low prices to public sector buyers.

Developing countries that participate in private sector innovation—typically with their own institutions as subcontractors, but not entirely so—will be positioned to more quickly learn about and have access to the technical progress that is critically important to driving improvements in health.

NOTES

1. Technical progress was defined in this study, as in the literature on economic growth, as an unexplained residual. In the cited study, technical progress was the rate of infant mortality decline after controlling for improvements in levels of education and income and increases in physician availability. Hence, technical progress encompasses increased utilization of better drugs and vaccines, diffusion of knowledge to guide individual behavior, and, potentially, better ways of organizing health systems.

2. Most discussions of health system development neglect the role of R&D; the World Health Organization (1999) is an exception.

3. Much of the material in this and the following section was drawn, with only minor modification and updating, from the report of the Ad Hoc Committee (which was chaired by the author of this chapter.)

4. Two good examples of public-private partnerships (the "PPPs") are the International AIDS Vaccine Initiative and the Medicines for Malaria Venture.

REFERENCES

Ad Hoc Committee on Health Research Relating to Future Intervention Options. 1996. *Summary of Investing in Health Research and Development.* Document TDR/Gen/96.2. Geneva: World Health Organization.

Jamison, Dean T. 1999. "Health and Development in the 20th Century." In Dean T. Jamison, Andrew Creese, and Thomson Prentice, and others, *The World Health Report 1999: Making a Difference.* Geneva: World Health Organization.

Jamison, Dean T., Martin Sandbu, and Jia Wang. 2004. "Why Has Infant Mortality Decreased at Such Different Rates in Different Countries?" Working Paper 21, Disease Control Priorities Project. Fogarty International Center, National Institutes of Health, Bethesda, Md.

TDR (UNDP, World Bank, World Health Organization Special Programme for Research and Training in Tropical Diseases). 1995. *Tropical Disease Research: Twenty Years of Progress.* Twelfth Programme Report. Geneva: World Health Organization.

World Health Organization. 1999. *Making a Difference: World Health Report, 1999.* Chapter 3. Geneva.

CHAPTER 17

Using Resource Profiles

Anders Anell

Health care delivery entails combining many resource inputs to provide a mix of services that will satisfy overall objectives and priorities. This sounds simple, but it is not, for a number of reasons. First, providers have to respond to an extraordinary array of immediate health problems. Second, health care relies heavily on human resources, and the quality of care ultimately depends on their skills, training, and motivation. Thus, investments in facilities and equipment have to be balanced against investments in human capital—education and training. Third, the financial resources that pay for health care are often collected and pooled by a third party not directly involved in providing care. This third party could be a ministry or central board of health, a provincial government, a not-for-profit sickness fund, or a commercial insurance company. While each approach is quite different, they all depend on the third party to act as a "good agent" on behalf of individuals in buying services from various providers. Fourth, good health has become close to a right in modern society, raising the question, with ever expanding possibilities to treat and prevent bad health: How should priorities be set and implemented?

The need to overcome the challenges of resource allocation in health care is greatest among middle- and especially low-income countries. Health care delivery in low-income countries is confronted by a nearly bottomless pit of health problems and extreme shortages of physicians, trained nurses, medicines, and equipment. The importance of balancing and promoting efficient use of available resources is clear, and so, too, are the negative consequences in terms of life years lost if this objective is not met. In practice, however, problems of inefficiency seem to be more pronounced in low-income countries (World Health Organization [WHO] 2000). Working morale is often low owing to inadequate pay and poor working conditions. Facilities and equipment are often not fully operational because capital investments and recurrent costs are poorly balanced. Institutions that promote accountability for overall objectives and transparency of actual resource allocations are usually weak.

In this chapter, data and resource profiles from selected low- and middle-income African and Latin American countries are presented to illustrate the importance of a multidimensional approach for the measurement and monitoring of health care resources.

CLASSIFICATION OF RESOURCES AND TYPICAL IMBALANCES

Reinhardt (1998) highlights the importance of distinguishing between the management of real health care resources (personnel, equipment, pharmaceuticals, and other real resource inputs) and the money transfer that these real resources receive from the rest of society. Anell and Willis (2000), borrowing this logic, develop a simple classification of different types of real and monetary resources. They also discuss the dynamic link between real and monetary resources and interdependencies across different types of real resources using data from six high-income countries.

In this chapter, the same type of analysis is extended to two groups of low- and middle-income countries. Although income is much lower, the principal problem of resource allocation is the same. First, resources from society should be allocated to health care as long as the marginal value of health services is greater than the value of resources in alternative uses. Second, resources within the health care systems should be allocated across different types of services and resource inputs so that their marginal value is equalized and output thereby maximized. The appropriate mix of resources will vary across health care systems, depending on availability of resources, relative prices of different resource inputs, and the nature of health problems to be solved. Low-income countries can afford only a minimum of advanced health care technologies, for example, patented drugs and expensive diagnostic equipment, because the prices of these inputs are very high compared with the price of, for example, consumables or drugs produced in the domestic market.

In practice, imbalances between different types of services and resource inputs seem to be the rule rather than the exception. This is equally true for high-, middle-, and low-income countries. Focusing on conditions in low- and middle-income countries, some typical problems are highlighted below.

The Influence of Past Investment Patterns

Resource allocation in health care is often heavily influenced by past investments in physical infrastructure and human resources. There are numerous reports of a persistent gap between the existing and preferred structure of resource allocation (WHO 2000). Too much has been invested in secondary hospital services and too little in primary health care and public health programs. Additional imbalances in health care resources usually exist between urban and rural areas.

Investments and Recurrent Costs

Investments in highly visible physical infrastructure have often been made with little regard to cost-effectiveness and the possibility of covering operation and maintenance costs. To make matters worse, multi- or bilateral agencies have often supported these investments (Lee 1998).

Difficulties in Adjusting to Medical and Technological Advances

The optimal mix of resource inputs is strongly linked to the availability of effective health care interventions (Weisbrod 1991). A new effective intervention within a specific disease area may completely alter the need for different types of resources. The fast progress of knowledge related to diseases and health care interventions implies that providers need to adapt continuously to new options and demands. In practice, health care systems are often slow to restructure services, facilities, and human resources to reflect technological advances.

Human Resource Problems

A well-balanced mix of different types of trained personnel is needed so that individuals, and all human resources, can perform at their best. In practice, both low- and middle-income countries often experience shortages of skilled human resources devoted to health care, especially in the public sector. Inadequate pay and poor working conditions are frequently reported problems in low-income countries (Berckmans 1999), suggesting resource imbalances. Imbalances that have a negative effect on working conditions are particularly problematic, because they affect not only the present performance of the health care system but also possibilities for attracting future human resources.

Shifting investment and purchasing patterns to favor an equitable distribution of cost-effective and essential services will no doubt encounter difficulty. Available resource inputs are usually not balanced toward this end. Specific interventions may be needed to increase or decrease intake for selected educational programs and create new programs to train health professionals, matching the curricula to specific functional needs. The same adjustment process applies for other types of resources. Correctly allocating resource inputs therefore requires not only data about actual resource levels, but also a set of references that can indicate whether there is "too much" or "too little" of each type of input. Since the correct level is hard to determine, a practical alternative is to compare present levels of resources with those in other countries with similar income levels. In the following sections, resource profiles from a selection of low- and middle-income countries are presented to illustrate an approach that may meet this objective.

DATA

Data have been compiled for a group of low- and middle-income countries. Burkina Faso, Malawi, Mali, Niger, and Tanzania are the low-income African countries. The Dominican Republic, Ecuador, El Salvador, Guatemala, and Peru are the middle-income Latin American countries. Selections were based on region, similar income levels (World Bank classification), and availability of data.

Countries in the two groups face similar and difficult conditions for allocating resources in health care but are heterogeneous in other dimensions such as political and socioeconomic context, demography, health problems, and organization of health care financing and delivery.

Data collection was problematic for all countries studied, particularly for the African group. As in many other low- and middle-income countries, African households pay a large proportion of health care expenditures directly to providers, and public expenditures in different forms are supplemented by donor contributions. This mix of financing sources makes the analysis of total health care expenditures more difficult, and estimates of private expenditure often require expensive household surveys. Moreover, records of real resource use are generally scarce and often outdated or of questionable validity. In this chapter, easily available data from World Bank and WHO databases were used. The reader should bear in mind that the principal aim is to illustrate an approach to resource measurement, not to make definitive statements about differences across the countries.

For the Latin American group, the analysis is limited to six variables representing both monetary and real resource measures (table 17.1). The three monetary measures are health care expenditures as a proportion of gross domestic product (GDP), total health care expenditures per capita, and public health care expenditures per capita. The three real measures are physicians, nurses, and beds per capita. Reliable data for nurses per capita were not available for the African group, so the analysis is limited to the other five variables (table 17.2).

CONSTRUCTION OF HEALTH CARE RESOURCE PROFILES

A desirable feature of expenditure data is that measures of resource use are condensed into a single number. Simultaneous comparison of an array of different resource measures, such as those presented in tables 17.1 and 17.2, is more

TABLE 17.1   Selected Health Care Expenditures and Resource Measures in Five Middle-Income Latin American Countries

Expenditure/measure	Dominican Republic	Ecuador	El Salvador	Guatemala	Peru
Expenditures (percentage of gross domestic product)	6.5	3.6	8.3	4.4	4.4
Expenditures per capita, 1998 (in international dollars)	240	119	343	168	197
Public expenditures per capita, 1998 (in international dollars)	68	55	146	80	112
Physicians per 100,000 people, ca. 1997	215.6	169.6	107.1	93.3	93.2
Nurses per 100,000 people, ca. 1997	29.9	70.1	34.9	27	115.2
Beds per 1,000 people, ca. 1995	2	1.6	0.8	1.1	1.3

Sources: WHO 2001, Annex Table 5, 2002; Pan American Health Organization (PAHO) 1998.

**TABLE 17.2   Selected Health Care Expenditures and Resource Measures
in Five Low-Income African Countries**

Expenditure/measure	Burkina Faso	Malawi	Mali	Niger	Tanzania
Expenditures, 1998 (percentage of gross domestic product)	4.1	6.3	4.3	2.6	3.0
Expenditures per capita, 1998 (current U.S. dollars)	9	11	11	5	8
Public expenditures, 1998 (percentage of gross domestic product)	1.3	2.8	2.1	1.2	1.3
Physicians per 100,000 people, 1993–98	3.8	*2.8*	6.3	3.3	4.1
Beds per 1,000 people, 1992–98	1.4	1.3	0.2	0.1	*0.9*

Note: Data *italics* are older than 1995.
Source: Health, Nutrition, and Population Stats, World Bank 2002.

demanding. Spider-web diagrams can facilitate increased understanding, however, by summarizing information in a graphical format.

Based on the data in tables 17.1 and 17.2, spider-web diagrams for the two
country groups were constructed (figures 17.1 and 17.2). To facilitate intragroup
comparison, the data are normalized to the maximum value for the group. For
example, El Salvador spent the highest proportion of GDP on health care (8.3
percent) so the value for El Salvador in this category was set to 1.00, the
"resource frontier." The value for Ecuador, for example, was then calculated to
3.6/8.3, namely 0.43.

The resource frontier in no way reflects best practice or the preferred position.
The procedure is intended only to provide information about the relative importance of different types of resources for a single country in comparison with the
maximum for a defined group of countries. This approach is used as a second-
best alternative, because information about "right" levels is usually not available. The definition of the resource frontier thereby heavily depends on the
selection of countries and will possibly change as new countries are added to the
group or as existing ones are omitted.

Resource Profiles for Five Middle-Income Latin American Countries

The health care resource profiles for the Dominican Republic, Ecuador, El Salvador, Guatemala, and Peru are presented in figure 17.1a–e, respectively. Several
interesting features can be noted. For example, while El Salvador defines the
resource frontier for all the expenditure measures, the underlying real resources
(physicians, nurses, and beds per capita) are lower than in the other four countries. In terms of real resources, El Salvador is similar to Guatemala, which operates
its health care system with considerably less transfer of purchasing power from the
society. In a previous National Health Accounts study it was noted that a high percentage of public health care spending in El Salvador went to labor compensation
and operating expenditures of facilities (Partnership for Health Reform 1998).

**FIGURE 17.1a–e   Selected Health Care Expenditures and Resource Measures
for Five Middle-Income Latin American Countries**

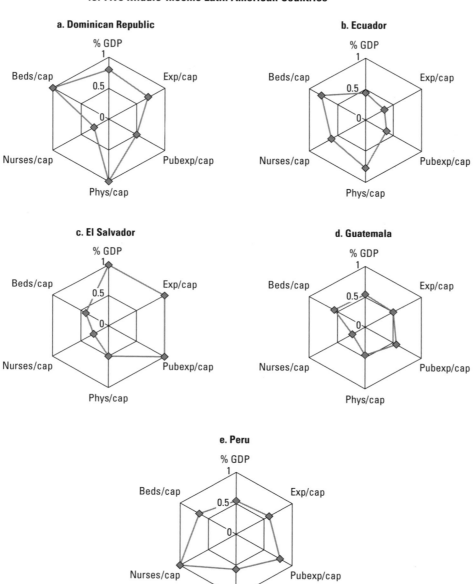

%GDP = health care expenditures as a percentage of gross domestic product; Exp/cap = health care expenditures per capita in
international dollars; Pub%GDP = public health care expenditures as a percentage of gross domestic product; Phys/cap =
physicians per capita; Beds/cap = beds per capita.
Note: Data are for 1997, or latest available data, normalized by the group maximum (see text).
Source: Calculations from data in table 17.1.

All countries in the group rely heavily on private, out-of-pocket funding for health care. Reliance on private funding is particularly striking in the Dominican Republic, 72 percent private, compared with 57 percent in El Salvador, 54 percent in Ecuador, 52 percent in Guatemala, and 43 percent in Peru (calculated from table 17.1). The relatively high use of private funding can also be seen in the resources profiles, as "exp/cap" (total expenditures per capita) for the Dominican Republic is closer to the resource frontier than the "pubexp/cap" (public expenditure per capita). The converse is true of Peru with its relatively high use of public funding. The Dominican Republic and Peru display completely different patterns in terms of real resources. The Dominican Republic has more physicians and beds per capita, while Peru has more nurses. In fact, these two countries define the resource frontier for these three real resource measures. This pattern of resource use is quite possibly related to the private–public mix in funding. Private, for-profit services have grown rapidly in the Dominican Republic, and surveys among users report a favorable opinion of private services in comparison with public facilities (PAHO 1998: 235). Nearly one third of the poorest citizens of the Dominican Republic are reported to use private clinics (Partnership for Health Reform 1998). The combination of an expanding economy, low public funding, and lack of trust in the public health system seems to have encouraged private purchasing power to favor physicians providing curative services.

In all five countries, the availability of resources varies across urban and rural areas. In Guatemala, 80 percent of physicians, 56 percent of professional nurses, and 50 percent of nursing aides are located in the metropolitan region, while 65 percent of the population lives in rural areas (PAHO 1998: 302). The availability of physicians in the metropolitan region, in fact, is about three times higher than the average number reported in profile b, figure 17.1. The same pattern is reported for Ecuador, with about twice as many physicians per capita in the mountains than in the Amazon region (PAHO 1998: 255). Also in the Dominican Republic, El Salvador, and Peru, there are wide variations in available resources across regions, to the detriment of rural and less-developed areas with a higher proportion of poor people. Separate resource profiles for different regions within countries could be used to summarize the existence and size of such variances.

Resource Profiles for Five Low-Income African Countries

Health care resource profiles for Burkina Faso, Malawi, Mali, Niger, and Tanzania are presented in figure 17.2a–e. Profiles are simpler than the profiles for the Latin American countries, because data for nurses per capita could not be found for the group. Furthermore, some of the data used are fairly old (marked in table 17.2), and the reported number of beds per capita in both Mali and Niger seem unreasonably low in comparison with the levels in Burkina Faso, Malawi, and Tanzania. These data problems also mean that it is more difficult to compare profiles and explore potential explanations for differences. Gaps in the availability of health care systems data for low-income African countries have been noted

FIGURE 17.2a–e   Selected Health Care Expenditures and Resource Measures for Five Low-Income African Countries

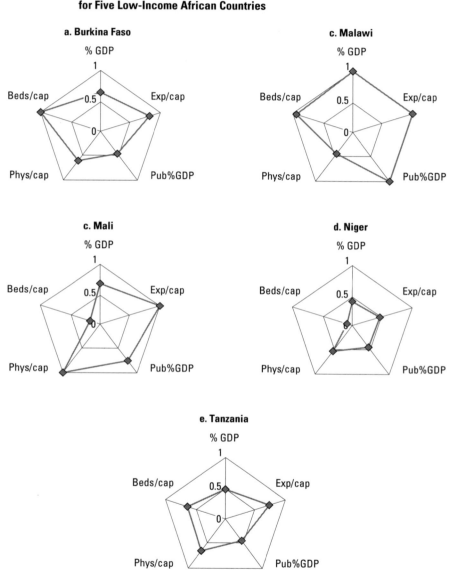

%GDP = health care expenditures as a percentage of gross domestic product; Exp/cap = health care expenditures per capita in international dollars; Pub%GDP = public health care expenditures as a percentage of gross domestic product; Phys/cap = physicians per capita; Beds/cap = beds per capita.
Note: Data are for 1998, or latest available data, normalized by the group maximum (see text).
Source: Calculations from data in table 17.2.

elsewhere (Peters and others 2000) and hinder not only comparison of resource profiles but also improvement in the management of the health care sector.

Like the Latin American countries, the five African countries also report wide differences in resource use. Similar to conditions in the Latin American countries, the dependence on private funding is high, although there is considerable variation. For instance, Burkina Faso is more dependent on private funding than the other four. A major difference between the two country groups is that the selected low-income African countries operate at resource levels that are significantly lower than in the middle-income Latin American group. All countries in the African group are also associated with economic slowdown, falling life expectancy, extremely poor living conditions for a majority of the population, and severe shortages of health professionals, drugs, and other supplies.

Three different countries define the resource frontier for the group of African countries: Malawi for "%GDP" (total health care expenditures as a percentage of GDP) and "pub%GDP" (public health care expenditures as a percentage of GDP); Malawi together with Mali for "exp/cap" (total health care expenditures per capita); Mali for "phys/cap" (physicians per capita); and Burkina Faso for "beds/cap" (beds per capita). Tanzania and especially Niger operate at a lower level of resource use on all five measures. For Burkina Faso, Malawi, and Mali, the relative importance of different types of resources is mixed. Malawi reports higher expenditures than the other four countries in the group, but a fairly low concentration of physicians. Malawi's public spending on health has historically been high relative to other Sub-Saharan countries and countries elsewhere with comparable GDP per capita (Picazo 2002). For Mali, the reported number of beds per capita is very low (as in Niger) and may be associated with poor availability and accuracy of data.

An uncertain link between health spending measures and outputs of health services for African countries was noted in a previous study. In comparing high-, middle-, and low-income African countries, McCarthy and Wolf (2001) found a positive association between spending levels and output measures defined by access and immunization rates. But the link was found to be unstable, and some low-income countries outperformed some middle-income countries with lower spending levels but higher access and immunization rates. These results further highlight the importance of managing not only health expenditures, but also the mix of real resources, in order to reach an optimal performance in terms of health output and outcome.

DISCUSSION

The annual purchasing power transferred from society to finance the provision of health care is an important determinant of the output and performance in the health care sector. The link between health expenditures, output, and performance is far from straightforward, however, and depends greatly on incentives and the management of real resources. The measurement of health care resources should consequently not only focus on patterns of expenditures, but also identify the levels and use of real resources such as physicians, nurses, beds, facilities, and health care technology.

Construction and comparison of resource profiles may be seen as a supplement to national health accounts and their main purpose as to facilitate the identification of potential imbalances across resource inputs. While resource profiles do not provide normative answers to questions about the optimal mix of resource inputs, they may identify relevant questions that should be analyzed in greater detail. They also highlight the fact that management of expenditures cannot replace management of the dynamic link between expenditures, real resources, and, ultimately, performance.

In a simple illustration using data from two groups of low- and middle-income countries, wide variances in resource use were detected and several issues for further analysis identified. Alternative approaches include comparison of resource profiles across regions in a specific country or longitudinal comparison within a specific country or region. The profiles can also be further developed and refined. Potentially fruitful directions include development of additional real resource measures of particular relevance for low- and middle-income countries or inclusion of data on output and performance.

Although resource profiles may facilitate the identification and enhanced understanding of existing and potential problems of imbalances, other interventions are needed to prevent or to overcome problems. The vested interests created by past investment and resource allocation patterns are probably the most important obstacle when implementing new directions for investment and purchasing. Past policies, including rigid budget-line thinking and separate planning for investments, recurrent costs, and human resources, need to be replaced by a strong commitment to cost-effectiveness and other explicitly defined objectives that guide decisions on what services to fund. If purchasers limit their funding to essential and cost-effective health services, an important signal will be sent to providers of services that they must organize their activities and balance their resource inputs accordingly.

REFERENCES

Anell, A., and M. Willis. 2000. "International Comparison of Health Care Systems Using Resource Profiles." *Bulletin of the World Health Organization* 78(6): 770–78.

Berckmans, P. 1999. *Initial Evaluation of Human Resources for Health in 40 African Countries.* Geneva: World Health Organization, Department of Organization of Health Services Delivery.

Lee, K. 1998. "Symptoms, Causes and Proposed Solutions." In B. Abel-Smith and A. Creese, eds., *Recurrent Costs in the Health Sector: Problems and Policy Options in Three Countries.* Document WHO/SHS/NHP/89.8. Geneva: World Health Organization.

McCarthy, F. D., and H. Wolf. 2001. "Comparative Life Expectancy in Africa." Policy Research Working Paper 2668. World Bank, Development Research Group, Public Service Delivery, Washington, D.C.

PAHO (Pan American Health Organization). 1998. *Health in the Americas,* vol. 2. Washington, D.C.

Partnership for Health Reform. 1998. "National Health Accounts: Summaries of Eight National Studies in Latin American and the Caribbean." Special Initiatives Report No. 7. Abt Associates Inc., Partnership for Health Reform, Bethesda, Md.

Peters, D. H., A. E. Elmendorf, K. Kandola, and G. Chellaraj. 2000. "Benchmarks for Health Expenditures, Services and Outcomes in Africa during the 1990s." *Bulletin of the World Health Organization* 78(6): 761–69.

Picazo, O. F. 2002. "Better Health Outcomes from Limited Resources: Focusing on Priority Setting in Malawi." Africa Region Human Development Working Paper Series. World Bank, Africa Region, Human Development Sector, Washington, D.C.

Reinhardt, U. E. 1998. *Accountable Health Care: Is It Compatible with Social Solidarity?* London: Office of Health Economics.

Weisbrod, B. A. 1991. "The Health Care Quadrilemma: An Essay on Technological Change, Insurance, Quality of Care, and Cost Containment." *Journal of Economic Literature* 24: 523–52.

WHO (World Health Organization). 2000. *The World Health Report. 2000. Health Systems: Improving Performance.* Geneva.

———. 2002. "Estimates of Health Personnel around 1998." Geneva. www.who.int/whosis.

World Bank. 2002. HNP Population Statistics. Washington, D.C. http://devdata.worldbank.org/hnpstats.

PART V

Supply, Demand, and Markets

CHAPTER 18

Single-Payer Health Insurance Systems: What Are the Advantages?

Gerard F. Anderson and Peter Sotir Hussey

Most countries have health insurance systems to protect their people against the financial risks of illness and to help them obtain appropriate medical and preventive care. All health insurance systems have mechanisms for collecting and pooling revenues, spreading risk, and purchasing health services. The way the health insurance system is organized profoundly affects the equity, efficiency, and organization of the health care delivery system.

Health insurance systems have been broadly classified into two groups, based on the number of insurance pools:

- *Single-payer systems.* In single-payer systems, one organization—typically the government—collects and pools revenues and purchases health services for the entire population. All citizens are included within a single risk pool. Single-payer insurers have monopsony power in purchasing health services.

- *Multiple-payer systems.* In multiple-payer systems, several different organizations perform all four functions for specific segments of the population. Their pools of insureds have potentially different health risks, and consumers can choose their own insurer.

This chapter briefly compares single-payer and multiple-payer systems and then concentrates on the organization and operation of single-payer health insurance systems. Single-payer systems can be classified into four generic models: regional private, regional public, central private, and central public. These models differ in the extent of centralization of financing and administration (regional or central) and in the ownership of health care providers (mainly public or mainly private). The locus of financing and administration affects the way revenues are generated, benefits are determined, and the system is regulated. The ownership of health care providers affects the purchasing relationship between insurers and providers. These differences are summarized in table 18.1.

DIFFERENCES BETWEEN SINGLE- AND MULTIPLE-PAYER SYSTEMS

This section focuses on four interrelated topics:

- *Revenue collection,* the process of collecting health revenues through taxation, premiums, out-of-pocket payments, or other methods

TABLE 18.1   Single-Payer Health Insurance Systems, Four Models

Model	Financing and administration	Provider ownership	Country example
Regional private	Decentralized	Mainly private	Canada
Regional public	Decentralized	Mainly public	Sweden
Central private	Centralized	Mainly private	Taiwan, China
Central public	Centralized	Mainly public	United Kingdom

Source: Author's compilation.

- *Risk pooling,* the aggregation of health insurance revenues for groups of individuals to protect individuals from the full cost of health care in the event of illness or injury

- *Purchasing,* the system by which insurers procure health services from providers for their beneficiaries

- *Social solidarity,* the sense of unity, interdependence, and community among members of a society that can be affected by mutual participation in a health insurance system.

Three other topics are also discussed for which there may be differences between single- and multiple-payer systems: provision of public health, incentives for innovation, and administrative costs.

Revenue Collection

Revenue collection is a primary function of health insurance. The organization of the insurance system influences how equitably this task is carried out, how efficiently revenues are collected, and the amount of revenue that can be raised (Schieber and Maeda 1997).

Equity. Revenues are generally collected through some combination of general taxes, payroll taxes, other taxes, and donations in the public sector and, in the private sector, premiums and out-of-pocket payments. The choice of revenue collection mechanisms determines the degree to which insurance systems are financed progressively or regressively. In progressive financing arrangements, the proportion of income contributed rises with income level, so that the affluent pay proportionately more than the poor. Regressive financing is the converse: the poor contribute proportionately more than the rich. Flat taxes represent the same proportion of income for every individual regardless of actual income.

Income taxes are typically the most progressive financing mechanism: higher earners usually pay higher income tax rates. Payroll taxes are usually flat taxes: regardless of actual income, each individual pays the same rate (although the upper limits on the maximum amount payable can make them regressive). Payroll taxes do not typically tax assets, making them more regressive, particularly in countries where assets make up a large proportion of wealth (that is, developing countries). Premiums and out-of-pocket payments are the most regressive financing options. Regardless of income, each individual pays the same price, which represents a greater proportion of income for the poor than for the affluent.

Through progressive financing arrangements, insurance systems can subsidize the costs of health care for low-income individuals. Single-payer systems accomplish this within the single risk pool through progressive taxation. Some multiple-payer insurance systems redistribute funds through subsidies such as interpool transfers and contribution exemptions for certain groups (for example, the elderly or the unemployed). For example, in Japan, transfers are made to the insurance pool of elderly individuals. The other insurance pools each contribute an equal amount per beneficiary to the elderly insurance pool. In addition, the central and local governments contribute 30 percent of the revenues of the elderly insurance pool (Ikegami 1996).

Economic efficiency. A tradeoff exists between the redistribution of revenues via taxation and the economic efficiency of the financing system (Schieber and Maeda 1997). Inefficiencies can arise from changes made by individuals and firms in reaction to a tax. For example, employers may alter their hiring behavior when faced with a tax to finance health insurance for their employees. This economic cost of taxation must be weighed against equity and other considerations when designing an optimal taxation system for raising health care revenues (Schieber and Maeda 1997). The administrative costs of collecting revenue must also be considered. The same impact on employment could be generated in a multiple-payer system, however, by a government mandate that all employers must provide their employees with health insurance. Economists and policymakers disagree widely on the relative magnitude of the employment effect of a mandate or a tax.

Aggregate level of funding. In some countries, government's ability to collect health insurance revenues is limited by the level and distribution of per capita income, the capacity to collect taxes, and the openness of the economy (Schieber and Maeda 1997). (This issue is further discussed below.)

ADVANTAGES OF SINGLE-PAYER SYSTEMS: REVENUE COLLECTION

Single-payer systems usually have an advantage over multiple-payer systems in the efficiency of collecting revenues, overall cost control, and capacity to subsidize health care for low-income individuals.

Efficiency in revenue collection. Single-payer health insurance systems collect revenue mainly through existing tax-collection mechanisms. Therefore, their collection costs are usually lower than those of multiple-payer systems with separate collection systems (World Health Organization [WHO] 2000).

Cost control. The overall funding for single-payer health insurance systems is typically determined through an annual budgeting process, giving government officials tight control over aggregate health expenditures from year to year. In multiple-payer systems, aggregate spending is more difficult to monitor and control, because different insurers may use different utilization monitoring, payment, and information systems. This can lead to cost shifting, where one insurer pays more than another for a similar product.

Close government control over aggregate spending in single-payer insurance systems may open the way for political determination of total health expenditure. In some countries such as the United Kingdom, some analysts say that it leads to underinvestment in health care (Klein 2001). Others observe that politicians may be more likely to increase health spending in election years (Cookson and Maynard 2000). The responsiveness of spending levels to political concerns was seen in the recent commitment to a major expansion of health care resources in the United Kingdom (Klein 2001).

Subsidization of low-income individuals. As described above, single-payer insurance systems tend to be more progressively financed than multiple-payer systems. Progressivity effectively provides a subsidy to low-income individuals.

ADVANTAGES OF MULTIPLE-PAYER SYSTEMS: REVENUE COLLECTION

Multiple-payer systems allow the health care resource pool to include other sources, when the government's own ability to collect taxes is limited. These systems may also be more sensitive than single-payer systems to individuals' preferences for their insurance coverage.

Government's ability to collect taxes. Government's ability to collect taxes is often limited by the large number of workers who earn income in the "informal economy," widespread tax evasion, and other related factors that limit the tax base. As a result, government revenues may not be sufficient to fund a universal single-payer insurance system, and community-based pools and other alternative mechanisms may be necessary to collect sufficient revenues. This issue is particularly relevant to low- and middle-income countries.

Responsiveness to individuals' preferences. Multiple-payer systems may be more sensitive than single-payer systems to individuals' specific demands for health services and better able to tailor their services and prices accordingly. Individuals can be given a choice regarding how much they are willing to spend on health insurance. For example, some insurers could provide unrestricted access to a wide variety of benefits and charge higher premiums, while other insurers could provide a low-cost alternative by restricting the set of providers and limiting the benefit package.

Risk Pooling

Health insurers pool revenues to protect individuals from the financial risks associated with the use of medical services. Numerous studies show that health expenditures are highly concentrated in a small proportion of the population (Light 2000). Insurance spreads these risks across a pool of individuals. Unpredictable risks become more predictable as the size of the pool grows, owing to the law of large numbers. The insurance pool size can vary from a system where all revenues go into a single pool (single-payer insurance), to a system where each individual has a medical savings account. *Medical savings accounts*—prepaid, personal health care accounts often subsidized through a tax incentive—do not spread the financial risk of illness across individuals. They may be preferred by individuals who are not averse to taking risk. Singapore is one country that has adopted medical savings accounts.

ADVERSE SELECTION

The uncertainty of health risks can contribute to the problem of adverse selection in health insurance systems. *Adverse selection* occurs when one party to a transaction uses an information advantage strategically against the interests of the less informed partner (Belli 2001). For example, a person selling a used car that needs maintenance may conceal that information and charge a higher price than the buyer would pay for a "lemon" (Akerlof 1970). The uninformed buyer, however, will assume that every car is a "lemon." The same principle applies to health insurance. Sicker individuals are more likely than the healthy to want to buy health insurance, but insurers cannot afford to insure only sick people. Insurers therefore attempt to identify sick people. In a system with multiple insurers and a choice of health insurance contracts, high-risk individuals will tend to buy more complete insurance coverage than low-risk individuals, who will opt for low-cost, low-coverage, catastrophe policies—or no insurance at all.

Insurers attempt to correct this information asymmetry by screening potential members for risk *(cream skimming)*. For example, individuals with preexisting conditions may not be offered a policy that covers that condition. Groups of high-risk individuals—such as smokers or workers employed in an industry with high occupational safety hazards—may have to pay higher premiums than otherwise similar individuals. Collecting data for evaluating risks can be expensive for insurers, which adds to the administrative costs of insurance without providing any benefit to individuals or society.

Unchecked risk selection can lead to a "premium death spiral" where insurers incurring a loss on high-risk individuals are forced to raise their premiums. In response to the higher premiums, low-risk individuals will opt out of the insurance pool for a lower cost alternative. The high-risk individuals remain, continuing to drive up the expected costs of the insurance pool and necessitating further premium increases. This cycle continues until the policy hits the "death" part of the spiral—the insurer stops offering the insurance policy. The premium death spiral has been observed, for instance, in the Federal Employees Health Benefits Plan in the United States (Newhouse 1994).

PREVENTING RISK SELECTION

Among the methods that can be used to try to prevent risk selection and the resulting death spiral are formation of risk pools unrelated to health, use of risk adjusters to redistribute resources among pools, and regulation. These methods can have the disadvantages of requiring considerable data, being expensive to operate, and being only partially effective.

Formation of nonhealth-related risk pools. Large insurance pools with a diverse risk structure have the ability to subsidize individuals with high expected utilization from others with little expected utilization. These risk pools need to be formed for a reason other than insuring against the financial risk of illness in order to be effective. Large employee groups, for example, are likely to include individuals with different exposures to health risk, because employment—not health insurance—is the primary reason for the pool's existence.

Use of risk adjusters. A second way to mitigate adverse selection is by redistributing resources among insurance pools on the basis of their risk structure. Measures that predict utilization are commonly known as *risk adjusters*. Risk adjusters can theoretically predict 15 to 20 percent of the variance in expenditures at the individual level, although most of them in use can explain only 10 percent (Cutler and Zeckhauser 2000; Newhouse 1994).

There are four main groups of risk adjusters: demographic information such as age and gender, prior utilization, actual utilization, and active medical conditions such as diabetes (Cutler and Zeckhauser 2000). When choosing a risk adjuster, policymakers must evaluate its predictive power, the ability of insurers to collect the data, the ability of respondents to manipulate the data to their advantage *(gaming)*, and incentives created by the risk-adjustment system.

Age and gender are the most commonly used risk adjusters. They are most resistant to gaming by insurers and are easiest to collect, but unfortunately they are weak predictors of actual utilization (van de Ven and Ellis 2000). Other methods have better predictive power, but the data required to operate the system are more difficult to collect, and some methods are more subject to gaming.

Although experience with use of risk adjusters other than age and gender is limited (Cutler and Zeckhauser 2000), experience in the competitive multiple-payer system in the Netherlands and the Medicare program in the United States shows that the implementation of good risk adjusters is "a long way from theory to practice" (Medicare Payment Advisory Commission 2002; van de Ven and others 1994).

Regulation. A third way to prevent adverse selection is through regulation. For example, insurers may be limited in the types of information they are allowed to collect about potential beneficiaries. They may be mandated to have open enrollment periods. The way premium levels are set can also be regulated. Insurers may be restricted from individually rating each person. Instead, insurers must offer community rates (the same rate for everyone) or community rates by class (for example, the same rate for everyone of a certain age or gender).

In response to these types of regulations, insurers can be expected to use other methods to attract good risks, such as benefits design—for example, a spa benefit may tend to attract young, healthy beneficiaries. A more sinister approach is to place the enrollment office on the second story of a building that does not have an elevator or access for the handicapped.

ADVANTAGES OF SINGLE-PAYER SYSTEMS: RISK POOLING

In multiple-payer insurance systems, insurers need to collect information on the individuals or groups of individuals covered in order to set premiums and coverage appropriately. Collection and analysis of these data can be expensive. Risk-adjustment methods are important. In addition, data collection leads to issues of personal privacy; insurers have an incentive to collect as much personal information as possible, while patients will want to protect some information from insurers. In single-payer systems, less data collection on individuals is necessary.

To prevent insurers from selecting only good risks in multiple-payer systems, regulations are required. For example, governments can regulate the types of information that insurers can collect or mandate an open enrollment period. In single-payer systems, no regulations are needed to prevent adverse selection.

Redistribution between risk pools in a multiple-payer health insurance system can be used to attenuate risk selection. As discussed earlier, interfund transfers can be made on the basis of the risk structure of each insurance pool through the use of risk adjusters. As described above, risk adjusters are not currently adequate to prevent adverse selection. In single-payer systems, the use of risk adjustment is not necessary to completely mitigate the effects of risk selection.

ADVANTAGES OF MULTIPLE-PAYER SYSTEMS: RISK POOLING

In multiple-payer systems, insurers can design insurance packages to provide services that are appropriate for certain risk groups. Specific insurance products can be tailored to meet specific needs and wants of specific types of individuals. For example, insurers could offer case-management benefits to insurance pools containing a high proportion of persons with chronic conditions. Other insurance pools could offer unrestricted access to specialists or coverage of alternative therapies. Insurance products can also be tailored to an individual's level of risk aversion. For example, less risk-averse people may prefer a medical savings account or plan with a high deductible, while the more risk averse may prefer a more comprehensive benefit package with little or no cost sharing.

In multiple-payer systems, groups of individuals who engage in healthy behaviors can be financially rewarded through lower insurance contributions. For example, an insurance policy could be offered exclusively to nonsmokers.

Purchasing

A third main role of health insurers is purchasing health services and supplies for their beneficiaries. Insurers can purchase services from public or private providers by using a variety of payment arrangements that place financial risk on a continuum from the provider (capitation) to the insurer (fee for service). The fundamental goal of purchasing is to achieve the optimum balance between effective incentives and acceptable risk for the provider.

In single-payer systems, the insurer is generally in a stronger bargaining position relative to providers than insurers in multiple-payer systems owing to the insurer's monopsony power. The monopsony power creates options for single-payer purchasing, such as global budgets and negotiated payment rates, that might not be possible in multiple-payer systems. Multiple-payer systems can, however, approximate the single-payer systems in different ways in terms of purchasing. For example, all-payer rate setting can be used in multiple-payer systems to negotiate uniform provider payment rates, as in the Republic of Korea and Germany.

ADVANTAGES OF SINGLE-PAYER SYSTEMS: PURCHASING

In purchasing health services, single-payer insurance systems have greater purchasing power than multiple-payer systems. They also have a greater ability to regulate what health services and products are available through activities such as technology assessment and pharmaceutical formularies.

Purchasing power. In single-payer insurance systems, there is little or no competition among purchasers. Single-payer insurers can use monopsony power in purchasing health services. For example, single-payer insurers can negotiate physician and hospital payment rates and buy pharmaceuticals in bulk. Savings are thus accrued at the expense of providers and drug companies, which may consider payments too low to continue providing high-quality care or adequate research and development.

Technology assessment. Technology assessment is the determination of the value of technologies to inform the allocation process. Policymakers may have different priorities for allocating new and established technologies, but common considerations are efficient use, obtaining the greatest health gains per unit of cost (Cookson and Maynard 2000); aggregate cost control, because medical technology is considered to be a primary driver of health spending growth (Newhouse 1993); and an equitable distribution of medical technologies.

Technology assessment is applied to allocation decisions in three main ways: approval processes, insurance reimbursement policies, and clinical guideline development and application. Single-payer systems, given their monopsony power in the health services market, may be better positioned than multiple-payer insurers to influence technology allocation through these mechanisms.

For example, in the United Kingdom, a single public agency—the National Institute for Clinical Excellence (NICE)—compiles guidelines for the effective use of health care technologies. Adherence to these guidelines can be easily adopted throughout the entire National Health Service through the benefit package, because a single, centrally set benefit package applies to every citizen. Capital budgets are allocated annually from the Ministry of Health to regional Health Authorities, allowing further central control over the proliferation and distribution of medical technology. In addition, another public agency, the Commission for Health Improvement, periodically audits providers to ensure compliance with NICE guidelines.

Formularies. A single-payer insurer can use its monopsony power to limit aggregate pharmaceutical costs and influence population drug utilization patterns through selective coverage of pharmaceuticals. Formularies can be used to limit the use of drugs with unproven effectiveness or to encourage the substitution of generic equivalents to brand-name products. For example, in Australia the cost-effectiveness of new drugs is considered before the drugs are eligible for reimbursement by the national insurance system under the Pharmaceutical Benefits Scheme.

ADVANTAGES OF MULTIPLE-PAYER SYSTEMS: PURCHASING

Multiple-payer insurance systems can provide people with a choice of insurance product, whereas single-payer systems do not. Multiple-payer systems also have a greater ability to selectively contract with providers and they are more likely to set higher prices for providers.

Consumer choice of insurer. In a multiple-payer health insurance system, the possibility of consumer choice of insurer could make insurers more responsive to people's preferences. Multiple-payer systems may be able to devise purchasing mechanisms and provider incentives that complement the preferences of beneficiaries (Zweifel 2001). For example, different people may have different preferences on unrestricted access to specialists, free choice of primary physician, provider payment methods, or levels of deductibles and coinsurance.

Selective contracting with providers. In a multiple-payer health insurance system, insurers can selectively contract with certain providers to provide a specialized level of service for their beneficiaries. For example, to provide an affordable benefit package, insurers could selectively contract with hospitals and physicians charging low rates. In Switzerland, individuals can pay higher premiums for better hospital amenities (van Doorslaer and others 1999). Insurers could also contract with higher quality, higher priced providers to offer a high-end option to beneficiaries. Single-payer health insurance systems that have attempted to implement contracting of health care providers, as the United Kingdom, have seen little change in historical relationships between purchasers and providers (Le Grand 1999; Tuohy 1999).

Another related issue to consider is that in single-payer insurance systems, doctors and other health care workers are often considered civil servants. Civil service rules can introduce rigidity to the process of adjusting the supply of health care labor to meet needs.

Quality of care. In wielding their monopsony power, single-payer insurers may pay doctors and other health professionals lower salaries, undersupply other inputs, or otherwise cause conditions leading to lower quality care. If the payment rates do not allow provision of services desired by some consumers, parallel markets may develop for these services. These could take the form of a black market, or a sanctioned parallel market that could draw resources from the health insurance system. For example, substantial informal markets for health services have developed in some former Soviet republics (Preker, Jakab, and Schneider 2001). Australia has enacted policies promoting a parallel private health care market to reduce public expenditures (Hall 1999). In some countries doctors see public patients during certain hours and private patients during others, perhaps giving more attention to their private patients to the detriment of the public patients. Doctors may actually prefer long waiting times in order to have a steady stream of private patients. These parallel markets detract from the equity of access to the health care system. Moreover, they could undermine the effectiveness of the public system.

Social Solidarity

Social solidarity refers to a sense of unity, interdependence, and community among members of a society. Though variously defined, most definitions involve the idea of society's common interests' overriding individual interests (Ashcroft, Campbell, and Jones 2000). In addition, solidarity often includes a sense of charity, for example, a shared sense of responsibility for providing health care to specific groups such as the elderly, the poor, or people with chronic conditions.

In the case of health insurance, a common concept of solidarity involves all members of a society making a fair financial contribution in return for guaranteed equal access to needed health care (Houtepen and ter Meulen 2000). Solidarity is therefore strongly tied to an idea of distributive justice (Rawls 1971, p. 336). In this case, access to health care is considered a positive freedom— something that people have a right *to*, as opposed to having freedom *from*—that should be distributed equally among similar individuals. This concept is supported by the U.N. Committee on Economic, Social and Cultural Rights.[1]

However, these values are by no means shared by all societies, giving rise to a broad array of national concepts of solidarity in the area of health care. For example, the United States could potentially be considered to be violating the United Nations' right to health care based on the distribution of health care resources.[2] The German health care system is guided rhetorically by a notion of social solidarity: everyone is guaranteed insurance coverage. Nonetheless, the well-off are allowed to opt into private insurance coverage, which gives them better access to health care because providers are paid higher rates.

ADVANTAGES OF SINGLE-PAYER SYSTEMS: SOCIAL SOLIDARITY

Single-payer health insurance systems spread the financial burden around more equitably than multiple-payer systems. Single-payer systems are financed more progressively than multiple-payer systems, which may increase solidarity between richer and poorer segments of the population. Single-payer systems can also foster citizens' trust in their government's ability to protect their welfare, enhancing their view of the legitimacy of the government.

ADVANTAGES OF MULTIPLE-PAYER SYSTEMS: SOCIAL SOLIDARITY

People have a sense of solidarity with others of the same community, profession, class, ethnicity, religion, or lifestyle. This solidarity could contribute to building "social capital," or features of social organization such as trust in others and civic participation, which can be used as a resource to help overcome social problems. Allowing the better off to opt out of the single-payer insurance system may enhance social solidarity in a normative sense, by securing the political support of high-income earners for the public insurance system.

OTHER SINGLE-PAYER ISSUES

Investment in public health. Multiple-payer insurers often do not expect to receive returns on investments in preventive health care. Because many beneficiaries are expected to change insurers within a few years, the insurer offering those benefits will not collect the long-term returns. In single-payer systems, investments in preventive care can lead to long-term savings due to a healthier population. In multiple-payer systems, the same result might be possible if the government provides more services as part of a public health program or mandates that all insurers provide a certain preventive benefit.

Incentive for innovation. The lack of competition between insurance bodies may inhibit innovation in single-payer insurance systems. Managed care principles and many other developments in the organization and administration of insurance were developed in the United States, where competition between insurers is strong. Single-payer systems may become rigid and reluctant to change.

Administrative costs. Single-payer insurance systems may achieve economies of scale in claims processing and other similar operations. Similarly, providers may have lower operating costs if all claims are processed by a single insurance agency using common forms. Multiple-payer insurers could reduce operating costs by consolidating administrative functions—for example, using a uniform set of claims forms—but this could diminish competitive forces. Countries such as Korea have integrated their administrative functions into a single entity while still having independent insurers.

TWO OPTIONS FOR REFORMING SINGLE-PAYER INSURANCE SYSTEMS

Some countries are modifying their health insurance system while preserving the single-payer nature by expanding the voluntary private health insurance market. Two countries that are increasing the role of private health insurance are South Africa and Australia. The Czech Republic and some other countries are abandoning their single-payer system in favor of a multiple-payer system. Both options for reforming single-payer health insurance systems are discussed below.

Expanding the Role of Private Insurance

Expanding the role of private insurance alongside a universal single-payer insurer is one way of balancing the tradeoffs between single- and multiple-payer insurance systems. All citizens would be entitled to the single-payer insurance policy, with the option of buying extra benefits from private insurers. Private insurance coverage can accommodate consumer needs that are not met by the single-payer insurer. The purchase of private coverage is likely to be skewed toward higher-income individuals, creating multiple tiers in the health insurance system. This influences equity of access to care and social solidarity.

Private insurance can exist alongside universal single-payer insurance in three ways: substitutive, complementary, or supplementary (Mossialos and Thompson 2001). *Substitutive* private insurance can be offered to eligible individuals in lieu of the national single-payer insurance option. Eligibility can be based on income (as in Germany and the Netherlands), employment status (the self-employed in Germany and the Netherlands), or occupation (civil servants in Spain and Germany) (Mossialos and Thompson 2001). *Complementary* private insurance can cover services not included in the single-payer insurance benefits (as in Canada). *Supplementary* private health insurance can be used to provide improved coverage of services also covered by the national single-payer insurer, for example, access to private providers without waiting lists for elective surgery (as in the United Kingdom).

South Africa is an example of an upper-middle-income country with a single-payer system alongside a substantial supplementary private insurance system. The public system serves mainly lower-income individuals, although it is available to all and paid for by all through taxes (van den Heever 1998). Private insurance covers mainly higher income, employed individuals who purchase it in addition to public coverage. The public system covers about 82 percent of the population (van den Heever 1998), but private insurance accounts for 60 percent of health spending, revealing a discrepancy between publicly and privately funded care (Schneider and Gilson 1999).

The South African government has enacted reforms to combine the centrally controlled public system with a managed, supplementary private insurance market. This involves increased regulation of the private insurance market in such areas as enrollment, benefits, and grievance procedures to mitigate adverse selection. In addition, private insurers will be required to pay for care beneficiaries receive in public facilities. These reforms aim to solidify the private sector's position as a supplement to the public single-payer system.

Australia is an example of a high-income country that has attempted to stimulate the market for supplementary private insurance alongside the national single-payer insurer. The private share of health care revenues is among the highest in the industrial world (Hall, Lourenco, and Viney 1999). Private insurance coverage, regulated by legislation, mainly provides access to private hospital treatment (Hall, Lourenco, and Viney 1999). Since 1995, the Australian government has passed three major reforms to encourage expansion of the private health insurance market. These reforms were a government-provided rebate of 30 percent of private health insurance premiums; the introduction of selective provider contracting in the private insurance market; and a switch from community rating to age-specific premium rating. These initiatives may have spurred expansion of private health insurance coverage.

The Australian private insurance market faces several obstacles to success as a strong supplement to the national insurance program. The first is adverse selection. Some observers point to rapidly increasing private health insurance premiums, which have grown faster than total health spending, as a potential cause of selection problems (Hall, Lourenco, and Viney 1999). Private insurance coverage in Australia is heavily skewed toward higher-income individuals (Willcox 2001).

A second challenge in supplemental private insurance is the scope of coverage. Private coverage often does not cover any difference between providers' actual charges and the scheduled charge, leaving patients with substantial out-of-pocket payments (Hall, Lourenco, and Viney 1999).

These examples show two efforts to strengthen a single-payer insurance system through a supplementary private insurance system. Countries with single-payer systems could use private insurance to supplement the finances of the health system through the private sector. However, the private insurance system could detract from the public system, creating multiple tiers of access to care.

Transforming a Single-Payer to a Multiple-Payer Insurance System

The Czech Republic, a former Warsaw Pact country, had a central, public single-payer system until the early 1990s. In the 1990s, the Czech health insurance system was transformed to a multiple-payer, employer mandate system with government coverage of special populations (Massaro, Nemec, and Kalman 1994). After years of socialism, other former Warsaw Pact countries have also been looking to markets to organize the welfare functions of the state (Kornai and Eggleston 2001).

Czech citizens are now served by 10 insurance providers, although 75 percent of the population is still enrolled in the plan that had been the sole provider of health insurance (Jack 2000). Insurance revenues, previously collected mainly through general taxation, are now raised through payroll taxes. These insurance payments have no relation to an individual's expected health insurance costs (Jack 2000).

Czech citizens have technically been given a choice of insurer, but they have little incentive to exercise their newly acquired consumer power. This is because national legislation regulates specific aspects of insurers' operations, eliminating most differences that consumers could use to choose from among competing plans. Benefit packages, beneficiary contributions, and provider payment rates are all set by the government (Jack 2000). Health risks enrolled and efficiency of operations are the main areas in which insurance plans can differ. To counteract adverse selection, a rudimentary risk-adjusted redistribution of revenues is conducted via a central fund, based solely on the proportion of beneficiaries over age 60 (Jack 2000).

The Czech reforms illustrate one way a single-payer system can be transformed into a multiple-payer system while potentially avoiding the problems of adverse selection. Through regulation and basic risk adjustment, Czech insurers have a reduced basis on which to select good health risks. However, age is an unlikely predictor of most health care use.

Although it is difficult to evaluate the administrative, allocative, and technical efficiency of Czech health insurers, they seem to be performing fairly well (Jack 2000). However, the risk-adjustment process has weakened insurers' incentives to collect revenues, because they can expect to recoup only a fraction of their contributions to the central fund, depending on the age structure of their beneficiary pool (Jack 2000). To further complicate the picture, other reforms have been enacted in the market for health *care* as opposed to health *insurance*. These reforms, including provider payment policies and choice of primary care physician, could have been implemented within a single-payer system as well.

CONSIDERATIONS SPECIFIC TO LOW- AND MIDDLE-INCOME COUNTRIES

Several characteristics particular to low- and middle-income countries must also be considered in the reform or design of a health insurance system. These characteristics will be outlined in the areas of financing, risk pooling, purchasing, and social solidarity.

Financing

Ability to raise public revenues. Low- and middle-income countries are able to raise less than half as much public sector revenue as a share of gross domestic product (GDP) compared with industrial countries (Schieber and Maeda 1997). Low-income countries raise a median of 19 percent of GDP in government revenues. In middle-income countries, this figure is 30 percent. In comparison, high-income countries raise a median of 44 percent of GDP in government revenues (Schieber and Maeda 1997). Low- and middle-income countries may have greater difficulties financing a single-payer insurance system, which relies primarily on public revenues.

Taxation. Low- and middle-income countries rely less than industrial countries on income taxes and corporate taxes and raise a greater share of public revenues through sales taxes and other indirect taxes (Schieber and Maeda 1997). Indirect taxes are generally regressive, because the poor spend a higher proportion of their income than the better-off on goods and services. The degree of regressivity can be moderated by targeting indirect taxes toward higher-income individuals through, for example, sales taxes on luxury goods such as cars. Income taxes are not a good source of revenue in many low- and middle-income countries owing to factors including the amount of income earned in the informal economy, lack of urbanization, high degree of income inequality, widespread tax evasion, and limited tax administration capacity (Schieber and Maeda 1997). Industrial countries rely primarily on general taxation to fund single-payer health insurance systems.

Risk Pooling

Mandatory insurance enrollment. Single-payer insurance systems in high-income countries typically have mandatory enrollment that includes the entire population. Low- and middle-income countries, with a higher share of rural and agricultural workers and other workers outside the formal economy, may have difficulty ensuring compliance with an insurance mandate for the entire population.

Adverse selection. Adverse selection presents a long-term threat to the viability of microinsurance pools and any other multiple-payer insurance system without adequate safeguards. Low- and middle-income countries face a difficult dilemma. They must balance two feasibility concerns: insufficient financial and administrative capacity to establish a single insurance pool, and adverse selection with multiple insurance pools. One compromise that has been advanced is the formation of multiple insurance pools with an eye toward building the capacity needed for a future single-payer system (WHO 2000). For example, an insurance pool covering only public sector employees could later be expanded to include the entire population. This, however, could encounter practical difficulties such as having to reduce the public sector benefits to make health insurance affordable for the rest of the population.

Purchasing

Out-of-pocket payments generally represent a much larger share of health spending in low- and middle-income countries than in industrial countries. In addition to being undesirable because of their highly regressive nature and lack of risk spreading, high levels of out-of-pocket payments may also undermine the payment incentives of the insurance system's purchasing arrangements (Ensor 2001). For example, a hospital collecting user per-diem charges from patients may not attempt to shorten stays in response to per-admission insurance payments.

Social Solidarity

Social solidarity can be compromised by income disparities, diversity of health needs, and high out-of-pocket payments. Low- and middle-income countries may have greater disparities in income, resources, and health status among their populations than high-income countries.

Most low- and middle-income countries also rely more heavily on out-of-pocket financing than high-income countries. Because the income elasticity of demand for health services is generally greater for poorer individuals, out-of-pocket payments may lead to better access to care for the rich than for the poor.

CONCLUSIONS

There is no universal paradigm for designing health insurance systems. Countries vary greatly in their priorities, populations, development, and systems of government. In this chapter, we have described four models of single-payer health insurance systems, contrasted these single-payer systems with multiple-payer systems, and outlined special considerations for low- and middle-income countries. The discussion has shown that each of the two major types of health insurance system—single-payer and multiple-payer—has strengths and weaknesses. Countries deciding on the reform or development of their health insurance system must evaluate these strengths and weaknesses against their own priorities and needs, political and economic constraints, and administrative capabilities.

NOTES

1. *The Economist* (2001). "Righting Wrongs." August 18, 2001.

2. *The Economist* (2001).

REFERENCES

Akerlof, G.A. 1970. "The Market for 'Lemons': Quality Uncertainty and the Market Mechanism." *Quarterly Journal of Economics* 84(3): 488–500.

Ashcroft, R. E., A. V. Campbell, and S. Jones. 2000. "Solidarity, Society and the Welfare State in the United Kingdom." *Health Care Analysis* 8: 377–94.

Belli, P. 2001. "How Adverse Selection Affects the Health Insurance Market." HNP Working Paper 2574. World Bank, Washington, D.C.

Cookson, R., and A. Maynard. 2000. "Health Technology Assessment in Europe: Improving Clarity and Performance." *International Journal of Technology Assessment in Health Care* 16(2): 639–50.

Cutler, D. M., and R. J. Zeckhauser. 2000. "The Anatomy of Health Insurance." In A. J. Culyer and J. P. Newhouse, eds., *Handbook of Health Economics*. New York, N.Y.: Elsevier.

Ensor, T. 2001. "Health Economics in Low Income Countries: Adapting to the Reality of the Unofficial Economy." *Health Policy* 57(1): 1–13.

Hall, J. 1999. "Incremental Change in the Australian Health System." *Health Affairs* 18(3): 95–110.

Hall, J., R. A. Lourenco, and R. Viney. 1999. "Carrots and Sticks—The Fall and Fall of Private Health Insurance in Australia." *Health Economics* 8: 653–660.

Houtepen, R., and R. ter Meulen. 2000. "New Types of Solidarity in the European Welfare State." *Health Care Analysis* 8: 329–40.

Ikegami, N. 1996. "Overview: Health Care in Japan." In N. Ikegami and J. C. Campbell, eds., *Containing Health Care Costs in Japan*. Ann Arbor: University of Michigan Press.

Jack, W. 2000. "The Purchase of Medical Care in the Czech Republic: Provider Payment Mechanisms in Practice." Draft HNP Working Paper. World Bank, Washington, D.C.

Klein, R. 2001. "What's Happening to Britain's National Health Service?" *New England Journal of Medicine* 345(4): 305–08.

Kornai, J., and K. Eggleston. 2001. *Welfare, Choice and Solidarity in Transition: Reforming the Health Sector in Eastern Europe*. Cambridge: Cambridge University Press.

Le Grand, J. 1999. "Competition, Cooperation, or Control? Tales from the British National Health Service." *Health Affairs* 18(3): 27–39.

Light, D. 2000. "Sociological Perspectives on Competition in Health Care." *Journal of Health Politics, Policy, and Law* 25(5): 969–74.

Massaro, T. A., J. Nemec, and I. Kalman. 1994. "Health System Reform in the Czech Republic." *JAMA* 271(23): 1870–74.

Medicare Payment Advisory Commission. 2002. *Report to the Congress: Medicare Payment Policy*. Washington, D.C.

Mossialos, E., and S. M. S. Thompson. 2001. "Voluntary Health Insurance in the European Union." London School of Economics Discussion Paper 19. May.

Newhouse, J.P. 1993. "An Iconoclastic View of Health Cost Containment." *Health Affairs* 12 (suppl): 152–71.

———. 1994. "Patients at Risk: Health Reform and Risk Adjustment." *Health Affairs* 13(1): 132–46.

Preker, A. S., M. Jakab, and M. Schneider. 2001. "Erosion of Financial Protection in Health Systems of ECA Transition Economies." HNP Working Paper. World Bank, Washington, D.C.

Rawls, J. 1971. *A Theory of Justice*. Cambridge, Mass.: Harvard University Press.

Schieber, G., and A. Maeda. 1997. "A Curmudgeon's Guide to Financing Health Care in Developing Countries." In G. Schieber, ed., *Innovations in Health Care Financing*. Washington, D.C.: World Bank.

Schneider, H., and L. Gilson. 1999. "Small Fish in a Big Pond? External Aid and the Health Sector in South Africa." *Health Policy and Planning* 14(3): 264–72.

Tuohy, C. H. 1999. *Accidental Logics: The Dynamics of Change in the Health Care Arena in the United States, Britain, and Canada*. New York, N.Y.: Oxford University Press.

The Economist. 2001. "Righting Wrongs." August 18, 2001.

van de Ven, W. P. M. M., and R. P. Ellis. 2000. "Risk Adjustment in Competitive Health Plan Markets." In A. J. Culyer and J. P. Newhouse, eds., *Handbook of Health Economics*. New York, N.Y.: Elsevier.

van de Ven, W. P. M. M., R. C. J. A. van Vliet, E. M. van Barneveld, and L. M. Lamers. 1994. "Risk-Adjusted Capitation: Recent Experiences in the Netherlands." *Health Affairs* 13(4): 121–36.

van den Heever, A. M. 1998. "Private Sector Health Reform in South Africa." *Health Economics* 7: 281–89.

van Doorslaer, E., A. Wagstaff, H. van der Burg, T. Christiansen, G. Citoni, R. Di Biase, U. G. Gerdtham, M. Gerfin, L. Gross, U. Hakinnen, J. John, P. Johnson, J. Klavus, C. Lachaud, J. Lauritsen, R. Leu, B. Nolan, J. Pereira, C. Propper, F. Puffer, L. Rochaix, M. Schellhorn, G. Sundberg, and O. Winkelhake. 1999. "The Redistributive Effect of Health Care Finance in Twelve OECD Countries." *Journal of Health Economics* 18: 291–313.

Willcox, S. 2001. "Promoting Private Health Insurance in Australia." *Health Affairs* 20(3): 152–61.

WHO (World Health Organization). 2000. *The World Health Report 2000—Health Systems: Improving Performance*. Geneva.

Zweifel, P. 2001. "Multiple Payers in Health Care: A Framework for Assessment." Expert report submitted to the World Bank. World Bank, Washington, D.C.

CHAPTER 19

Multiple Payers in Health Care: A Framework for Assessment

Peter Zweifel

When it comes to health care, both consumers and governments suspect that they are not getting their money's worth. Governments point to a high and often rising share of health care expenditure in the gross domestic product (GDP). However, it is not clear at all whether simply reducing this share would be in the interest of consumers and voters, who in their daily lives do not seek just to keep expenditure low but to obtain "value for their money," a favorable ratio between benefits and cost. This ratio may attain its optimal value even at a high cost, as evidenced by the example of private transportation, where many individuals willingly pay 10 percent of their income or more to be able to drive a car. One way to improve the ratio of benefits to cost is to choose payment systems that give providers of health care services the right incentives.

As a matter of principle, either a multiple-payer or a single-payer system for financing health care may convey the right incentives to providers. All economic theory says is that the optimal choice of a payment system importantly depends on the amount of information available to the (prospective) patient. This topic is treated in the second part of this chapter. It starts out with the case of full information, then considers the case of asymmetric information with regard to provider effort only, and ends by considering the most difficult case of asymmetric information both with regard to effort and type of provider. In each case, the optimal payment function is stated and discussed.

However, it turns out that the prospective patient as the uninformed principal is unlikely to find these optimal functions for the physician (or any health care provider) because he or she does not know crucial parameters in the formulas. This failure opens a market for complementary agents, introduced in the third part of the chapter.

Competing health insurers as complementary agents are likely to be associated with multiple-payer systems, while governments as complementary agents are tempted to use their monopsony power to reduce public health care expenditure.

The fourth section is dedicated to a survey of future challenges for health care systems. The choice of a complementary agent and the concomitant payment system should be made in view of these challenges. A final assessment will reveal that governments acting as complementary agents have a comparative advantage in managing challenges that originate domestically, such as aging and the increasing number of one-person households. However, competitive health insurers as complementary agents will be especially able to adjust to challenges emanating from globalization and changing medical technology. Thus, multiple-payer systems hold the promise of keeping the incentives of services providers aligned with changing asymmetries in their relations with patients. The chapter concludes with a summary and an outlook.

THEORETICAL BACKGROUND

The objective of this section is to show that very different payment systems are optimal for the prospective patient, depending on the amount of information available about the service provider's level of effort exerted and level of ability ("type"). This paves the way for the argument that insurers acting on behalf of their clients should negotiate a choice of payment systems. Following a short review of the case of no information asymmetry, asymmetry with regard to provider effort is discussed and related to medical care. Finally, information asymmetry with regard to both effort and type is considered.

The Case of Full Information

The case of full information is described in elementary textbooks of economic theory. Here, the patient can be seen as a purchaser of health care services under a budget constraint. To achieve the maximum health effect, he or she must observe the condition (Zweifel and Breyer 1997, chapter 7.3.3.3):

$$\frac{p_1}{p_2} = \frac{\partial H/\partial M_1}{\partial H/\partial M_2} \qquad (1)$$

Here, p_1 is the fee for the health care service M_1, and similarly for p_2. On the right-hand side of equation 1 is the ratio of two marginal productivities, with $\partial H/\partial M_1$, for example, symbolizing the marginal productivity of health care service M_1 with regard to health status. This optimality condition is nothing but the requirement that the ratio of factor prices be equal to the ratio of marginal productivities. There may be cases where the (prospective) patient can estimate these marginal productivities. For example, the health condition may be well defined, and the health care provider's main task will be simply to issue or fill a prescription. However, the following two cases seem far more relevant for health care.

Asymmetric Information with Regard to Effort Only

Economic theory uses principal-agent theory to model the relationship between a patient and a health care provider (Grossman and Hart 1983; Holmström 1979).

CONTROLLING PROVIDER BEHAVIOR THROUGH PAYMENT

The patient, acting as the principal, seeks to devise a payment scheme that avoids both the tendency toward "flat of the curve medicine," induced by fee-for-service payment, and the tendency toward underservicing, induced by a fixed payment that fails to reward performance (Rodwin 1993).

The difficulty of finding such a payment scheme can be seen from figure 19.1. It displays density functions defined over outcomes of medical treatment in terms of health outcomes θ, $f(\theta|a_0)$ and $f(\theta|a_1)$. Specifically, the density function given a_0 obtains if the provider expends little effort for his or her patient, making unfavorable outcomes (indicated by low values of θ) rather likely. If physician effort is $a_1 > a_0$, favorable outcomes become more probable. Nevertheless, bad outcomes such as θ_s cannot be excluded with certainty. Because the patient, lacking medical knowledge, cannot really judge effort, he or she is constrained to using outcome θ as a basis for payment. An optimal payment function $p^*(\theta)$ can bring about an optimal outcome in expected value only—a modest standard, considering that in surgery, for example, an individual typically deals with a particular surgeon once in his lifetime.

FIGURE 19.1   Health Outcomes Due to Provider Effort

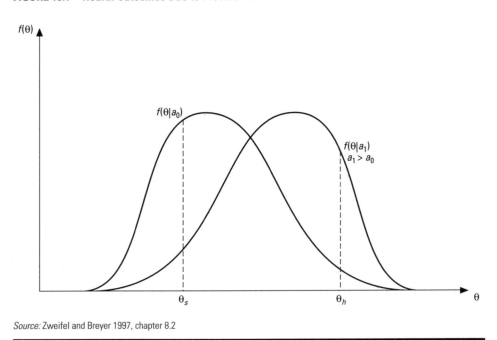

Source: Zweifel and Breyer 1997, chapter 8.2

CONCLUSION 1: *In the physician-patient relationship, opportunity for control by the patient typically is limited to the choice of a payment function that promises to provide the physician with optimal incentives on average.*

Choice of Payment Function in the Case of Medical Care

Assuming that the principal (the patient) maximizes his or her expected utility through choice of the optimal payment function $p^*(\theta)$, the optimal function satisfies the condition (Levinthal 1988; Rogerson 1985):

$$\frac{u'^P[\theta - p*(\theta)]}{u'^A[p*(\theta)]} = \lambda - \mu \cdot \frac{\dfrac{\partial f(\theta \mid a^*)}{\partial a}}{f(\theta \mid a^*)} = \lambda + \mu \cdot E, \text{ with } E := \frac{\dfrac{\partial f(\theta \mid a^*)}{\partial a}}{f(\theta \mid a^*)} \quad (2)$$

The left-hand side of equation 2 is a ratio of marginal utilities. Its numerator denotes the marginal utility of the principal (the patient), evaluated at his or her claim to the benefit, $[\theta - p * (\theta)]$. Its denominator symbolizes the marginal utility of the agent (the physician), evaluated at his claim to the benefit, $p^*(\theta)$. Since marginal utility of the patient decreases with increasing net benefit ($u''^P < 0$ due to risk aversion), a high value on the left-hand side of equation 2 indicates a payment function that strongly benefits the physician. Conversely, if the left-hand side of equation 2 takes on a low value, the major share of the benefit from the transaction goes to the patient.

The right-hand side of equation 2 contains the objective determinants of the optimal sharing rule $p^*(\theta)$:

- The term $\lambda > 0$ is a fixed amount, designed to motivate the physician to conclude the offered contract. A high value of λ occurs if failure to contract would have important consequences for the patient in terms of his or her health. In this situation, a capitation payment may be optimal for the patient. For a case study from Thailand, see Mills and others (2000).

- The second term corresponds to the incentive component of the fee. It consists of two parts. The first is the Lagrange multiplier $\mu > 0$, which indicates the effect that failure to provide the right incentives to the agent would have on the principal. It takes on a large value if any deviation of physician effort from optimality (as determined by the physician) has a great impact on the utility of the patient. The second component shows the stochastic effectiveness of the physician's treatment. A high value of $\partial f(\theta \mid a^*)/\partial a$ indicates that additional physician effort would move a great deal of probability mass in the density function defined over health outcomes. Indeed, $\partial f(\theta \mid a^*)/\partial a$ may be interpreted as the amount of shift in the distribution of health outcomes in figure 19.1 if physician effort marginally increases, for example, from a_0 to a_1. This shift is normalized by dividing through by the initial value of the density function given effort level a^*, $f(\theta \mid a^*)$.

Whereas this structuring of the contract has intuitive appeal, the patient's ability to identify such a scheme remains doubtful. In fact, he or she would have to estimate two parameters to be able to identify the optimal amount of incentive payment in the contract. The first indicates the extent to which a violation of incentive compatibility would affect the patient's welfare patient (multiplier μ). Estimating this parameter requires knowledge of the consequences that would obtain if the physician had marginally less interest in concluding the contract. The second factor is crucial. It reflects the effect of medical activity on the distribution over possible health outcomes. The more the physician is able to shift the distribution of health outcomes to higher values of θ (figure 19.1), the higher should be the incentive component (E in equation 2).

Both quantities are extremely difficult for a patient to estimate, with the possible exception of a chronically ill person, who has at his disposal repeated observations under side conditions held about constant. As a rule, therefore, the patient will be unable to identify the optimal degree of incentive payment in his or her contractual relationship with the physician. As a consequence, physician effort will generally assume a suboptimal value, often resulting in too unfavorable an outcome of treatment.

CONCLUSION 2: *Under asymmetry of information regarding effort, chances for the patient as the principal to identify such a scheme are minimal, causing treatment outcomes to be suboptimal. In particular, he or she lacks the information with regard to effectiveness of the contribution to the improvement of his or her health status.*

Asymmetry of Information Regarding Both Effort and Type

Sometimes, a prospective patient is not satisfied with having a contract with a particular health care provider, but would like to be sure of access to a good or the best provider available. Indeed, some providers accomplish much more than others with the same amount of effort. Because the prospective patient typically cannot find out which type is which, the asymmetry of information is compounded, existing not only with regard to effort but also type. Under these conditions, Laffont and Tirole (1993, chapter 1.4) derive the following optimality condition:[1]

$$p(\hat{\beta}, C) = p*(\hat{\beta}) - \left[1 - \frac{\kappa}{1+\kappa} \cdot \frac{F[\beta]}{f[\beta]} \cdot \psi''[e*(\beta)] \right] \cdot (C - C*[\hat{\beta}]), \text{ with} \qquad (3)$$

$$p*(\hat{\beta}) = \psi'[e*(\beta)] + U*(\beta).$$

This condition may be interpreted as follows:[2]

- The left-hand side of equation 3, $p(\hat{\beta}, C)$, symbolizes the payment function for a provider type who signals to be type $\hat{\beta}$ and has observed cost C of service. This already points to the problem that signaled and true type (that is, the effectiveness with which the provider can reduce cost through additional effort, similar to the marginal effectiveness E in terms of improved outcomes in the second section, above) need not coincide. However, for the payment function to be truly optimal, it must induce providers to reveal their true type (the "revelation principle").

- The first term on the right-hand side, $p^*(\hat{\beta})$, symbolizes the optimal payment function if the type of the health care provider is known (which still signaled to be $\hat{\beta}$). As stated in the second line of equation 3, it must cover the psychic marginal cost $\psi'[e^*(\beta)]$ that occurs if the provider exerts the optimal amount of effort e^*. This optimal value clearly depends not on the signaled type $\hat{\beta}$ but true type β. In addition, however, there is the rent $U^*(\beta)$, which is designed to ensure participation. Contrary to the parameter in equation 2, however, $U^*(\beta)$ does not go to all providers equally. Specifically, it is an informational rent received by the more effective types who are not recognizable as such but need to be attracted by a payment that exceeds their true psychic marginal cost.

- The second term of equation 3 shows how deviations from cost targets $C^*[\hat{\beta}]$—which again depend on signaled type—are dealt with. As argued below, the multiplier in square brackets is positive but smaller than one. This means that cost overruns $(C - C * [\hat{\beta}] > 0)$, while causing a deduction from payment, are not fully charged to the provider. This has nothing to do with risk aversion (the parties to the contract are assumed risk neutral) but takes into account the fact that a "steep" payment function would also contain powerful incentives for less-effective providers to contribute to output. Cost savings optimally are not fully credited to the provider either.

- Finally, the multiplier showing the extent to which deviations from cost targets are credited or debited is one minus an attenuation that is the product of three factors:

  (1) Attenuation is the higher, the higher κ, with κ indicating the amount of inefficiency associated with financing the payment in question. This can occur through tax revenue or contributions to health insurance. In the latter case, it amounts to the loading contained in the premium for health insurance.
  (2) The second component is $F[\beta]/f[\beta]$, showing the frequency of providers up to level β compared with the frequency at that level, thus the relative frequency of less-effective types. The higher this frequency, the larger the attenuation effect—designed to prevent less-effective types from exerting too much effort.
  (3) The third factor is the increase of marginal cost $\psi''[e^*(\beta)]$. It shows that it would not make much sense to induce much effort on the part of agents whose marginal cost rises sharply with additional effort.

CONCLUSION 3: *Under asymmetry of information regarding both effort and type, optimal payment schemes for health care services contain additional parameters that are not easily observed. Thus, chances for the patient as a principal to identify such a scheme are even slighter, causing treatment outcomes to be more suboptimal still.*

Preliminary Implications for the Multiple-Payer Issue

Conclusions 2 and 3 point to a tradeoff. On one hand, multiple payers hold the promise of negotiating remuneration schemes with health care providers that are attuned to the severity of the information asymmetry. On the other, multiple payers may not negotiate in the interest of their clientele and may not base their remuneration schemes on the parameters discussed above, although competition for clients will restrict these tendencies. As soon as premiums do not fully reflect true risk, however, competition induces insurers to use different schemes merely for *cream skimming* (that is, risk-selection activities).

A single payer, by way of contrast, typically establishes one uniform remuneration scheme, which saves transaction costs, especially for health care providers. Except for low-income countries, this argument does not carry too much weight anymore because several computerized medical billing systems now enable a physician or a hospital to bill according to many different payment systems. The crucial argument in favor of one single payer thus seems to be the opportunity to exert monopsonistic power. This means that the payer can negotiate lower fees because the providers lack an alternative (apart from leaving health care or the country). Given low estimated money price elasticities for demand for medical care, lowering fees should result in lowered health care expenditure.

COMPLEMENTARY AGENTS: THEIR OBJECTIVES AND CONSTRAINTS

The provider–patient relationship as the basic element of all health care systems was found to be deficient in the previous section when reviewed in the light of economic theory as soon as there is asymmetry of information regarding effort, type, or both. Accordingly, a market for complementary agents promising to correct this deficiency may be expected to emerge in health care.

Tasks of a Complementary Agent

Within this framework, two different functions of complementary agents can be distinguished, namely the provision of information and the negotiation of contracts with providers of services.

- *Provision of information.* To determine the optimal payment scheme, knowledge of effectiveness of medical treatment was found to be crucial in the preceding section. The complementary agent could theoretically limit its activities to providing this information while leaving identification and negotiation of the payment function to the patient.

- *Negotiation of contracts.* Even if a potential patient did have sufficient information to evaluate the stochastic effectiveness of a health care provider, negotiation of the contract is usually costly. Therefore, complementary agents are considered in their role as negotiators in the following.

Given a demand for the services of a complementary agent, which institutions (existing or new) can be expected to meet it? The transaction cost generated in their creation and generated or saved in their use may serve as a guide to explain why certain solutions have proved economically viable while others have not come into existence (Williamson 1985, chapter 1).

The transaction cost argument points above all to medical associations, whose officers, themselves physicians, could assess a member's effectiveness at low cost. In addition, they are engaged in the negotiation of fee schedules in most countries outside the United States.

However, the same argument also applies to private and social health insurers, who routinely collect information that could be used to gauge the effectiveness of providers of medical services while being their negotiating partners. Yet, as Havighurst (1988) notes, in the United States, insurers have been hesitant to implement, for example, second opinion or quality monitoring programs, arguably due to lack of competition.

Because most individuals have a labor contract, the employer also qualifies as a possible complementary agent. Indeed, it was Henri Kaiser, owner of a large construction firm, who "invented" the health maintenance organization by hiring his own physicians to ensure medical care for his employees who were working at remote sites in the United States. However, many a risk-averse employee may shy away from having his employer organize medical care for him, fearing the possible flow of medical information from hired physicians to the employer, who would then be in a position to easily recognize any loss of productivity caused by deterioration of his/her health.

Finally, every citizen has an implicit contract, as it were, with his/her government. Political institutions such as elections and a parliament serve to limit transaction costs involved in charging the government with an additional function, namely to provide information on the quality of medical care, negotiate fee schedules, or hire physicians and run hospitals on behalf of voters. However, the cost of actually using the government as a complementary agent may be deemed too high by a majority of citizens, preventing them from entrusting these functions to public officials.

Types of Complementary Agents in Health Care

There may well be additional future alternatives in the market for complementary agents. However, instead of speculating about them, we now draw

CONCLUSION 4: *Five types of complementary agent are likely to prevail in present health care systems: medical associations, private health insurers, social health insurers, employers, and the government.*

MEDICAL ASSOCIATIONS AS COMPLEMENTARY AGENTS

Medical associations have to perform two tasks (Feldstein 1996, chapters 3, 4; Schulenburg 1987; Zweifel and Eichenberger 1992). They should safeguard and enhance their members' reputations and limit competition among them (table 19.1). The first task provides a motive to take on the role of a complementary agent in order to relieve the basic physician–patient relationship of some of the deficiencies discussed above.[3]

In many developing countries, professional associations seem to act as an important complementary agent, since neither private nor social insurance (which is usually limited to the formal sector) has the necessary information or resources for negotiation. This situation typically results in a multiple-payer system as in Lebanon, where for open-heart surgery, the Ministry of Health pays 8 million Lebanese pounds, the National Social Security Fund 7.2 million, with private health insurers varying (Cotterill and Chakraborty 2000).

EMPLOYERS AS COMPLEMENTARY AGENTS

Employers can profit in several ways from assuming the role of complementary agent in the health care sector. One is reduced employee turnover, an important objective in industries where hiring a new worker entails a great deal of job-specific investment. By purchasing employee health care from a specific

TABLE 19.1   Complementary Agents: Objectives and Examples

Complementary agent	Objectives of the complementary agent	Countries where complementary agents are important
Medical association	• Conserve reputation of members	Australia
	• Prevent competition among members	Germany
		Lebanon
Employer	• Reduce employee turnover	United States (health maintenance organizations)
	• Improve knowledge of employee productivity	Yugoslavia (before 1985)
Private insurer	• Achieve competitive advantage	Netherlands
		Switzerland
		United States
Social health insurer	• Foster solidarity	Canada
	• Keep within the budget	Czech Republic
		France
		Spain
		Sweden
		Thailand
Government	• Accept risks associated with free labor market	China
	• Win votes	Great Britain
		Italy
		Portugal

Source: Author's own compilation.

group of physicians and hospitals, an employer makes a change of jobs costly. Arranging for health insurance giving access to specific provider groups has the same effect. However, to retain the more productive workers, employers have an interest in monitoring health status as an indicator of productivity. Medical information becomes quite valuable, and many employees may fear leakages of medical information. This fear may well be a reason employers are not the main complementary agent in any western country (table 19.1). The former Yugoslavia (before 1985), where enterprises purchased medical care for their employees, probably came closest to assigning an important role to employers as complementary agents. Because there is a multitude of employers in a market economy, the resulting system is multiple payers almost by definition. However, payment functions are likely to vary, too. Because employers compete for (productive) workers, they cannot deviate from worker preferences when acting as a complementary agent. Contracts negotiated with provider groups will therefore reflect both the different health conditions of employees and the incentive conditions of physicians and hospitals.

PRIVATE HEALTH INSURERS AS COMPLEMENTARY AGENTS

Private health insurers have an interest in performing as complementary agents provided that this service gives them a competitive advantage over competitors. Creating payment schemes that tie physicians more strongly to the interests of patients may enhance a private insurer's competitive advantage. At the same time, however, health insurance undermines clients' interest in the choice of payment function because it largely protects them from the financial consequences of suboptimal incentives in contracts. Therefore, insurers often prefer not to interfere with pricing (for example, in the United States and in Switzerland) or to settle for fee schedules negotiated by social health insurers (Germany).

As could be expected, when private insurers are important as complementary agents, multiple-payer systems prevail. In the United States, most providers derive a substantial part of their income from both managed care networks (which usually pay a capitation) and governmental programs such as Medicare (for the aged) and Medicaid (for the poor). In Switzerland, several sick funds have introduced managed care alternatives, where providers are paid a capitation. However, the great majority of physicians continue to derive most of their incomes from fee-for-service practice.

SOCIAL HEALTH INSURERS AS COMPLEMENTARY AGENTS

In only a few countries do social health insurers compete with each other. They therefore enjoy considerable liberty to pursue two objectives. The first is to foster solidarity, which means that the stochastic income redistribution brought about by private insurance is replaced by a systematic redistribution according to, for example, age, gender, and income. Their second objective is to keep within their budget because this helps insulate the government's budget from the vagaries of the economy. In this way, politicians may use the budget strategically to ensure reelection by favoring decisive voter groups (Van Dalen and Swank 1996).

In some countries, social health insurers have extensive authority, especially in the domain of fee negotiations, making them important complementary agents in the health care sector (table 19.1). Instances in point are the Czech Republic (Jack 2000), France and, especially, Canada with its uniform national health insurance (Evans 1983). All of them seek to avoid multiple payers in an attempt to keep fees (and public health care expenditure) low. In France, the Securité Sociale even plays two medical associations against each other.

THE GOVERNMENT AS COMPLEMENTARY AGENT

The deficiencies of the physician–patient relationship may be seen as a market failure, suggesting remedial action by the government. Indeed, political decisionmakers, especially in western industrial countries, have been inclined to take over the role of complementary agent in health care. Citizens of countries with market economies are challenged to make a living in a free labor market full of risks. Because good health greatly increases the probability of success in the labor market, this challenge was sweetened by promising everyone equal access to health care (table 19.1).

The continued interest of politicians in acting as complementary agents of (potential) patients lies in gaining votes (Feldstein 1996, chapter 2). Acting as negotiators, they have leeway to shift rents to voter groups decisive for (re)election. Usually, the details of negotiation are delegated to medical associations and (social) health insurers. Only in a few cases (for example, China, Great Britain, Italy) does government intervention go as far as to assume responsibility for actually delivering health care services. Quite generally, governments have a wide choice of actions at their disposal, such as the power to impose fee schedules and upper limits on medical incomes.[4]

Of course, governments seek to implement single-payer systems. This is achieved to a great extent in China, although some private, out-of-pocket payment is likely to occur (Yip and Eggleston 1999). This constitutes a second, unofficial source of health care finance. In Great Britain, physicians working for the National Health Service have the right to operate a limited number of private beds, whereas their Italian colleagues may split their work week between public and private practice. Therefore, multiple payers in fact slip in. However, the opportunity to negotiate payment schemes with tailor-made incentives on behalf of consumers is not used by the private insurers, presumably due to lack of competition.

Single- versus Multiple-Payer Systems: Preliminary Evidence

The complementary agents, their objectives, and constraints were described above and related to their preferred type of payment system. These hypotheses appear in table 19.2, where the predicted payer system is listed for each complementary agent.

TABLE 19.2   Complementary Agents and Single- versus Multiple-Payer Systems

Complementary agent	Predicted payer system	Actual payer system (examples)
Medical association	Multiple	Multiple (Australia)
		Multiple (Germany)
		Multiple (Lebanon)
Employer	Multiple	Multiple (United States)
		Single (former Yugoslavia)
Private insurer	Multiple	Multiple (United States)
		Multiple (Netherlands)
		Multiple (Switzerland)
Social health insurer	Single	Single (Canada)
		Single (Czech Republic)
		Multiple (France; Mutuelles)
		Single (Spain)
		Multiple (Sweden; health districts)
		Single (Thailand)
Government	Single	Single (China)
		Single (Great Britain)
		Multiple (Italy; health regions)
		Single (Portugal)

Source: Author's own compilation.

Medical associations, employers, and private insurers were predicted to opt for multiple-payer systems. In the first case, the opportunity for price discrimination may be the decisive motivation; for the other two, the competitive pressure of the market leads them to look for new ways to better align consumer and provider incentives. The examples cited are in accordance with predictions, with the exception of the former Yugoslavia, where worker-managed firms were conceived as autonomous units providing health care in a nonmarket environment.

With regard to the second group, comprising social health insurers and governments as complementary agents, the predicted choice is single-payer systems. This is borne out in most cases. One exception is Sweden, where some health districts have been experimenting with purchaser models, resulting in different payment systems within the country. Italy is another exception (this time in the governmental camp), because several regions have attained wide autonomy with regard to health care. Thus, both levels and modes of payment of providers differ somewhat within the same country.

CONCLUSION 5: *Among the five complementary agents considered, medical associations, employers, and private insurers are predicted to prefer multi-payer arrangements;*

social insurers and governments, single-payer arrangements. These predictions are largely confirmed by the available evidence.

A Case Study: The Czech Republic

The Czech Republic's experimentation with provider payment systems illustrates the importance of providing favorable incentives through the choice of remuneration (Jack 2000). In 1992, all Czech citizens were enrolled in a single statutory general health insurance company. Private insurers were permitted to enter the market in the following years, but the general health insurance company maintains a dominant market position, covering about 75 percent of the population. Contributions are based on the insured's wages, similar to Germany. However, an insurer receives only 40 percent of an individual's compulsory contribution, whereas 60 percent comes from a central fund.

Thus, private health insurers have little autonomy, stifling competition for members. Moreover, because providers are reimbursed on a uniform point-based scale administered by the Ministry of Health, chances are slim that insurers, through a choice of payment system, give health care providers the right incentives. As shown above, the optimum payment function importantly depends on the type of information asymmetry, which is not compatible with the uniformity imposed by the Ministry of Health. Recent developments are characterized by rising general practitioner fees and hospital admission rates. Some observers suspect that this is due to overuse, overreporting, or both. In all, experience in the Czech Republic seems to drive home the point that, under a uniform payment system for health care providers, important advantages of (potential) competition between health insurers may be lost. The Czech choices of complementary agents seem to favor social health insurance rather than competing private health insurers.

FIVE MAJOR CHALLENGES

Five major challenges confront health care systems throughout the world: new illnesses, an aging population, growing numbers of one-person households, technological change, and opening up to international competition.

- *Emergence of new illnesses.* The human immunodeficiency virus/acquired immunodeficiency syndrome pandemic is the single most important disease challenge, certainly for most African countries but also some Asian and Latin American countries.

- *Aging of the population.* Most countries will be confronted with an increase in their dependency ratio.[5] Among the industrial countries, this increase will be most marked in the case of Germany where by the year 2050, 100 active persons will have to support no fewer than 42 aged persons, compared with 26 at present (Weber and Leienbach 1989). However, this development also characterizes countries as different as China and the Czech Republic, with China (but also, for example, Thailand) expecting a doubling of the dependency ratio between 2000 and 2020. By 2050, Asia as a whole will likely have reached a value of 24 percent, comparable to France in 1990 (Bougaarts 1998).

- *Increasing number of one-person households.* The frequency of one-person households in industrial countries has been growing dramatically since about 1960 (Roussel 1986), and a similar trend can be expected for middle-income countries (United Nations 1997).

  This individualization has a direct impact on the demand for health care services, as illustrated by a simple thought experiment (Zweifel and Breyer 1997, chapter 9.3). A couple living together is likely to fall back on services provided by third parties only if both partners are ill. The probability that this combined event will occur is lower than the probability that just one person will fall ill. The two partners thus provide mutual protection from health risks, causing them to rely on formal health care less often than two single individuals. Thus, growing prevalence of one-person households is likely to fuel demand for medical care.

- *Technological change in medicine.* There is good reason to expect the pace and direction of technological change in medicine to depend on the extent of health insurance (Newhouse 1981). Yet health policymakers cling to the notion of exogenous technological change in medicine, a viewpoint adopted here, for simplicity. Indeed, much of this change occurs internationally, spilling over into the domestic health care sector. Its cost implications are obvious.

- *Opening up to international competition.* As in the production of other goods and services, countries have comparative advantages in the production of health care services. Because transportation was costly until well into the 20th century, social health insurers imposed the principle of local treatment, resulting in almost no international trade in medical services. Factor mobility as fostered by the European Union is apt to increase international competition in the health care sector. Physicians and dentists have had the right to locate freely within the European Union since the mid-1970s, a freedom accorded to dependent workers as well since 1992. Mobility will continue at a low rate, however, as long as the protection afforded by health insurance stops at the border of the country of origin. In practice, it takes full portability of health insurance to give workers an opportunity to choose between national offers of medical treatment. These considerations reduce the importance of international competition as an issue for the health care sectors of low- and middle-income countries.

Implications of These Challenges for Single versus Multiple Payers

These five challenges have implications for the choice between single- and multiple-payer systems at two levels. First, they affect the relative importance of the three degrees of information asymmetry distinguished above. If these challenges were to result in the predominance of one of these three types, a single-payer system would become more attractive (provided that it corresponds to the predominant category). If these challenges can affect information asymmetry either way, however, they would favor the multi-payer alternative. Second, the complementary agents considered do not have equal capabilities to cope with these challenges. If governments, for example, are better able to deal with them than other complementary agents, they are likely to increase the domain of their preferred payment scheme, the single-payer alternative. If competitive health insurers, say, have the comparative advantage in meeting these challenges, however, the domain of multi-payer systems is likely to increase in the future.

Direct Consequence of Future Challenges

The emergence of new illnesses initially shifts the weight toward the most severe asymmetry of information, the combination of uncertainty about both effort and type. This calls for an adjustment of remuneration schemes in favor of attenuated incentives, where providers can rely heavily on cost reimbursement. Aging, associated with a prevalence of chronic conditions, tends to reduce information asymmetry, making fee for service the appropriate alternative. The growing share of one-person households, however, results in the treatment of minor health losses within the health care sector. Because knowledge about the type of provider is less decisive in this case, this challenge should make the intermediate degree of asymmetry more important. If marginal effort of the service provider does not make much difference (low value of E in equation 2), a fixed payment in the guise of capitation may increasingly become optimal. In contrast, technological change in medicine boosts the value of E, calling for bonus payment for excellent outcomes. Finally, the opening up of health care systems to international competition does not seem to have any immediate implication for the different degrees of information asymmetry.

In sum, these future challenges have disparate influences on the different degrees of information asymmetry. This motivates

CONCLUSION 6: *Some of the five future challenges considered reduce the severity of information asymmetry; some of them increase it. This causes uncertainty about the optimal payment system, conferring some advantage on multiple-payer systems.*

Indirect Consequences of Future Challenges

In this section, the comparative ability of the different complementary agents to cope with future challenges is considered first. Because different agents prefer different payment systems (table 19.2), a prediction can be derived about the likely future importance of multiple- relative to single-payer systems.

To simplify the analysis, the challenges are grouped into two categories. The first group comprises those of domestic origin: the emergence of new illnesses, the aging of the population, and the increased share of one-person households.

The second group consists of challenges exogenous in origin: technological change in medicine and opening up to international competition between health care systems.

Medical associations, acting as complementary agents, are prepared to deal with the domestic challenges. Their members can easily organize the redistribution of medical care required by the emergence of new illnesses and aging. With regard to the exogenous challenges, the associations stand ready to ensure the adoption of new medical technology. However, because protecting their members from competition is one of their missions, medical associations cannot easily cope with an opening up of their domestic markets.

In contrast, *employers* are little prepared, acting as complementary agents, to deal with the domestic challenges that call for redistribution that clashes with their own quest for systems with favorable incentives (Clarke and Darrough 1983). The exogenous challenges match their know-how much better: assessing and monitoring use of new technology and profiting from possibilities of international procurement. This know-how will be valuable if international competition in the health care sector intensifies. So far, however, employers have not been strongly engaged in health care issues,[6] and they cannot be counted upon to become active in the near future.

Competitive *health insurers* will have an advantage as complementary agents because most of the challenges considered do not run counter to the objectives of insurance companies, which moreover have the expertise to deal with most of them. The emergence of new illnesses is an exception because insurers shy away from covering risks they cannot (yet) calculate. However, when it comes to managing technological change in medicine, private insurers can be expected to objectively weigh the benefits and costs (reflected in the extra premium) of including a new therapy in their benefit plans. Admittedly, such an unbiased weighing on behalf of consumers comes about only under pressure from competition, after disbanding national cartels still in existence.

The agents of *social health insurance* have the instruments to deal with domestic challenges that call for redistribution. However, exogenous challenges run counter to their mission of budget balance (technological change) or their domestic orientation (increased international competition).

Finally, *governments* can use their powers to impose any redistribution they deem necessary to confront domestic challenges. These powers are not useful, however, whenever the health care sector has to adjust to technological change in medicine or to intensified international competition.

In sum, no single complementary agent appears to be best prepared to deal with all the emerging challenges. In countries where domestic challenges such as new illnesses loom large, reliance on social insurers and the government may increase in the future. Indirectly, this tendency will enlarge the domain of single-payer systems (table 19.2). If, however, international challenges such as new medical technology are deemed crucial, competitive health insurers have a comparative advantage as complementary agents, entailing an increased importance of multiple payers (and multiple-payment schemes to the extent that they are permitted to compete on this score).

CONCLUSION 7: *The future challenges of domestic origin favor social insurers and governments as complementary agents and, with them, single-payer systems. Those of international origin favor competitive insurers and possibly medical associations and, with them, multiple-payer systems.*

Final Assessment

On efficiency grounds, a case can be made for having three basic payment systems, reflecting the three degrees of information asymmetry distinguished above. The existence of multiple-payer systems increases the chance of having of this choice of payment schemes. Whether this case is strengthened or weakened by the future challenges considered depends on the relative importance of the direct and the indirect effects. The direct effect of these challenges seems to be that differentiated payment schemes will become more appropriate in the future, because the degree of information asymmetry may change unpredictably. However, the indirect effect through a complementary agent may deal with some types of challenges better than with others. If the domestic challenges predominate, social insurers and governments have the advantage as complementary agents, and this efficiency advantage translates into a tendency in favor of single-payer systems. If international challenges are of primary importance, direct and indirect effects point in the same direction. Competitive health insurers can deal with those challenges while also preferring multiple-payer systems that go along with multiple-payment schemes.

CONCLUSIONS

Applying economic principal–agent theory to the provider–patient relationship leads to the conclusion that the patient, acting as the principal, generally lacks the knowledge to identify the payment scheme that indirectly controls provider effort in an optimal way. In most cases, his or her information seems insufficient to estimate crucial parameters determining the optimal payment function in the presence of asymmetrical information. This failure creates a market for complementary agents whose task is to provide the patient with the necessary information, or negotiate the payment scheme on his/her behalf, or both. Medical associations, employers, and private health insurers are complementary agents associated with multiple-payer systems, whereas social health insurers and governments favor single-payer systems. The domain of these alternatives will be affected by challenges confronting health care systems, including new illnesses, aging of the population, increasing numbers of one-person households, technological change in medicine, and the opening up of health care sectors to international competition. These challenges have disparate impacts on the different degrees of asymmetry of information, calling for flexibility with regard to payment systems that may come about in multiple-payer systems. However, there is an indirect impact as well, because these challenges favor some complementary agents while putting others at a disadvantage. When the challenges are domestic in origin, social insurers and governments are well prepared to handle them; accordingly, the domain of single-payer systems should increase. For challenges of international origin, private health insurers and possibly medical associations (and with them, multiple-payer systems) have the advantage. Since multiple-payer systems typically go along with multiple-payment schemes, there is a chance to improve matching of contract provisions in health care with the different degrees of information asymmetry, with the promise of an efficiency gain.

NOTES

1. Contrary to equation 2, which determines optimal output-augmenting effort, equation 3 is about cost-reducing effort. However, in view of the duality relationship between output maximization and cost minimization, this difference does not really matter. Indeed, Laffont and Tirole (1993, p. 135ff) show that a high value of effort e goes along with a high value of output.

2. For the provider, effort has (marginal) cost regardless of whether it is performance improving (a in equation 2) in the second section] or cost reducing (e in equation 3). The difference in notation is retained for easier reading of the original literature.

3. A formal modeling of the choice of a dominant complementary agent is beyond the confines of this paper, but see Zweifel, Lehmann, and Steinmann (2002) for such an attempt.

4. These powers are not at the disposal of a social health insurer as a contractual partner of providers. For this reason, it makes sense to distinguish between social insurance and the government.

5. The dependency ratio is defined as the number of 65-year-olds and older relative to the number of persons aged between 15 and 64 years.

6. This need not be a disadvantage, since associating health insurance with the work place is becoming increasingly problematic, because it hampers labor mobility, as evidenced by U.S. experience.

REFERENCES

Bougaarts, J. 1998. *Dependency Burdens in the Developing World*. New York, N.Y.: Population Council.

Breyer, F., and F. Schneider. 1992. "Political Economy of Hospital Financing." In P. Zweifel and H. E. Frech III, eds., *Health Economics Worldwide*, pp. 267–85. Dordrecht, Netherlands: Kluwer.

Clarke, F. H., and M. N. Darrough. 1983. "Optimal Employment Contracts in a Principal-Agent Relationship." *Journal of Economic Behavior and Organization* 21(4): 69–90.

Cotterill, P., and S. Chakraborty. 2000. "Lebanon Provider Payment Case Study." Revised final draft prepared for the World Bank. World Bank, Washington, D.C.

Evans, R. G. 1983. "The Welfare Economics of Public Health Insurance: Theory and Canadian Practice." In Lars Söderström, ed., *Social Insurance,* pp. 71–104. Amsterdam: North Holland.

Feldstein, P. J. 1996. *The Politics of Health Legislation. An Economic Perspective,* 2nd ed. Chicago: Health Administration Press.

Grossman, S. J., and O. D. Hart. 1983. "An Analysis of the Principal-Agent Problem." *Econometrica* 51: 7–45.

Havighurst, C. C. 1988. "The Questionable Cost-Containment Record of Commercial Health Insurers." In H. E. Frech III, ed., *Health Care in America,* pp. 221–58. San Francisco, Calif.: Pacific Research Institute.

Holmström, B. 1979. "Moral Hazard and Observability." *Bell Journal of Economics* 10(1):74–91.

Jack, W. 2000. "The Purchase of Medical Care in the Czech Republic: Provider Payments Mechanisms in Practice." Draft prepared for the World Bank. World Bank, Washington, D.C.

Laffont, J. J., and J. Tirole. 1993. *A Theory of Incentives in Procurement and Regulation.* Cambridge, Mass.: MIT Press.

Levinthal, D. 1988. "A Survey of Agency Models of Organizations." *Journal of Economic Behavior and Organization* 9: 153–85.

Mills, A., S. Bennett, P. Siriwarangsen, and V. Tangcharoensatkien. 2000. "The Response of Providers to Capitation Payment: A Case-Study from Thailand." Draft report submitted to the World Bank. World Bank, Washington, D.C.

Newhouse, Joseph P. 1981. "The Erosion of the Medical Marketplace." In R. M. Scheffler, ed., *Advances in Health Economics and Health Services Research* 2, pp. 1–34. Greenwich, Conn.: JAI Press.

Rodwin, M. A. 1993. "Medicine, Money and Morals." *Physicians' Conflicts of Interest.* Oxford: Oxford University Press.

Rogerson, W. 1985. "The First-Order Approach to Principal-Agent Problems." *Econometrica* 53: 1357–68.

Roussel, L. 1986. "Evolution récente de la structure des ménages dans quelques pays industriels" [Recent Development of Household Structure in Some Industrial Countries]. *Population* 41(6): 913–34.

Schulenburg, J. M. 1987. "Verbände als Interessenwahrer von Berufsgruppen im Gesundheitswesen" [Associations as Agents for the Professions in the Health Care Sector]. In L. Männer and G. Sieben, eds., *Der Arbeitsmarkt im Gesundheitswesen* [Labor Markets in Health], pp. 317–418. Gerlingen: Bleicher.

United Nations. 1997. "World Population Monitoring." United Nations Commission on Population and Development, New York.

Van Dalen, H. P., and O. H. Swank. 1996. "Government Spending Cycles: Ideological or Opportunistic?" *Public Choice* 89: 183–200.

Weber, S., and V. Leienbach. 1989. *Soziale Sicherung in Europa* [Social Security in Europe]. Baden-Baden: Nomos.

Williamson, O. E. 1985. *The Economic Institutions of Capitalism.* New York, N.Y.: The Free Press.

Yip, W., and K. Eggleston. 1999. "Provider Payment Reform in Hainan, China." Report submitted to the World Bank. World Bank, Washington, D.C.

Zweifel, P., and F. Breyer. 1997. *Health Economics.* New York, N.Y.: Oxford University Press.

Zweifel, P., and R. E. Eichenberger. 1992. "The Political Economy of Corporatism in Medicine: Self-Regulation or Cartel Management?" *Journal of Regulatory Economics* 4: 89–108.

Zweifel, P., H. Lehmann, and L. Steinmann. 2002. "Patching Up the Physician-Patient Relationship and Choice of Complementary Agents. In Björn Lindgren, ed., *Individual Decisions in Health,* pp. 207–233. London: Routledge.

CHAPTER 20

Influencing the Demand Side of Purchasing

Tim Ensor and Stephanie Cooper

Much public health spending, supposedly targeted to help the poor and vulnerable, instead benefits the better-off, according to a growing body of evidence (chapter 2, Gwatkin, this volume). Statistics point to persistent differences in access to health and health care between rich and poor groups (Wagstaff 2000), and substantial barriers to access for the poorest (Sachs 2001).

Many prospective patients are accustomed to making choices among private providers, without considering treatment at public facilities. Spending on public health facilities is often low, they are sparsely distributed and, once there, patients have to negotiate a maze of informal exchanges before receiving treatment. An average British citizen who falls ill goes to a general practitioner or a nearby hospital emergency department where referral is a normal part of treatment. An average Bangladeshi in a similar situation has a myriad of confusing choices to make. A rural resident may have to decide whether to go to a local subdistrict or union health center, a facility run by a nongovernmental organization (NGO), a minimally trained village doctor, or a local drug store (where the owners, qualified pharmacists or not, offer advice). Reaching the nearest district hospital can mean hiring a rickshaw and then paying for a bus ticket. Tight household finances can force choices about which household members receive treatment. Every day thousands of sick people have to navigate through these complex decisions in Bangladesh.

The supply of services is only one factor in the decisionmaking process. Service quality could undoubtedly be better in most countries, but many of the reasons for unequal and poor access lie on the demand side. Health services of reasonable quality are often there, but few use them. Just as important as the physical and financial accessibility of services is knowing what providers offer and how best to use self- and practitioner-provided services and cultural norms of treatment. The importance of demand-side barriers is illustrated in a survey of obstetric choices in Bangladesh (Barkat and others 1995 reported in Piet-Pelon, Rob, and Kahn 1999) where demand factors were found to be all of the most important reasons for not seeking emergency obstetric care (table 20.1).

Despite the importance of demand-side barriers, health policy and resource allocation are often directed mainly toward improving the supply side. Most government planning models have historically been supply driven, with staff size and capacity of facilities determining funding flows. Attention switched to population determinants of health care need with the development of resource

TABLE 20.1   Reasons for Not Seeking Care in Obstetric Emergencies in Bangladesh

Issue		Percent
Education	Do not know about emergency problems	59.5
Financial	Financial costs are relatively high	45.5
Information	Do not know about the availability of specific service at the facility	39.3
Social/cultural	Required medicines not always available	38.2
Social/cultural	In-laws object	35.6
Social/cultural	Religion does not permit going outside of the house, especially during pregnancy	35.3
Social/cultural?	Shyness	32.3
Distance	Facility too far from home	28.3
SUPPLY	Doctor not available when needed	25.2
Distance	Poor communication facilities	17.8
Family	Husband objects	17.0
SUPPLY	Difficult to get admission	14.1
SUPPLY	Attitude of service providers to clients not very friendly	5.6

Source: Adapted from Barkat and others 1995; issue added by author.

allocation formulas (Van de Ven and Ellis 2000). Allocations increasingly take into account the needs of small geographic areas, but most of the funding is still allocated to health care facilities and practitioners.

DEMAND-SIDE BARRIERS

Most of the standard economic frameworks of health care utilization model a supply and demand side.

An Economic Model of Demand

Supply includes factors derived from the health care production function that interact to produce effective health care services (figure 20.1). These include knowledge of technology, management, and input (factor) prices. Access at point of delivery is rationed by the official price, waiting time, or other mechanism such as a referral by a gatekeeper (for example, a general practitioner or a triage nurse). On the demand side, the economic literature is dominated by adaptations of the Grossman model that analyze individual investment and consumption decisions to improve health and use health care (Grossman 2000). Demand is influenced by factors that determine whether an individual identifies illness and is willing and able to seek appropriate health care.

Income is possibly the most important demand-side factor. Because address-ing income inequalities is primarily the realm of economic and social policy,

FIGURE 20.1   Supply and Demand for Health Care

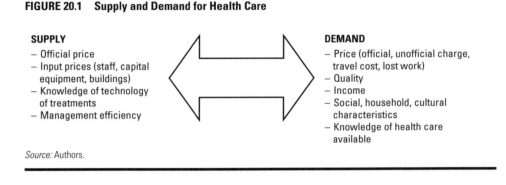

SUPPLY
- Official price
- Input prices (staff, capital equipment, buildings)
- Knowledge of technology of treatments
- Management efficiency

DEMAND
- Price (official, unofficial charge, travel cost, lost work)
- Quality
- Income
- Social, household, cultural characteristics
- Knowledge of health care available

Source: Authors.

however, income will not be discussed here except where it interacts with other demand factors.

Education and information are key determinants of demand, and, where they are inadequate, many health care markets fail. Because individuals often do not recognize their need for health care and the best available treatment options, an agent to guide decisionmaking is desirable. In most, but particularly low-income, countries, a wide variety of people fill this role—family members, traditional healers, community workers, unqualified birth attendants, midwives, pharmacists, and, occasionally, a doctor.

Besides the direct cost of medical care, a second important group of demand-side factors contribute to the price of treatment. Most important are distance and opportunity costs of work forgone to obtain treatment.

Another group of factors relates to the cultural and social acceptability of obtaining treatment. Influenced by the community, family, or religious affiliation, these factors may outweigh all others. A family wealthy enough to afford health services, for example, could still refuse to spend money to treat a particular family member.

Education and Information

Education, often measured by level or duration of schooling, is the most important correlate of good health (Grossman and Kaestner 1997). In Pakistan, for example, maternal schooling is the most important factor in determining child survival (Agha 2000). Mehrotra (2000) suggests that a high education base is a major determinant of above-average social development.

As a determinant of health care utilization, education is a complex variable. Education can improve individuals' ability to improve their own health by lifestyle changes rather than reliance on health services. There is also much evidence that better basic education can, through general improvements in literacy and specific health studies, increase desired and actual use of health services. Studies across a number of countries, for example, indicate the importance of maternal education on the use of obstetric services (Cleland and Van Ginneken 1988; Raghupathy 1996).

Education provides consumers with the basis for evaluating their own or a dependant's need for treatment. Information on the best places to seek care is also required. Although it is sometimes suggested that individuals cannot assimilate information on treatment options, work in Tanzania challenges this assumption (Leonard 2002; Leonard, Mliga, and Marian 2001, p. 43.). These studies suggest that, far from being passive consumers, patients actively seek out both the best-known provider and the best facility for each illness. Perceptions of quality accord well with technical evaluations.

The importance of misinterpreting health messages given out by health workers is clear from many studies. One, examining the reasons for choosing delivery sites in Uganda, suggests that, when told during antenatal care that "there are no problems," women often take this as a sign that the delivery will be normal and that attendance at a facility is therefore not required (Amooti-Kaguna and Nuwaha 2000). In Uganda, people think obtaining drugs, not the consultation, is the main reason for going to a clinic, and demand for antenatal care is thought to be low because medicines are not routinely dispensed (Ndyomugyenyi, Neema, and Magnussen 1998).

FINANCIAL AND DISTANCE BARRIERS

Location and distance costs often inhibit service utilization. In studies reviewed, transport makes up 28 percent of total patient costs in Burkina Faso, 25 percent in northeast Brazil, and 27 percent in the United Kingdom (Frew and others 1999; Sauerborn, Bodart, and Essomba 1995; Souza and others 2000). In Bangladesh, transport is the second most expensive item for patients after medicines (CIET Canada 2000).

In Vietnam, distance is a principal determinant of how long patients put off seeking care (Ensor and San 1996). In Zimbabwe, up to 50 percent of maternal deaths from hemorrhage can be attributed to the absence of emergency transport (Fawcus and others 1996). Distance is also a reason women choose to deliver at home rather than at a health facility (for example, in the Philippines [Schwartz, Akin, and Popkin 1993], Uganda [Amooti-Kaguna and Nuwaha 2000], and Thailand [Raghupathy 1996]). Yet, the women living farther away from a facility are the most vulnerable ones in an emergency. Distance may also have a differential impact across income groups. Qualitative evidence in Vietnam suggests that poorer households usually have access to inferior transport in the event of illness (Segall and others 2000).

Consuming health care can be time intensive. Both patients and relatives may have to give up work (or leisure) for long periods to receive treatment. This is an important cost to individuals, especially at harvest time and other peak periods of economic activity. Convenient opening hours, an indicator of the importance of taking time off from work, are important in determining service use in both Vietnam and Ghana (Bosu and others 1997; Segall and others 2000).

Opportunity costs vary for different groups. In Pakistan, for example, compliance is better among the economically inactive, because they are more likely to have time to go for treatment (Khan and others 2002). In Uganda, poorer patients will travel great distances searching for better facilities, perhaps because their opportunity costs (see below) are lower (Akin and Hutchinson 1999). Similar results are borne out in studies of the private sector in India, where quality (a supply variable) often overrides the distance cost and leads to complex and lengthy search strategies (Bhatia and Cleland 1999; Shenoy, Shenoy, and Krishnan 1997). These findings must, however, be balanced by the lower opportunity costs of obtaining care that is also a product of low income.

Financial barriers may also interact with other demand barriers. In Kazakhstan, for example, the education of the head of household or the care seeker is an important determinant of the willingness to travel long distances to obtain treatment (Thompson, Miller, and Witter, 2003).

Social and Cultural Barriers

The Voices of the Poor cross-country study finds general agreement that men invariably receive preferential access to health care over women (Narayan 1997). In Bangladesh, India, and Côte d'Ivoire (but not in Peru, where the opposite result is reported) females are much more likely to visit health care facilities and benefit from public and household health care expenditure (Begum and Sen 2000; Booth and Verma 1992; Gertler and van der Gaag 1990). In India, the bias toward boys is reduced when the household head is more highly educated (Booth and Verma 1992). These differences are related to both cultural patterns and social factors within the household and the community.

Cultural norms such as purdah restrictions can prevent women from seeking health care outside the home for themselves and their children (Rashid and others 2001). This barrier, often higher when men provide services, has been offered as a reason why Asian women living in western countries make little use of health services (Whiteford and Szelag 2000). Such restrictions may also interact with other barriers. In India, distance poses a bigger barrier for women than men with similar incomes (Vissandjee, Barlow, and Fraser 1997). This may be because it is culturally unacceptable for women to leave their homes for long periods or could reflect less access to household resources to pay for transport.

Other examples of culture as a barrier to using services is the perception among the Alur people of Uganda and the Bariba tribe of Benin that help with delivery indicates "weakness" (Bhatia and Cleland 2001; Ndyomugyenyi, Neema, and Magnussen 1998). Another is the unacceptability of modern contraception among men in parts of Pakistan (Casterline, Sathar, and Haque 2001).

In a related issue, men often make decisions for women on care seeking. In Senegal, for instance, men make more than 50 percent of decisions on female treatment (Post 1997). This is particularly important because male decisionmakers often spend less than women on social items, according to a study in Bangladesh, South Africa, Indonesia, and Ethiopia (Quisumbing and Maluccio

1999). In many South Asian societies, the mother-in-law dominates decisions on childbirth and pregnancy-related care, particularly in early marriage. Thus, whether a woman is delivered at home by a family member or a traditional birth attendant or at a health facility depends on the mother-in-law's beliefs (Piet-Pelon, Rob, and Khan 1999). At the community level, the traditional birth attendant is also vital in influencing demand. In Rajasthan, more than 90 percent of women who did not obtain referral care were advised against it by the traditional birth attendant (Hitesh 1996).

Increasing demand is thus far more complex than simply providing health education or information. Quisumbing and Maluccio (1999) find that educational differences between male and female members are crucial in determining who has most influence in a household. In India, women who cannot contribute through superior education or earnings maintain their status through household chores, which may militate against their receiving care in the event of illness (Ramasubban and Rishyasringa 2000). This reinforces opportunity cost as a factor in reducing demand, not by loss of income but by loss of position within the household hierarchy.

Intervening to Reduce Barriers

An extensive review of the literature on the nature and impact of demand-side interventions was carried out, based on a structured search of key electronic databases, Web sites of international agencies and NGOs, and key informant contacts with researchers working in related fields (Ensor and Cooper 2002, p. 63).

Why Intervene?

The overview in the previous section indicates that demand-side barriers are important in influencing use of services and, ultimately, access to good health. Two further questions arise: Should these barriers be reduced through intervention and, if so, how?

There are two principal justifications for intervening to reduce demand barriers:

- To correct market imperfections arising from incorrect, inadequate, or asymmetric information or incomplete markets.

- To reduce social inequity.

MARKET IMPERFECTIONS

Individuals may not fully realize they need medical care to prevent serious disease, not just when they are sick. They also need information on the range of services for appropriate treatment and the specific facility likely to deliver the services most cost-effectively. Finally, some markets may be insufficiently developed, particularly those that spread risk through insurance or loans.

Educating individuals, households, and communities is a way of dealing with information gaps that lead to inadequate demand and market failure (table 20.2). Developing insurance or loan mechanisms to spread demand-side costs is a way of addressing the market failure of inadequate capital and insurance markets, a common problem in low- and middle-income countries.

SOCIAL EQUITY

A second justification for intervention is on the grounds of social equity. Some groups have fewer resources than others because of either the society's underlying income distribution or differences in intrahousehold or community bargaining power. This could justify interventions to target resources toward the needy who cannot access services.

Subsidies for service or improving supply-side access to services can be a response to either the efficiency (lack of information or markets) or the equity question. Reducing demand-side costs to individuals can mitigate information market failures and stimulate demand (table 20.2). Selective cost reductions can address equity concerns through a subsidy-based reallocation of resources. These subsidies are different in that one group targets the poorly informed, while the other targets the poor and other socially disadvantaged groups.

A difficulty in evaluating evidence on demand-barrier impact is that the many confounding factors make causation from a particular intervention hard to attribute.

TABLE 20.2   Types of Intervention to Correct Demand Barriers

	Information imperfections	Increase ability to pay	Supply side
Lack of knowledge			
• Education	Fill knowledge gaps	Stimulate demand through general cost reduction	
• Information			
• Culture	Educate communities and households		Deliver culturally sensitive health care services
Uncertainty		Develop insurance, loans, and prepayment schemes to finance costs	
Equity			
• Distance costs		Reallocate resources through targeted subsidies for the poor	Bring services to communities, more flexible opening hours
• Opportunity costs		Develop patient payments, loan funds	
• Intrahousehold		Target subsidies	

Source: Authors.

Ideally, the intervention should be implemented when few other factors are changing or when these factors can be measured and their confounding impact adjusted.

A striking aspect of this research was that much has been written about barriers, but far less on means of reducing them. Still fewer studies documented evidence of the impact of the interventions. The next sections will review interventions targeted at maternal health and family planning, two areas where interventions have been widely used, followed by other more general interventions.

Maternal Health and Family Planning

The concept of demand barriers is well recognized in the literature on maternal health, formalized in the delays model (Maine 1997). This model classifies three barriers to accessing care: delay in deciding to seek care, delay in getting to the facility, and delay in obtaining appropriate care once at the facility. The first two delays can be classified as demand barriers. A variety of interventions have been conducted to overcome these delays. Many of them were implemented through the Prevention of Maternal Mortality (PMM) network, but there is also evidence from a variety of other sources.[1]

Interventions to improve education and information frequently center on training community educators. These are usually women living in the target communities who can convince families they need maternal care and facilitate admission to a hospital in an emergency. Three such schemes in Nigeria, Sierra Leone, and Ghana all led to a substantial increase in hospital admissions for normal and complicated deliveries (Kandeh and others 1997; Nwakoby and others 1997; Opoku and others 1997). An NGO in Bangladesh trained traditional birth assistants to advise women on referral and help them get to the hospital (Barbey and others 2001). A non-PMM education initiative in Malawi reported a threefold increase in use of hospitals or clinics for postpartum care and a doubling in delivery care (Gennaro and others 2001). Another educational campaign in Kebbi State, Nigeria, reported an increased awareness of obstetric complications but no impact on referrals (Gummi and others 1997). In the Nigerian case, a decline in real incomes and other factors were thought to confound the positive impact on use, but no attempt was made to adjust for them.

A variety of interventions facilitated transport. One intervention, in northwest Nigeria, worked with transport unions to provide reliable and affordable transport (Shehu, Ikeh, and Kuna 1997). A seed fund for the cost of fuel was set up and replenished with contributions from users. Drivers were trained to be respectful to their passengers by avoiding smoking, talking loudly, or showing impatience. A project in Sierra Leone provided radios to call vehicles to take women to the hospital in obstetric emergencies (Samai and Sengeh 1997). Both interventions report a substantial increase in the numbers of people going to the hospital.

One non-PMM project implemented community education, transport, and training for traditional birth assistants in Indonesia, Bolivia, and Guatemala to promote use of essential obstetric care (Kwast 1995, 1996). Although no results are reported for the Javanese interventions, substantial increases in referrals are reported in both Guatemala and Bolivia. The projects were intended to highlight the improvements that community level (demand-side) interventions could make in referrals and maternal mortality. The studies provide no information on intervention costs.

Another group of interventions has helped develop community loan funds, used by people who have to pay for transport and other health care costs. Obstetric admissions doubled in one district that had developed loan funds but did not change in nonintervention communities (Fofana and others 1997). Of the six communities targeted, only two, under strong leadership, succeeded in establishing funds. Other loan projects were evaluated in Ekpoma, Cross River State, and Zaduna in Nigeria (Chiwuzie and others 1997; Essien and others 1997; Olaniran and others 1997). The evaluation concentrated solely on the number of loans made and their repayment (more than 93 percent) within the first year. The project is considered a success within these narrow parameters, although concerns have been raised about fund depletion and possible interest rate increases to offset default costs. Fifty-eight percent of the project money was spent on loans, implying a relatively high administrative cost. Because start-up and ongoing costs are not separated, however, the recurrent costs of administration are difficult to measure.

Establishing maternity waiting homes near district hospitals is another intervention used to overcome distance barriers. Two such interventions, in Zimbabwe and Ethiopia, report high use of hospitals and low complication rates for deliveries (Poovan, Kifle, and Kwast 1990; Spaans, van Roosmalen, and van Wiechen 1998). No attempt was made to check for possible selection bias arising from certain types of women using these facilities. In Ghana and Zaire, similar interventions were less positively received, largely because the facilities were located in desolate surroundings and lacked good facilities for preparing meals (Hildebrandt 1996; Post 1997). These studies emphasize the importance of consulting with the community on the potential intervention before making an investment.

Many of the efforts to stimulate demand for family planning services focus on service delivery within the community. The strategy, "community-based delivery," takes supplies into potential users' villages and even their homes. This strategy may help to overcome a multiplicity of demand-side obstacles, including ignorance of family planning products, cultural reluctance by men and women to seek contraceptives in public facilities, and minimization of demand-side costs. It may also motivate people to use other services. In India, for example, family planning workers help promote demand for child health services, at the same time offering family planning advice (Srivastava and Bansal 1996).

One review of community delivery in Africa suggests a generally positive impact on contraceptive prevalence (Phillips, Greene, and Jackson 1999). Little attention, however, was given to cost-effectiveness or sustainability of such schemes.

Doorstep delivery of family planning services to rural households in Bangladesh has significantly increased the contraceptive prevalence rate, but is considered unnecessarily expensive (Arends-Kuenning 1997). Delivery has been shifted to community clinics (Government of Bangladesh 1998). What impact this will have on use of services is not yet known.

Other Care

The important influence of transport networks on demand is recognized by the growing number of social protection projects that are financing local road upgrades. Examples were found, for example, in World Bank social protection projects in Argentina, Burundi, Georgia, Madagascar, and Vietnam (World Bank project Web site http://www.care.org/programs/). However, only one project (Burundi) specifically mentions investment in roads as a way of improving access to health care.

The proliferation of community insurance schemes theoretically offers a way of addressing demand-side barriers by incorporating transportation costs into the benefit package. Yet, only one of the recent reviews of community schemes mentions that those costs are covered. The one exception is a scheme in Samburu district, Kenya, which covers transport costs up to US$60 a year for a household premium of US$5 a year (Macintyre and Hotchkiss 1999). The scheme is evaluated only in terms of numbers of members, and no evidence is offered of the effect on use.

Interventions covering users' indirect opportunity costs have been stimulated by a growing appreciation that the need to present regularly for therapy is one inhibitor of continued treatment. Payments may compensate patients for time off work, travel, and general inconvenience.

Treatment of tuberculosis is well suited to this type of intervention because it is intensive, and the externalities of nontreatment are significant. Farmer and others (1991) identified 26 separate schemes across low-, middle-, and high-income countries that offer inducements, including food and transport subsidies, for clinic attendance. One project in Haiti makes financial payments to cover travel, nutrition supplementation, and income lost during treatment. All patients treated recovered, whereas 46 percent of those in the control group still had the disease after one year.

POLICY DISCUSSION AND RESEARCH IMPLICATIONS

The importance of demand-side factors in determining access to services can be seen from discussion so far. The findings suggest that this is an underresearched area, but one with potentially substantial policy implications.

How far policymakers might extend the boundaries of public health care expenditures to include activities that reduce demand-side barriers is a core issue. Many of the interventions reviewed were funded primarily by NGOs, although many of the PMM interventions received moderate cofunding from local governments. Health ministries often finance some demand-side interventions (behavioral change, information, and education), but such spending usually accounts for a small part of the budget, an estimated 3 percent, for example, in Bangladesh (Ministry of Health and Family Welfare 2001). Wider interventions to assist, for example, with transport costs are often not considered. The development of poverty reduction strategies, stimulated by the HIPC[2] initiative, may prompt creative thinking about the ways funding can be used to improve access for the poor. Initiatives to reduce demand barriers are an important ingredient of such strategies.

If health sector purchasers—whether health ministries, insurance funds, NGOs, or donors—are to target demand barriers, they need a strong evidence base. This raises a series of research considerations concerning the need for more rigorous studies of demand and combined supply and demand strategies, an explicit focus on poverty, and choice of realistic behavioral models.

More Rigorous Studies of Demand

Though still fragmented, evidence is increasing on which supply-side measures work in the delivery of medical care. Similar evidence on effectiveness and cost-effectiveness of demand-side interventions is scanty or nonexistent. Treatment of many of the interventions in both the published and unpublished literature was largely descriptive with limited evaluation, particularly the PMM studies. Most evaluations did not control for confounding factors. Cost information is scarce. Few studies differentiate between capital and recurrent costs or provide sufficient information for even a rudimentary cost-effectiveness analysis.

Combined Supply and Demand Strategies

The limitations of demand-side strategies must be recognized. Creating demand is no substitute for improving supply. No one will be convinced to use poor-quality health services. This is confirmed by some of the evidence reported in this chapter that people bypass local facilities and travel long distances for good care. It was also recognized in the design of the PMM interventions, which first ensured the supply of good maternal health care before stimulating demand. Another limitation relates to the scope of the health sector, as traditionally defined by the remit of a typical health ministry. Money can be spent to train doctors or improve a clinic, but budget flexibility may not extend to improving a rural road even if poor transport is the main barrier to increasing utilization. Successful demand strategies often require assistance both from donors and ministries responsible for other sectors.

Focus on Poverty

Another aspect lacking in most studies is an explicit focus on interventions that target the demand barriers that most affect the poor. Few interventions differentiate between their impact on poor and nonpoor groups. This is important, considering that many interventions are designed to reduce financial barriers, which are likely to be higher for the poor. Many interventions target entire communities to enlist general community support in order to reduce maternal deaths. In this case, a direct targeting approach would be inappropriate. Yet, policymakers still need information on who actually benefits from an intervention if they want to concentrate resources on the people least able to afford health services.

Some interventions are designed for specific vulnerable groups. Interventions to increase compliance in tuberculosis treatment, for example, may benefit vulnerable groups disproportionately as well as having a wider public health function. Yet, evaluation data on the beneficiaries would still be useful if only to convince governments and donors of the desirability of the interventions.

Choosing the Right Model of Behavior

A further issue is whether the most appropriate model of patient decisionmaking is used when designing interventions. One illustration relates to interventions designed to increase use of obstetric services and reduce maternal mortality. Some interventions are designed to get women to the hospital in an emergency. Others are intended to develop the general transport services available to men and women for both emergency and nonemergency care.

A household faces two main choices before a woman in that household gives birth. It can transport the woman to the hospital in plenty of time, perhaps to a maternity waiting home until the onset of labor. This reduces the likelihood of severe complications or death, but the household incurs a cost for travel and waiting prior to admission to the hospital. In this case, the loss to the household is the financial cost of taking the woman to the hospital. Alternatively, the household can plan for a home delivery with a traditional birth attendant or relative, taking the woman to the hospital only in an emergency. (A third "choice" exists—no medical care—perhaps the only option for deeply impoverished families.) The loss to the household is a combination of the financial cost of the trip and the increase in likelihood of medical damage arising from the delay weighted by the probability of an emergency.

Which option is chosen depends on a gamut of demand-side variables, including income, costs of the options, knowledge of treatment options, and household decisionmaking. Policy interventions influence the relative loss and may alter the household choice, sometimes in unexpected directions. If, for instance, a household places a low value on a female member's health and, with little wealth, has a high marginal utility of income, subsidizing the cost of emergency transport may make the household more likely to delay sending the woman to the hospital, avoiding the certain costs and relying on subsidized transport in an emergency. If society places high value on maternal health and wishes to correct perceived intrahousehold inequality in resource use, subsidizing nonemergency transport and maternity waiting homes may be a more effective policy. This example, though only one possible scenario, illustrates the perverse incentives that could arise if policy is based on an ill-thought-out model of reality.

NOTES

We are grateful to a large number of people and organizations for providing information on demand-side barriers and initiatives. In particular: Jayshree Balachander, Oona Campbell, Ramon Abel Castano-Yepes, Lesong Conteh, Kiran Dev Pant, Priti Dave Sen, Nel Druce, Maria Goddard, Davidson Gwatkin, Sara Joseph, Barbara Klugman, Jack Langenbrunner, Kenneth Leonard, Benjamin Loevinsohn, Di McIntyre, Adilet-Sultan Meimanaliev, Kate Marsden, Anne Mills, Valeria Oliveira-Cruz, Kris Prenger, Dzhamilya Sadykova, Rachel Tolhurst, Catriona Waddington, Pongsadhorn Pokpermdee, Christian Aid, and CARE International. The World Bank provided funding to carry out this research.

1. Initially the PMM project was supported by the School of Public Health, Columbia University, but since 1996 it has become a permanent regional body with headquarters in Accra.

2. A World Bank debt relief program for Heavily Indebted Poor Countries (HIPC).

REFERENCES

Agha, S. 2000. "The Determinants of Infant Mortality in Pakistan." *Social Science and Medicine* 51: 199–208.

Akin, J. S., and P. Hutchinson. 1999. "Health-Care Facility Choice and the Phenomenon of Bypassing." *Health Policy and Planning* 14(2): 135–51.

Amooti-Kaguna, B., and F. Nuwaha. 2000. "Factors Influencing Choice of Delivery Sites in Rakai District of Uganda." *Social Science and Medicine* 50: 203–13.

Arends-Kuenning, M. 1997. "The Equity and Efficiency of Doorstep Delivery of Contraceptives in Bangladesh." Population Council, Policy Research Division, Dhaka.

Barbey, A., A. J. Faisel, J. Myeya, V. Stavrou, J. Stewart, and S. Zimicki. 2001. "Dinajpur SafeMother Initiative: Final Evaluation Report." CARE Bangladesh, Dhaka.

Barkat, A., J. Helali, M. Rahman, M., Majid, and M. L. Bose. 1995. "Knowledge, Attitude, Perception and Practices Relevant to the Utilization of Emergency Obstetric Care Services in Bangladesh: A Formative Study." University Research Corporation, Dhaka.

Begum, S., and B. Sen. 2000. "Not Quite, Not Enough: Financial Allocation and the Distribution of Resources in the Health Sector." Bangladesh Institute of Development Studies, Dhaka.

Bhatia, J. C., and J. Cleland. 1999. "Health Seeking Behavior of Women and Costs Incurred." In S. Pachauri, ed., *Implementing a Reproductive Health Agenda in India*. New Delhi: Population Council.

———. 2001. "Health-Care Seeking and Expenditure by Young Indian Mothers in the Public and Private Sectors." *Health Policy and Planning* 16(1): 55–61.

Booth, B. E., and M. Verma. 1992. "Decreased Access to Medical Care for Girls in Punjab, India—The Roles of Age, Religion, and Distance." *American Journal of Public Health* 82(8): 1155–57.

Bosu, W. K., D. Ahelegbe, E. Edum-Fotwe, K. A. Bainson, and P. K. Turkson. 1997. "Factors Influencing Attendance to Immunization Sessions for Children in a Rural District of Ghana." *Acta Tropica* 68: 259–67.

Casterline, J. B., Z. Sathar, and M. U. Haque. 2001. "Obstacles to Contraceptive Use in Pakistan: A Study in Punjab." Population Council, Policy Research Division, Islamabad.

Chiwuzie, J., O. Okojie, C. Okolocha, S. Omorogbe, A. Oronsaye, W. Akpala, B. Ande, B. Onoguwe, and E. Oikeh. 1997. "Emergency Loan Funds to Improve Access to Obstetric Care in Ekpoma, Nigeria." *International Journal of Gynaecology and Obstetrics* 59(suppl. 2): S231–36.

CIET Canada. 2000. "Service Delivery Survey: Second Cycle 2000 Preliminary Findings." CIET Canada, Dhaka.

Cleland, J. G., and J. K. Van Ginneken. 1988. "Maternal Education and Child Survival in Developing Countries: The Search for Pathways of Influence." *Social Science and Medicine* 27(12): 1357–68.

Ensor, T., and S. Cooper. 2002. "Resource Allocation and Purchasing: Influencing the Demand Side." Report to World Bank. University of York, Centre for Health Economics, York, United Kingdom.

Ensor, T., and P. B. San. 1996. "Access and Payment for Health by the Poor in Northern Vietnam." *International Journal of Health Planning and Management* 11(1): 69–84.

Essien, E., D. Ifenne, K. Sabitu, A. Musa, M. AltiMuazu, V. Adidu, N. Golji, and M. Mukaddas. 1997. "Community Loan Funds and Transport Services for Obstetric Emergencies in Northern Nigeria." *International Journal of Gynaecology and Obstetrics* 59(suppl 2): S237–44.

Farmer, P., S. Robin, S. L. Ramilus, and J. Y. Kim. 1991. "Tuberculosis, Poverty, and 'Compliance': Lessons from Rural Haiti." *Seminars in Respiratory Infections* 6(4): 254–60.

Fawcus, S., M. Mbizvo, G. Lindmark, and L. Nystrom. 1996. "A Community-Based Investigation of Avoidable Factors for Maternal Mortality in Zimbabwe." *Studies in Family Planning* 27(6): 319–27.

Fofana, P., O. Samai, A. Kebbie, and P. Sengeh. 1997. "Promoting the Use of Obstetric Services through Community Loan Funds, Bo, Sierra Leone." *International Journal of Gynaecology and Obstetrics* 59(suppl 2): S225–30.

Frew, E., J. L. Wolstenholme, W. Atkin, and D. K. Whynes. 1999. "Estimating Time and Travel Costs Incurred in Clinic Screening: Flexible Sigmoidoscopy Screening for Colorectal Cancer." *Journal of Medical Screening* 6: 119–23.

Gennaro, S., D. Thyangathyanga, R. Kershbaumer, and J. Thompson. 2001. "Health Promotion and Risk Reduction in Malawi, Africa, Village Women." *Journal of Obstetric, Gynaecologic and Neonatal Nursing* 30(2): 224–30.

Gertler, P., and J. van der Gaag. 1990. "The Willingness to Pay for Medical Care: Evidence from Two Developing Countries." World Bank Report 11595. World Bank, Washington, D.C. http://www.wds.worldbank.org/servlet/WDSContentServer.

Government of Bangladesh. 1998. "Project Implementation Plan, Health and Population Sector Programme." Dhaka.

Grossman, M. 2000. "The Human Capital Model." In A. J. Culyer and J. P. Newhouse, eds., *Handbook of Health Economics,* Vol. 1A. Amsterdam: North-Holland.

Grossman, M., and R. Kaestner. 1997. "Effects of Education on Health." In J. Behrman and N. Stacey, eds., *The Social Benefits of Education.* Ann Arbor: University of Michigan Press.

Gummi, F. B., M. Hassan, D. Shehu, and L. Audu. 1997. "Community Education to Encourage Use of Emergency Obstetric Services, Kebbi State, Nigeria." *International Journal of Gynaecology and Obstetrics* 59(suppl 2): S191–200.

Hildebrandt, E. 1996. "Building Community Participation in Health Care: A Model and Example from South Africa. *IMAGE: Journal of Nursing Scholarship* 28(2): 155–59.

Hitesh, J. 1996. "Perceptions and Constraints of Pregnancy Related Referrals in Rural Rajasthan." *Journal of Family Welfare* 42(1): 24–29.

Kandeh, H. B., B. Leigh, M. S. Kanu, M. Kuteh, J. Bangura, and A. L. Seisay. 1997. "Community Motivators Promote Use of Emergency Obstetric Services in Rural Sierra Leone." *International Journal of Gynaecology and Obstetrics.* 59(suppl 2): S209–18.

Khan, M. A., J. D. Walley, S. Witter, N. Imran, and N. Safdar. 2002. "Costs and Cost Effectiveness of Different DOT Strategies for the Treatment of Tuberculosis in Pakistan." *Health Policy and Planning* 17(2): 178–86.

Kwast, B. 1995. "Building a Community-Based Maternity Program." *International Journal of Gynaecology and Obstetrics* 48(suppl): S67–82.

Kwast, B. 1996. "Reduction of Maternal and Perinatal Mortality in Rural and Peri-Urban Settings: What Works?" *European Journal of Obstetrics and Gynaecology and Reproductive Biology* 69: 47–53.

Leonard, K. L. 2002. "Active Patients in Rural African Health Care: Implications for Welfare, Policy, and Privatization." Columbia University, New York.

Leonard, K. L., G. R. Mliga, and D. H. Marian. 2001. "Bypassing Health Centers in Tanzania: Revealed Preferences for Observable and Unobservable Quality." Columbia University, New York.

Macintyre, K., and D. R. Hotchkiss. 1999. "Referral Revisited: Community Financing Schemes and Emergency Transport in Rural Africa." *Social Science and Medicine* 49: 1473–87.

Maine, D. 1997. "The Strategic Model for the PMM Network." *International Journal of Gynaecology and Obstetrics* 59(suppl 2): S23–25.

Makinen, M., H. Waters, M. Rauch, N. Almagambetova, R. Bitran, L. Gilson, D. McIntyre, S. Pannarunothai, A. L. Prieto, G. Ubilla, and S. Ram. 2000. "Inequalities in Health Care Use and Expenditures: Empirical Data from Eight Developing Countries and Countries in Transition." *Bulletin of the World Health Organization* 78(1): 55–74.

Mehrotra, S. 2000. "Integrating Economic and Social Policy: Good Practices from High-Achieving Countries." UNICEF Innocenti Research Centre, Florence, Italy.

Ministry of Health and Family Welfare. 2001. "Public Expenditure Review of the Health and Population Sector Programme 1999/2000." Health Economics Unit and Management Accounting Unit, Dhaka.

Narayan, D. 1997. *Voices of the Poor: Poverty and Social Capital in Tanzania,* Environmentally and Socially Sustainable Development Studies and Monographs Series. Vol. 20. Washington, D.C.: World Bank.

Ndyomugyenyi, R., S. Neema, and P. Magnussen. 1998. "The Use of Formal and Informal Services for Antenatal Care and Malaria Treatment in Rural Uganda." *Health Policy Planning* 13(1): 94–102.

Nwakoby, B., C. Akpala, D. Nwagbo, B. Onah, V. Okeke, W. Chukudebelu, A. Ikeme, J. Okara, P. Egbuciem, and A. Ikeagu. 1997. "Community Contact Persons Promote Utilization of Obstetric Services, Anambra State, Nigeria." *International Journal of Gynaecology and Obstetrics* 59(suppl 2): S219–24.

Olaniran, N., S. Offiong, J. Ottong, E. Asuquo, and F. Duke. 1997. "Mobilizing the Community to Utilize Obstetric Services, Cross River State, Nigeria." *International Journal of Gynaecology and Obstetrics* 59(suppl 2): S181–89.

Opoku, S. A., S. KyeiFaried, S. Twum, J. O. Djan, E. N. L. Browne, and J. Bonney. 1997. "Community Education to Improve Utilization of Emergency Obstetric Services in Ghana." *International Journal of Gynaecology and Obstetrics* 59(suppl 2): S201–07.

Phillips, J. F., W. L. Greene, and E. F. Jackson. 1999. "Lessons from Community-Based Distribution of Family Planning in Africa." Working Paper 121. Population Council, Policy Research Division, New York.

Piet-Pelon, N. J., U. Rob, and M. E. Khan. 1999. *Men in Bangladesh, India and Pakistan.* Dhaka: Karshaf Publishers.

Poovan, P., F. Kifle, and B. E. Kwast. 1990. "A Maternity Waiting Home Reduces Obstetric Catastrophes." *World Health Forum* 11(4): 440–45.

Post, M. 1997. "Preventing Maternal Mortality through Emergency Obstetric Care." SARA issues paper. Academy for Educational Development, Support for Analysis and Research in Africa Project, Washington, D.C.

Quisumbing, A. R., and J. A. Maluccio. 1999. "Intrahousehold Allocation and Gender Relations: New Empirical Evidence." Policy Research Report on Gender and Development. Working Paper 2. World Bank, Washington, D.C.

Raghupathy, S. 1996. "Education and the Use of Maternal Health Care in Thailand." *Social Science and Medicine* 43(4): 459–71.

Ramasubban, R., and B. Rishyasringa. 2000. "Treatment Seeking by Women in Mumbai Slums." In *Reproductive Health in India: New Evidence and Issues.* Pune, Maharastra, India: Tata Management Training Centre.

Rashid, S. F., A. Hadi, K. Afsana, and S. A. Begum. 2001. "Acute Respiratory Infections in Rural Bangladesh: Cultural Understandings, Practices and the Role of Mothers and Community Health Volunteers." *Tropical Medicine and International Health* 6(4): 249–55.

Sachs, J., ed. 2001. *Macroeconomics and Health: Investing in Health for Economic Development.* Report of the Commission on Macroeconomics and Health. Geneva: World Health Organization.

Samai, O., and P. Sengeh. 1997. "Facilitating Emergency Obstetric Care through Transportation and Communication, Bo, Sierra Leone." *International Journal of Gynaecology and Obstetrics* 59(suppl 2): S157–64.

Sauerborn, R., C. Bodart, and R. Essomba. 1995. "Recovery of Recurrent Health Services Costs through Provincial Health Funds in Cameroon." *Social Science and Medicine* 40(12): 1731–39.

Schwartz, J. B., J. S. Akin, and B. M. Popkin. 1993. "Economic Determinants of Demand for Modern Infant-Delivery in Low-Income Countries: The Case of the Philippines." In A. Mills and K. Lee, eds., *Health Economics Research in Developing Countries.* New York: Oxford Medical Publications.

Segall, M., G. Tipping, H. Lucas, T. V. Dung, N. T. Tram, D. X. Vinh, and D. L. Huong. 2000. "Health Care Seeking by the Poor in Transitional Economies: The Case of Vietnam." Institute of Development Studies, University of Sussex, Brighton, United Kingdom.

Shehu, D., A. T. Ikeh, and M. J. Kuna. 1997. "Mobilizing Transport for Obstetric Emergencies in Northwestern Nigeria." *International Journal of Gynaecology and Obstetrics* 59(suppl 2): S173–80.

Shenoy, K. T., T. S. Shenoy, and T. N. Krishnan. 1997. "Determinants of Health Care Service Utilization in Kerala." *Journal of Clinical Epidemiology* 50 Supplement 1(2001): 45S.

Souza, A. C. T. D., K. E. Peterson, F. M. O. Andrade, J. Gardner, and A. Ascherio. 2000. "Circumstances of Post-Neonatal Deaths in Ceara, Northeast Brazil: Mothers' Health Care Seeking Behaviors during Their Infants' Fatal Illness." *Social Science and Medicine* 51(11): 1675–93.

Spaans, W. A., J. van Roosmalen, and C. M. van Wiechen. 1998. "A Maternity Waiting Home Experience in Zimbabwe." *International Journal of Gynaecology and Obstetrics* 61(2): 179–80.

Srivastava, R. K., and R. K. Bansal. 1996. "Please Use the Health Services—More and More." *World Health Forum* 17: 165–68.

Thompson, R., N. Miller, and S. Witter. 2003. "Health Seeking Behavior and Rural/Urban Differences in Kazakhstan." *Health Economics* 12(7): 553–64.

Van de Ven, W., and R. Ellis. 2000. "Risk Adjustment in Competitive Health Plan Markets." In A. J. Culyer and J. P. Newhouse, eds., *Handbook of Health Economics,* Vol. 1B. Amsterdam: North-Holland.

Vissandjee, B., R. Barlow, and D. W. Fraser. 1997. "Utilization of Health Services among Rural Women in Gujarat, India." *Public Health* 111: 135–48.

Wagstaff, A. 2000. "Socioeconomic Inequalities in Child Mortality: Comparisons across Nine Developing Countries." *Bulletin of the World Health Organization* 78(1): 19–29.

Whiteford, L. M., and B. J. Szelag. 2000. "Access and Utility as Reflections of Cultural Constructions of Pregnancy." *Primary Care Update* 7(3): 98–104.

PART VI

Legal and Regulatory Issues

CHAPTER 21

Law and Regulation

Frank G. Feeley

The simple concept of resource allocation and purchasing (RAP) soon ramifies into a complex structure upon investigation of the market interactions implied by the "purchasing" role. Looking at the impact of laws and regulations on the RAP model further complicates the analysis. Some laws governing the provision of health services—notably provider licensing and liability for professional negligence—predate modern concepts of risk pooling and purchasing and do not directly address the role of an "agent" purchasing services on behalf of patients. Such laws may constrain the actions of the RAP agent and perhaps should be modified in the light of RAP theory.

In systems with social or private health insurance, a variety of laws govern risk pooling and revenue collection roles as well as RAP behavior. These rules are particularly important if the statutory structure does not explicitly incorporate all of the population into a single risk pool or coverage scheme. Recent reforms in the regulation of South African health insurance schemes explicitly address abuses that can arise when only a portion of the population is included in insurance schemes and the government health service provides for uninsured individuals as well as for services not covered by the private RAP arrangements and too expensive for an individual to purchase out of pocket (Soderlund 1998, p. 197).

Rules governing risk pooling and revenue collection are dealt with elsewhere in this book. A note of caution is warranted in designing accompanying financial solvency requirements for RAP purchasers: Respect the differences between provider-based managed care schemes, where the provider incurs most or all of the financial risk, and schemes where the purchaser pays independent providers according to the amount of care delivered. To encourage the development of health maintenance organizations (HMOs) in the United States, the federal government passed a law in the 1970s changing some of the rules applied to this developing innovation. Financial solvency guarantees can be less stringent for provider-based managed care schemes, because the provider has the ability to expand output at modest marginal cost to meet medical demands in excess of expectations. The "pure" insurer, however, must pay out cash for each service and needs a larger financial cushion. Similarly, community finance schemes with modest benefit packages need less of a solvency guarantee than nationwide insurers. To demand too much in solvency guarantees will inhibit the development of potentially innovative schemes.

In this chapter, we focus on the laws and regulations that affect the purchaser's ability to act as an effective agent in buying health services. We look not only at laws already in place but also at laws that may be contemplated to regulate the purchaser's activity in:

- Deciding which services to purchase ("What to pay for")

- Selecting the providers that will offer the services and determining the conditions under which they will do so ("Whom to pay")

- Determining the amount and method of payment for services ("How much and how to pay").

A TYPOLOGY OF RAP ARRANGEMENTS

The RAP concept paper (chapter 1) recognizes a spectrum of purchasing arrangements that begins with systems integrating the financing and direct provision of care by ministries of health and runs through integrated nongovernmental HMOs to social health insurance, and to private and community health insurance. At the far end of this spectrum, individuals purchase health services with their own resources; no entity acts as an agent on their behalf to enhance efficiency, effectiveness, or equity. The area of interest lies in the part of the spectrum that begins with HMOs (where there is some blurring of the "purchaser" and "provider" roles) through to private and community health insurance. Under all these arrangements, a RAP agent makes decisions to purchase services on behalf of the patients. We ask how existing (and potential) laws can:

- Improve the ability of the agent to enhance the effectiveness and efficiency of care

- Enhance equity in the treatment of patients with varying medical needs and ability to pay for care

- Make services more responsive to individual patient needs.

One important element to consider in the legal analysis is the extent to which the RAP agent has concentrated purchasing power. If both the service provider and the patient have a wide choice of different RAP agents, each agent may exercise greater freedom to set the terms by which it purchases care. A disgruntled provider or patient may move to an alternative purchasing arrangement. But such fragmented arrangements have inherent problems in developing large risk pools or require complicated mechanisms to adjust for differences in risk and level inequalities in the ability to pay premiums.

If the RAP agent acts on behalf of most or all of the patients in a geographic region, it captures the broad pool of medical risks and may internalize some of the necessary resource transfers across groups (high and low income, well and sick, productive and dependent). But the power it has as a "single purchaser" must be subject to stricter rules on its purchasing behavior. At a minimum, it will be required to provide greater procedural protections for individuals damaged by a purchasing decision. If a RAP agent with monopsonistic power refuses to purchase covered services from a particular provider, that provider will be driven out of business, even though it complies with national licensing standards. Aggrieved providers will seek procedural protection of their economic interests, if not an outright guarantee of provider status as long as they are duly licensed. The purchaser may not refuse or withdraw a contract without adhering to published rules for such decisions or without a hearing before an impartial body. Implementing regulations should provide procedural protection without discouraging the RAP purchaser from making difficult decisions that will improve equity, efficiency, or quality. Procedures should permit community insurance schemes with a very small share of the relevant market a freer hand to contract with a small number of providers and in doing so leverage better prices or service levels for its patients.

What follows are brief discussions of the laws that *may* exist, or be adopted, in a country and their impact on the operation of an efficient RAP arrangement. In general, countries at the lowest levels of development show the least development of such laws and regulations, often having little more than a basic licensing law for physicians or inpatient hospitals. Such rules rarely specify more than minimum educational attainment (and occasionally "good moral character") in the case of physicians, or minimal standards for ownership and physical structure in the case of hospitals. No reference is made to laws that control investment or general corporate operations for all businesses, including health providers.

To obtain some idea of the issues in countries with a more elaborate legal infrastructure affecting health providers and purchasers, we draw on the available literature on regulation and health insurance in South Africa, Chile, and the Philippines. No pretense is made to a full-scale legal analysis in these countries or to an accurate description of the laws worldwide. Instead, we seek to set out here an annotated checklist for local legal analysis to serve those who ask: "Does my country have an effective RAP arrangement? Could it be improved, and what role might the law play in such improvements?"

REGULATING WHAT IS PURCHASED

The choice of efficient benefit packages and the definition of core or mandatory benefits in purchasing schemes are covered in chapter 3.

Covered Benefits

Many statutory schemes regulate the purchaser's flexibility in determining which services to purchase. There are several reasons for doing this:

- A defined minimum benefit package may establish a basis for competitive purchasing, or "managed competition" as envisioned by Einthoven (1993).

Purchasers must offer the same benefits and can compete on price and quality, not through subtle variations in the benefit package.

- Purchasers can be required to offer the benefits that the regulator deems cost-effective, having high externalities and public health benefits, or particularly important for social protection.

- Defined benefits can prevent private insurers from dumping high-cost cases on the public health care system, as has happened in South Africa (Soderlund and Khosa 1997, p. 349)

Required benefits may also be a form of "regulatory capture," in which provider groups mandate coverage by the purchasing arrangement so that they can expand the market for their services. Should psychotherapy (if covered) be limited to psychiatrists, or must purchasers also pay psychologists and social workers for the service? Sometimes patient and provider groups collaborate to mandate a benefit. For example, women's groups and obstetricians may lobby for coverage of family planning or infertility services.

As an economy grows and health care expenditures increase, the need to fix a reasonable minimum benefit package becomes greater. In the early stages of developing RAP schemes, a minimum benefit scheme may prevent poorer groups from achieving the benefits of risk pooling. In some African community health insurance schemes, only inpatient benefits are covered. A "sound" benefit package would seem to include both inpatient and outpatient benefits so as to prevent unnecessary hospitalization. The acceptable annual premium for a health financing scheme in a rural village may be enough for basic inpatient coverage but inadequate to cover one or two outpatient visits as well. Risk pooling in that market is better achieved without a mandated combination of outpatient and inpatient benefits. Other poor communities may choose to focus their premiums on obtaining local primary care and drug supplies and leave inpatient benefits to the government. Mandated benefit packages in such a circumstance can inhibit the development of RAP schemes.

Excluded Benefits

In addition to the positive requirement for a minimum benefit package, a government may want to limit the ability of a purchaser to exclude certain benefits for many other reasons:

- To prevent the purchaser from *cream skimming* a risk pool by denying benefits to those with chronic or congenital diseases.

- To reduce the burden on the public safety net (as in South Africa).

- To prevent deceptive marketing by insurance companies, which hide the exclusions in the small print of the insurance contracts.

- To enhance the level of economic protection provided by a RAP scheme.

Balanced against these reasons for limiting exclusions is the purchaser's need to make the health plan affordable. Thus, limits on exclusions are more acceptable as incomes rise, and patients demand broader coverage and can afford higher premiums. However, one form of exclusion must usually be permitted, but must always be closely regulated. This is the classic "preexisting condition" exclusion where a patient is not covered (for some period of time) for the costs of a medical condition existing at the time he or she joined the purchasing scheme. No risk pool will work if members can join only when they have immediate major medical needs. The purchaser must pool the resources, and medical needs, of the healthy and the sick.

Where RAP coverage is mandatory and continuous for all, it is reasonable to bar preexisting condition exclusions. Where coverage is optional, some other approach must be taken. The period of the preexisting condition exclusion can be limited. Or such exclusions can be banned if the patient has continuous coverage with other RAP schemes. Or all schemes can have an "open enrollment" period once each year, when they must accept all applicants, who must then stay enrolled for a fixed period of time. Whatever route is taken, this is one area in which laws governing RAP schemes should be clear and explicit.

Medical Necessity

Even the cleverest lawyers will lag behind the complexity of medical care and the advancing science of evidence-based medicine. It is impossible to draft a structural law, or even a regulation, that can comprehensively mandate benefits and define every permitted exclusion. There will always be cases in which a particular treatment may be of great benefit to one patient, yet of negligible benefit to another. The need to distinguish between such cases is usually accommodated by a stipulation that the purchaser pays only for "medically necessary" treatments. But what is medically necessary? Most statutory language provides a poor guide. In assessing the legal structure for a RAP arrangement, it is perhaps better to concentrate on an appeals mechanism (see below and the example of Chile), instead of trying to craft a definition that will apply to every RAP plan and every case.

Services Reserved to Other Parts of the Health System

Purchasers may try to avoid including in the benefit package services provided free by the government, particularly preventive services and treatment of infectious diseases such as tuberculosis. Where the government mandates that treatment for certain conditions occur in government-controlled institutions—as it does with psychiatry in Russia—a purchaser will often avoid including such services in the benefit package, for it would otherwise be forced to replace tax dollars with RAP funds.

Excluding these government services may be rational. In Africa, government is better in offering some primary care services such as vaccinations and prenatal care than in providing district hospital treatment for illness and accidents. Thus, it is reasonable to permit a community health insurance plan to require its members to use these government preventive services and reserve scarce premium dollars for other services where quality is available only with the payment of user fees. However, such an approach can fragment care. If clinical and preventive care take place at different sites, patients may not seek the preventive services that would lower treatment costs. Where most health care funding flows through RAP arrangements and not through direct government-provided services, it is usually desirable to require the RAP plans to include the full range of services, even though they could be obtained from government clinics. This is more likely to result in cost-effective and comprehensive care. In low-income countries where direct government funding is still a significant part of health spending and is focused on preventive and primary care, leaving to the purchaser the decision to exclude some government-provided services may be reasonable.

Nondiscrimination

Though not immediately apparent, laws that ban discrimination generally may have an impact on a RAP system's freedom to define covered benefits. If a country has a strong law barring discrimination against individuals with human immunodeficiency virus/acquired immunodeficiency syndrome (HIV/AIDS), does this mean that the RAP arrangement must cover antiretrovirals? Do laws mandating equal protection for women mean that a maternity benefit must be included in a RAP arrangement? If drug or alcohol abuse is considered a psychiatric condition, must treatment for these be covered to the full extent of any psychiatric benefit?

There is no single answer to this question. Sometimes the antidiscrimination statute may specify that it applies to medical benefits. More often a general principle is stated, and the implications for RAP arrangements are not thought through at the time of passage.

In performing a review of local laws that might affect a RAP scheme, the first step is to list existing antidiscrimination laws and identify any portions of these laws or implementing regulations that are specific to medical care benefits. If the laws are silent, the question must then be asked, "Should RAP arrangements accept this ambiguity or seek clarifying legislation? For the purchaser, the greatest freedom in designing a benefit package is desirable, and a scheme should not be required to provide a benefit that it cannot afford. At the moment, any argument by extension from AIDS antidiscrimination laws that a community financing scheme in Africa must cover antiretroviral drugs might render a scheme unmarketable, particularly where HIV prevalence is high and low-cost antiretrovirals are not yet available to scheme providers. In severely afflicted countries, the required premium could be beyond the capacity of potential members, unless external donors subsidize some of the AIDS treatment costs or make antiretroviral drugs available at reduced prices. Some community health financing schemes may want to cover maternity benefits, while others may consider them a predictable and "normal" expense and will choose a benefit package oriented more toward infectious diseases and accidents. Although it is true that this decision may reflect the prejudices of a group of older males who control the purchasing scheme, the expansion of community RAP arrangements will not be encouraged by preempting these decisions.

Where multiple RAP schemes develop in a poor country, leaving benefit decisions to the schemes is probably preferable to preempting benefit design through antidiscrimination legislation. Development of RAP schemes may be encouraged by a clear legal statement that the selection of a benefit package is *not* subject to litigation under antidiscrimination laws. However, where there are a few well-funded RAP schemes, it is likely that arguments for additional benefits (such as antiretrovirals) will be made under antidiscrimination statutes. In such cases, it may be better to have the decision subject to specific legislative action amending the minimum benefit package. The costs and benefits can then be publicly weighed, rather than attempting to achieve the same result through litigation of ambiguously worded antidiscrimination laws.

Appeals Process

At some point, any RAP arrangement must say "No" to payment for some services that could be offered by a medical provider. Certain well-established services (transplants) may be categorically rejected as exceeding the purchaser's ability to pay or as ineffective in relation to the cost (routine tonsillectomies). In addition, however, most purchasing arrangements will reserve the right to reject services that are not medically necessary, as discussed above. Should there be recourse for the patient who wants the service and the provider who is willing to offer it?

Many nascent purchasing arrangements have yet to encounter this issue, but they will as patient and provider sophistication increase. In Russia, for instance, the Federal Mandatory Health Insurance (MHI) Fund invested substantial effort in developing sanctions that insurers could impose on providers who denied services or delivered unnecessary services. The draft regulations also specified procedures for enforcement, but ignored the possibility that the insurer might prevent a patient from receiving a covered serviced (Federal Compulsory Health Insurance Fund 1999). But when asked if they were developing comparable procedures for aggrieved patients denied a service by the insurer, Federal Fund officials responded that they did not think this was needed. They had not considered that the insurer might deny payment for a service deemed unnecessary or that the patient might claim that the service needed was, in fact, a covered benefit. No patient appeals procedure was being developed.

Chile, which has an extensive private health insurance system coupled with a government safety net of social insurance, has a well-developed appeals mechanism that might be a model for other countries. Complaints against the private insurers (ISAPREs) can be filed with the responsible regulatory authority, and there is a well-defined process from initial complaint through informal dispute resolution to arbitration, where the burden of proof lies with the insurer. In 1997, the insurer won 28 percent of these contests, while the insured was fully or partially victorious in 59 percent (Jost 1999, pp. 15–16).

The appropriate level of patient protection and appeal will vary from society to society and will generally increase with the scope of the benefit and education of the covered population. For simple community financing schemes, a formal appeal process will be too expensive and perhaps unnecessary. But some avenue of appeal may benefit the community financing movement, particularly where the population is skeptical of other insurers that are perceived to shirk claim-payment obligations. Where medical care is expensive and large RAP schemes few, some avenue of patient appeal becomes imperative. The outlines of the appeal system should be included in a law structuring a single-payer arrangement, while general principles for appeals should be stated for more disparate RAP arrangements. The procedures should be as simple and swift as possible and should give due consideration to the purchaser's need for efficiency as well as the patient's desire for care.

REGULATING THE CHOICE OF PROVIDERS

The choice of providers is usually regulated by licensing of physicians and hospitals, and sometimes by antitrust and competition laws. Many West European countries try to control health care spending by limiting the supply of beds and expensive medical equipment. Some countries by law require the purchaser to accept any qualified provider.

Professional and Facility Licensing

Even the least developed countries usually have a law that requires licensing of physicians and hospitals. Often, medical associations are delegated the authority to license physicians. Licenses are frequently given for life and rarely withdrawn. Even if the government retains the licensing authority and requires periodic renewal, few physicians lose their license because of incompetent practice. Although the government retains the authority to license hospitals, the regulations are usually poorly developed and antiquated. Enforcement can be nonexistent or corrupt. In short, a purchaser will want to require that a provider hold a license, but this should not be the sole criterion for a provider's participation in a RAP arrangement.

One possible way of enforcing high standards is to add to the licensing requirement a stipulation that the provider hold further qualifications granted by self-regulatory bodies such as a society of specialist physicians. While the standards developed for such accreditation are likely more rigorous than government licensing regulations, enforcement and withdrawal of accreditation may be haphazard. One alternative, used in the Philippines, is to authorize the national purchaser to establish its own accreditation program (Hindle, Acuin, and Valera 2001). In the absence of such a statute, the purchaser can develop "conditions of participation" in its provider contracts that permit it to enforce standards of quality or performance. In Russia, this has resulted in a de facto incorporation into the health insurance program of outdated medical quality standards descended from the Soviet era. It would be better if Russian purchasers developed more modern evidence-based standards, but they generally defer to health authorities. No firm rule can be established for the "best" statutory structure, but it is advisable that the law either mandate or permit the insurer to enforce standards in addition to the minimums associated with professional licensure.

Monopoly and Competition

Antitrust and monopoly laws may limit RAP purchasing arrangements. The analysis will vary from country to country, depending on the governance of the RAP arrangement (public or private), the structure of the health care system, and the specific procompetition rules. In general, RAP purchasers should be free to choose providers in order to maximize efficiency and quality. If multiple purchasers operate in a market, the question of *tying*—locking a provider into a purchasing arrangement to the exclusion of other purchasers—may arise. If providers consolidate to increase their negotiating power with purchasers, a monopoly or oligopoly may be created to the detriment of consumers and purchasers. Yet, consolidation of providers may also permit desirable downsizing of an inefficient health system. No hard and fast rule on the application of antimonopoly laws is possible, but—"caveat RAPtor"—the purchaser should check competition laws before designing purchasing arrangements that exclude other purchasers or providers.

Certificate of Need and Planning Approval

Many countries in Western Europe attempt to control total health care spending by limiting the supply of expensive medical equipment or the construction or reconstruction of hospital beds. Even the United States experimented with a "Certificate of Need" law for health system investment, recognizing that medical costs obey Roemer's law, with utilization, and insurance payments, expanding with installed capacity

To understand the implications of such capacity control, one must first know if a population is served by a single or multiple RAP arrangements. If there is a single payer for the country or the region, it should play a role in the approval of major capital investment. In effect, this could even be delegated to the purchaser, which has the best knowledge of cost implications for any investment.

However, the providers, and the ministry of health, may object. They may want capacity to offer services that the purchaser does not want to pay for. This usually results in negotiations during the approval process. If approval is granted, the single RAP purchaser usually has little choice but to pay for services in the approved facility, unless the approval specifically exempts it from such obligation. As single-payer RAP arrangements develop, statutes delineating their role in the approval process are desirable.

Where multiple RAP arrangements (private insurers, community-based schemes, industry-based sickness funds) serve a single medical market, the questions become more complex. An individual purchaser cannot (and should not) control the planning decision, although it should have an opportunity to be heard in the approval process. But what happens once a decision is made and the new investment approved? Is each purchaser obligated to accept the new or expanded facilities within its provider network? For efficiency purposes, the answer should be "No." The purchaser should have the flexibility to decide if it can obtain care more efficiently by negotiating with a subset of approved providers. Perhaps it can obtain a lower price for a tertiary procedure by concentrating all its cases in a single location. But providers will argue that approval of the investment implies an obligation for each purchaser to pay for patients who reach the facility. Of course, the purchaser can still utilize gatekeeping arrangements to keep patients away from a facility it considers superfluous or expensive. Operationally, decisions will be simplified by a law that clarifies the purchaser's freedom to exclude (or not exclude) providers that otherwise have the necessary planning approvals

"Any Willing Provider"

"Any willing provider" laws, though usually seen as a reaction to the growth of the managed care movement in the United States, can become an issue wherever a purchaser seeks to trim its commitment to an excessive network of practitioners or facilities. Such laws state that the purchaser must accept as a provider any qualified practitioner willing to accept the general terms (for example, price, payment conditions) of a provider contract. The purchaser cannot selectively contract with providers in order to drive down prices or to limit capacity in the provider network so as to reduce unnecessary procedures performed to generate additional income. This is currently an issue in the Philippines, where the national health insurance system must accept all accredited providers, thus limiting its ability to negotiate more favorable rates in return for greater patient volume (Hindle, Acuin, and Valera 2001).

Lest this seem a problem peculiar to litigious American health providers, consider the circumstances of the former Soviet Union (FSU). Most cities have more hospitals and beds than necessary. If all the doctors currently practicing in the system were to seek to make a living through fee-for-service practice, the purchaser could not afford the total cost or would have to pay prices so low that the doctor could not make an acceptable wage (effectively what has happened). A purchaser—single or multiple—could achieve great efficiency benefits by contracting selectively with the best pieces of the existing health system. In fact, this has not happened in Russia and most of the FSU countries. Where insurers have been created, they have been under great pressure to include all providers in the payment scheme. A few have attempted to negotiate preferential arrangements for their insureds with the best facilities, but the purchasers have generally been ineffective in downsizing the system. If the opportunity exists and downsizing is necessary, a country should consider passage of a law specifically permitting purchasers to contract selectively.

REGULATING THE PURCHASING TRANSACTION

To protect consumers, some countries allow patients or their families to sue for negligent medical care. Some countries also set by law maximum and minimum prices for health care services and drugs and forbid direct payments. "Patient privacy" in the Internet age is an issue in industrial countries.

Liability for Professional Negligence

Countries in the Anglo-Saxon common law tradition permit a patient or his/her heirs to sue a medical provider for "breach of the duty of care" when he/she is injured (or killed) by deficient medical treatment. Other countries provide by statute for compensation for damages in the event of such professional malpractice. The frequency of litigation is a function of many factors besides the extent of malpractice in the medical care system. In India, damages resulting from physician and hospital negligence have been brought within the scope of the Consumer Protection Law to facilitate recovery by injured patients (Bhat 1996, pp. 267–68).

The first question to be asked of RAP arrangements and professional negligence is: Does the RAP purchaser have any role to play? If it has paid additional medical costs due to medical negligence, the purchaser has an economic interest in recovering these costs from a provider found liable for the injury. This could be accomplished by a simple statute that requires the inclusion of such costs in the allowable recovery and gives the insurer a lien on the recovery if the patient's claim is successful. The third-party purchaser may, however, want to waive recovery of such costs, thus reducing the volume of litigation and its cost to the health care system. If the purchaser is confident of its ability to select providers and eliminate the incompetent, it will want to use information about professional negligence in its decisions to grant or continue provider status.

Should the purchaser go beyond passive recovery of its costs or use information on professional negligence to take an active role in assisting the patient to recover? This occurs in the Russian MHI system, where the insurer seeks to position itself as the defender of the patient's interests. In addition to penalizing deficient providers and recovering the medical costs associated with negligent care, insurers do attempt to recover some damages on behalf of the patient. A third-party purchaser should have much greater expertise than a patient in assessing the quality of care and the extent of a provider's negligence. Using the purchaser to determine the level of a patient's recovery might be an administratively efficient way to replace the large frictional costs of individual case litigation. However, the extent to which patients will be willing to cede to an insurer the protection of their interests, and their right of recovery, will vary greatly. The number and amount of recoveries in the early years of the Russian MHI system were small (Federal Compulsory Health Insurance Fund 1999), and do not provide a basis for assuming that the third-party purchaser will be more zealous in protecting the damaged patient's interests than the common law system or the consumer protection law in India.

Determining Rates of Payment

Some countries have legislation that fixes maximum or minimum prices for health care services. In addition, where medical societies are powerful, they may influence fees by publishing suggested fee levels. Peer pressure (and self-interest) then motivates members to maintain these fee levels. Without entering the debate on the economic merits of price legislation, it is clear that such rules should not be applied to RAP arrangements. If the RAP purchaser can obtain prices below the statutory minimum, it should be allowed to do so. As long as quality and access are ensured by the purchaser, the patient will benefit. A purchaser might also want to pay above the maximum for a service, perhaps to guarantee quality or to encourage a provider to include supplementary services or bundle separate fees into a single price for a procedure or diagnosis.

In addition to the general question of minimum or maximum fees, special issues arise around incentives the purchaser may incorporate in its fee structure. Should a purchaser be allowed to offer the provider incentives (through capitation, fee withholding, or other mechanisms) to reduce the volume of services provided or obtained through referral? This has been a basic tool of the managed care industry in the United States, but was also used to some effect with fund-holding general practitioners in Britain and has been tried at various sites in Russia such as Maroyaroslavets rayon in Kaluga oblast and in Tula oblast. The economic principles behind RAP schemes suggest that the freedom to cut such "deals" should not be constrained. However, consumers and providers may believe that such incentives create an unacceptable conflict with the doctor's Hippocratic obligation to act in the patient's best interests. Indirect incentives (available to a more extensive system of providers, rather than an individual) will likely be preferable to those that directly increase a doctor's take-home pay by denying care. The general practitioner fundholding experiment used indirect incentives, where the practice benefited (by offering better facilities or supplementary services), but savings did not go directly into the physician's pocket. RAP system designers will find it difficult to dictate that there be no constraint on incentive structures, but they can lobby for greater freedom and must design the purchasing arrangement with these constraints in mind.

Enforcing Limits on Direct Patient Payment

Limits on direct patient payment must be enforced in any country that has a tradition of "gray market" health care payments and should be part of the statutory structure for any general RAP arrangement. Such a law makes it illegal for a provider to charge a patient for covered services unless such direct payments (for example, copayments and deductibles) are specifically permitted under the terms of the purchasing arrangement. Although this condition seems obvious, it is often overlooked. One of the reasons Korean health care costs grew so rapidly after the introduction of widespread health insurance was that there was no limit on charging for most services in addition to collecting the insurance payment. In effect, insurance just lowered the price to the consumer, thus increasing the demand and providing only modest financial protection to those with high medical need (Yang 1996, pp. 240, 246). Under the Philippines National Health Insurance scheme, the purchaser pays only a portion of hospital costs. When the scheme raised payments to reduce out-of-pocket costs and make scheme benefits more accessible for the poor, hospitals raised their prices and continued to collect the difference directly from the insured patients (Hindle, Acuin, and Valera 2001).

What sanction should be invoked if a provider is shown to demand illegal supplements to RAP payments? The simplest and most direct sanction is to terminate provider status in the RAP scheme. Where the RAP scheme is generous, and a single purchaser is responsible for the entire medical market, this should be sufficient to obtain provider compliance, unless the provider can survive on a "cash and carry" trade with the rich. Where the purchaser is one of many in the market, such a sanction may be insufficient. The provider may leave the RAP scheme and charge cash to the beneficiaries of schemes that pay poorly, while complying with the ban on supplementary payments where he or she deems the purchaser's allowance to be adequate. A stronger sanction (used by some U.S. jurisdictions) places the professional license at risk if the provider demands payments not authorized by the agreement with the purchaser. Such a sanction usually requires a more complicated legal process, but can be effective. The purchaser must have a carefully crafted contract with each provider and a clear definition of services that are *not* covered and supplementary payments that are allowed.

It is often argued that laws barring supplementary payments cannot, or will not, be enforced without a general understanding that the purchaser's payments and permitted supplements are "adequate." What is adequate depends on market conditions in the country and the expectations of practitioners. In some FSU countries, insurance payments are so low that cash supplements or "gifts" are considered inevitable. However, it would be better to shrink the provider network or limit the covered benefits and specifically permit certain supplementary payments instead of allowing the tradition of unregulated gray market payments to continue.

Privacy, Data, and Benefit Management

Conflicts between the privacy of medical records and a purchaser's "need to know" the details of the care purchased have been a concern in most industrial countries. There, privacy is a major consumer issue, and electronic claims processing systems enable purchasers to amass (and potentially misuse) a vast amount of medical information. However, as RAP arrangements become more sophisticated in newly industrializing and transitional economies, the same concerns will arise, particularly if providers are paid on a fee-for-service basis.

One way around the privacy concern is to capitate providers to provide all or a portion of the care needed by enrolled members. This puts the provider at risk of "excess utilization" and eliminates the need to report diagnoses and procedures to the purchaser. Such an approach has been tried with a number of community health financing schemes, which pass premiums through to a local provider that offers the full range of covered benefits.

In the absence of such capitation arrangements, the law should clarify the right of the insurer to obtain medical data needed to audit the quality and necessity of the care purchased. This can be done by statute or by having the patient sign a "limited release" at the time of treatment so that the provider will waive direct payment and bill the purchaser. In all countries, but particularly where the sophistication of claims processing is developing and the level of patient education low, language stating the following principles should be included in statutes that structure the RAP arrangement:

- The right of the purchaser to audit medical records

- The right of the purchaser, as a condition of payment, to obtain information routinely on patient diagnosis and services received

- The obligation of the purchaser to hold any patient information confidential and not to release it to employers or use it for any purpose other than the validation of claims.

Assessing the impact of the law on a RAP scheme is not simple. Additions or deletions from the statute book must take into account the nature of the RAP arrangement, the presence of single or multiple payers, the level of economic development and feasible premiums, and the existing capacity of the medical care system. But without the analysis outlined here, and the necessary actions by legislators and regulators, a law (or its absence) can derail the most carefully laid plans of economists and medical managers.

REFERENCES

Bhat, R. 1996. "Regulating the Private Health Care Sector: The Case of the Indian Consumer Protection Act." *Health Policy and Planning* 11(3): 265–79.

Einthoven, A. C., 1993. "The History and Principles of Managed Competition." *Health Affairs* 12 (suppl): 24–48.

Federal Compulsory Health Insurance Fund. 1999. "External Control of Health Care Quality in Mandatory Health Insurance System: Guidelines." English translation. Moscow.

Hindle, D., L. Acuin, and M. Valera. 2001. "Health Insurance in the Philippines: Bold Policies and Socio-Economic Realities." *Australian Health Review* 24(2).

Jost, T. S. 1999. "Managed Care Regulation: Can We Learn from Others? The Chilean Experience." *University of Michigan Journal of Law Reform* 32:863 et seq., Nexis printout.

Soderlund, N. 1998. "Possible Objectives and Resulting Entitlements of Essential Health Care Packages." *Health Policy* 45: 195–208.

Soderlund, N., and S. Khosa. 1997. "The Potential Role of Risk Equalization Mechanisms in Health Insurance: The Case of South Africa." *Health Policy and Planning* 12(4): 341–53.

Yang, B. M. 1996. "The Role of Health Insurance in the Growth of the Private Health Sector in Korea." *International Journal of Health Planning and Management* 11: 231–52.

CHAPTER 22

Quality-Based Purchasing in the United States: Applications in Developing Countries?

Peggy McNamara

Stakeholders in the global health care debate increasingly recognize the potential power of the purchasing function—whether led by national and regional governments, social insurance funds, community-based insurance organizations, employers, health plans, or consumers—to achieve not only efficiency and equity but also quality goals. Stakeholders from high-, middle-, and low-income countries are looking for the evidence base to guide future purchasing policies and practices. So, too, are representatives of the global health care community. No matter what it is called—quality-based purchasing, value-based purchasing, performance-based purchasing, responsible purchasing, or strategic contracting—the concept of leveraging payer clout to promote quality of care and improve health outcomes has a compelling logic and broad appeal.

CALL TO ACTION FOR U.S. EMPLOYERS

In 2001, the Institute of Medicine called for a strategic redesign of health care in the United States, citing more than 70 reports, in peer-reviewed publications, documenting serious quality of care shortcomings. Report authors call on purchasers to use their leverage to support the development of an information infrastructure to facilitate quality measurement and evidence-based practice and to establish payment incentives that support and reward high-quality care (Committee on Quality of Health Care in America 2001). Employers are by far the largest purchaser of health care in the United States. In 2000, employers bought health coverage for nearly two-thirds (64 percent) of the U.S. population (U.S. Bureau of the Census 2001). Are employers heeding the call to arms and accepting the mantle of quality-based purchasing?[1]

QUALITY-BASED PURCHASING BY EMPLOYERS

Some employers are interested in some indicators of quality and are incorporating them in a variety of purchasing strategies (Fraser and McNamara 2000). The indicators most frequently used by employers, however, are not the ones clinical experts and policymakers would select as most reflective of clinical or technical quality. Instead, to the extent employers incorporate quality indicators, they reflect "amenities" such as patient waiting times. Fraser and McNamara conclude that employers as a group are not acting as quality drivers—with the exception of a few well-resourced outliers.

McLaughlin and Gibson (2001) report little evidence to suggest that employers use performance data to change plan behavior or influence employee plan choice. McLaughlin and Gibson find employers more likely to use measures of consumer satisfaction and preventive care access than measures of clinical or technical quality.

Some analysts believe that employers view quality as a given and that they assume it is constant from provider to provider (Kindig 2001). A focus group of employee benefits managers residing in the Washington, D.C., metropolitan area supports this view (Gabel 2001). The employee benefits managers interviewed were surprised to hear statistics about provider error rates and nonadherence to selected clinical practice guidelines. None considered provider quality or safety markers in selecting a health plan for their employees. None indicated they had negotiated performance guarantees related to satisfaction, quality, or safety. None indicated that quality or safety were ever a factor in terminating a health plan.

Some analysts believe that employers think quality is the responsibility of health plans (versus employers), which have access to provider performance data and are, after all, in the business of health care (Hibbard and others 1997). In particular, managed care plans, which by definition selectively contract with a group of providers, are well situated, compared with their fee-for-service counterparts, to influence quality of care by choosing to contract only with providers that meet their quality criteria.

Do health plans, as buyers of provider services, pursue quality-based purchasing? Health plans in New York State do not use data from the statewide cardiac surgery reporting system, which provides hospital-specific and surgeon-specific data on risk-adjusted mortality following coronary artery bypass graft (CABG) surgery, to direct their enrollees or otherwise reward higher-performing providers (Chassin 2002). A broader review of the literature finds a lack of evidence that health plans shop for quality (Gold and others 1998).

To better understand the nature of plan-provider contractual provisions relating to quality circa 1999–2001, Sutton and Milet (2002) reviewed a sample of standard contracts.[2] They report that the most frequently used quality-assurance mechanisms focus on nonclinical attributes, many of them required to comply with state licensing requirements. Additional provisions suggestive of employer influence are the exception.

Some analysts think that expecting health plans to be guardians of quality is unrealistic. Hibbard and others (1997) make the point that, because health care costs are a dominant concern among employers and that employers hold plans accountable for costs, plans have insufficient incentive to selectively contract with high-quality hospitals and physicians.

We know that employers say that the cost of health plans matters to them, but do they send signals to plans that quality matters? After interviewing the leadership of 24 health plans, Scanlon and others (2000) conclude that employers exert only a minor influence on health plan activities to improve quality.

Some recent developments suggest a focus perhaps antithetical to quality-based purchasing. For example, a trend toward "tiered hospital plans," urged by some employers in response to rising health care costs, encourages patients to use lower-cost hospitals. Copayments vary by hospital according to the relative cost of the hospital care: higher copayments for higher-cost hospitals. To the extent higher-cost hospitals provide better care, employees' quality of care suffers under tiered hospital plans. A number of the large plans offer tiered hospital care, and some analysts predict most will do so within the next two years.[3]

BARRIERS TO QUALITY-BASED PURCHASING

Why is it that employers do not seem to be using their power in the health care market to demand high-quality care? A number of barriers undermine quality-based purchasing by employers. These include challenges inherent in the technical nature of medicine as well as market characteristics.

- *There is no consensus on a definition of quality.* Thousands of measures, indicators of care, and performance benchmarks have been developed to quantify and compare health care quality (Kindig 2001). Some indicators focus on structure, some on process, and others assess outcomes of care. What employers deem an important indicator of quality may be viewed as irrelevant by their employees.

- *Technology in medicine changes swiftly,* with a constant stream of new devices, drugs, and procedures. For example, between 1990 and 2000, nearly 1,000 new drugs were introduced into the U.S. market (Newhouse 2002). A best practice in one year may be outmoded and considered inferior care in subsequent years. The pace of technological change poses significant problems for providers in keeping up; the challenge for purchasers is even more overwhelming.

- *The task of assessing a provider's performance is difficult,* even if there is a consensus on quality (Newhouse 2002). Development of valid data on how specific plans and providers perform is a daunting task, requiring sophisticated technical expertise and significant resources.

- *An undersupply of providers can undermine certain quality-based purchasing strategies.* For example, selective contracting is difficult in markets where a small pool of providers can deliver most of the services.

- *Employer power is diffuse.* If no particular employer represents a threshold share of business in a particular market, health plans and providers may feel free to ignore them.

- *A lack of separation between the purchaser and provider functions results in role confusion.* In health care systems in which the same entity has responsibility for both purchaser and provider functions, because there is no purchaser independence, quality-based purchasing is difficult. While not relevant to employer purchasing and only relevant to a small portion of U.S. public sector purchasing, it is included here in the list of barriers because it can be a formidable challenge in certain developing countries.

EMPLOYER ACTIVISTS

Despite the body of evidence suggesting that U.S. employers as a group are passive purchasers of health care, at least when it comes to clinical or technical attributes of quality, anecdotal evidence suggests this may be changing. To say that a quality-based purchasing movement is underfoot may be an overstatement, but a small and seemingly growing number of leaders in the employer community are committing tremendous resources to overcoming the barriers in the pursuit of a quality-based purchasing agenda.

Cutting-edge employer-led initiatives are happening at the national, local, and company-specific levels. The Leapfrog Group, which includes more than 110 Fortune 500 companies and other organizations and represents 32 million covered lives, was formed partly in response to an Institute of Medicine publication (Kohn, Corrigan, and Donaldson 2000) that reported up to 98,000 Americans die every year from preventable medical errors in hospitals. This statistic ranks medical errors as a leading cause of death in the United States. The Leapfrog Group's goal is to trigger giant "leaps" forward in the quality and safety of hospital care. The initial set of leaps calls for hospitals to: (1) install a computer system linked to software designed to prevent prescribing errors by physicians entering medication orders; (2) staff intensive care units (ICUs) with physicians who have credentials in critical care medicine; and (3) perform certain complex medical procedures (for example, CABG) only if it performs a threshold number of the procedure.

These three leaps were selected partly because hospital performance on these indicators can be easily ascertained. Does the hospital have a computer system to prevent medication errors—yes or no? Is the ICU staffed by intensivists—yes or no? Does the volume of certain surgeries meet or exceed a certain threshold—yes or no? The Leapfrog Group asks all U.S. hospitals how they fare on these three criteria, and their responses—and nonresponses—are made available to the public via the Leapfrog Group's website. Not all hospitals participate and, at this point, few hospitals have fully implemented the three recommended practices

(Leapfrog Group 2002). To encourage adoption, some employers pay bonuses to hospitals that employ intensivists in their ICUs and have installed or begun to install a computerized prescribing system.[4] Some individual employer members of the Leapfrog Group educate their employees about the three criteria and encourage use of the website.

Another national, multiemployer effort is under way, headed by the National Business Coalition for Health (NBCH) and a subset of its nearly 90 local, employer-led health coalitions. Employer coalitions began to take off in the early 1980s as a vehicle to leverage employer purchasing power, because few employers on their own can invest the resources required to become sophisticated purchasers of health care (Zelman 1996). And few employers, on their own, represent a large enough share of a geographic market to effectively command the market to act in any particular way. While the coalition movement initially focused on cost containment to curtail spiraling employer costs (Bergthold and Solomon 1997), NBCH activities now are guided by a set of principles that incorporate the concept of quality (National Business Coalition for Health 2002).

Since 1997, NBCH has been working with its employer community to develop a common set of health plan quality specifications covering patient safety, chronic care management practices, and physician performance. The product of this collaboration, referred to as the "standardized health plan request for information (RFI)" or the "common RFI," advances the national quality-based purchasing agenda in several important ways. First, to the extent individual employer members of coalitions opt to use the quality specifications in the common RFI instead of crafting their own, they will help deliver a single, market signal to health plans and the providers with which they contract about quality attributes employers consider important. Second, NBCH has developed a computer-based tool for its membership that presents the responses received from plans that accept the common RFI. Individual employers can compare health plan responses and select the plan that best meets their needs. NBCH in aggregate represents more than 34 million covered lives, nearly one-fifth of the private U.S. insurance market. With this market clout, it is not surprising that more than a hundred plans responded to the common RFI in 2002 (National Business Coalition for Health 2002).

Local employer coalitions, most of them affiliated with NBCH, are independently breaking new ground in the area of quality-based purchasing. The Pacific Business Group on Health (PBGH), a coalition of 45 large employers based primarily in Northern California, uses both public reporting and payment incentives as strategies to promote quality of care. In terms of payment incentives, as part of the annual rate-negotiation process, PBGH establishes performance targets with each participating plan. Performance targets span measures of clinical quality, customer service, and member satisfaction. Plans must set aside 2 percent of their annual payments from employers—more than $10 million in 1996. If performance targets are not met, plans must repay employers from the funds set aside. The financial incentives are having an impact (see below).

Another local coalition, the Central Florida Health Care Coalition (CFHCC), representing 120 employers, has a somewhat different emphasis and strategy. Recognizing that, to consider practice changes, providers need comparative information on their own and their peers' performance, CFHCC has supported the development of a comprehensive data system of profiles and comparisons. Hospitals and physicians receive data on how they compare with the national average, for example, in terms of cesarean deliveries, pediatric asthma treatment, hysterectomies, and CABGs. The provider profiling strategy is having an effect (see below). Though not yet operational, the next phase of CFHCC's initiative will categorize physicians into one of three groups (platinum, gold, or silver), based on their performance compared with national standards. Physicians in the platinum category will receive higher payments than those in the gold and silver groups. "Platinum" physicians also will benefit from some nonfinancial rewards such as special dispensation from using formularies or adhering to precertification requirements (Bailit Health Purchasing 2002; Milbank Memorial Fund 2001).

Another 20 local employer coalitions—nearly one-fourth of NBCH's membership—are working with hospital performance data to develop comparative reports. Some are tapping existing administrative datasets available to the general public or purchased from a vendor, some are surveying hospitals about care processes and outcomes, others are surveying employees about their satisfaction with hospital care, and some are doing a mix of these. The target audience for the hospital performance data varies by coalition. Some performance reports are intended as a quality assessment and benchmarking tool exclusively for a provider audience; often these are referred to as *provider profiles*. Some are intended for employees' use in selecting providers; often these are referred to as *provider report cards*. In addition, hospital data are used by the employer group itself as part of the provider selection and contracting process.

Some very large employers devote significant resources to advance quality of care to tailor their own purchasing strategy. In 1996 the General Electric Corporation (GE) decided to apply the same quality-control processes it uses in its design of its new products and services to its health care purchasing practices. GE developed a health plan scorecard to assess performance in four areas, two of them member satisfaction and quality of care. If performance is not satisfactory, plan enrollment may be frozen or a plan contract may not be renewed. Portions of the scorecard are shared with employees during enrollment periods to influence their plan selection (Bailit Health Purchasing 2002; Milbank Memorial Fund 2001).

GENERIC EMPLOYER STRATEGIES TO PROMOTE HEALTH ACCOUNTABILITY FOR QUALITY

Several typologies have been advanced to help define and distinguish employers' efforts to promote quality (Bailit Health Purchasing 2002; Fraser and McNamara 2000; Midwest Business Group on Health 2003).

Perhaps the most basic distinction among employer approaches is whether the employer or employer group sees itself as an arbiter of quality on behalf of employees, or whether the employer sees its role as a purveyor of information to enable employees to act as their own arbiters. Said another way, employers can seek to influence quality of care by focusing their efforts on the supply side (that is, directly affecting health plan and provider behavior) or by focusing on the demand side (that is, directly affecting employee decisionmaking and indirectly affecting health plan and provider behavior). Employers who opt for the latter might not feel qualified to ascertain quality and might lack the resources to hire the necessary expertise, or they may have liability concerns associated with inserting themselves into the delivery paradigm (Fraser and McNamara 2000).

Regardless of which strategy an employer or group of employers may pursue, the most basic strategy—a prerequisite to any other employer strategy—is an effort to collect data or information to help tease out and identify high-performing providers according to the quality markers important to the employer. Some quality markers or indicators can be gleaned relatively easily from health plan self-assessments (perhaps in response to a request for information issued by employers) or from a government-sponsored plan report card. More sophisticated measures require more resource-intensive data collection, for example, a survey of employee satisfaction or a customized analysis of claims data or medical records. Table 22.1 provides a summary of employer strategies.

Supply-directed efforts can take several forms. Some employers prescreen plans according to their quality priorities and make only the subset that meets their criteria available to their employees. Some employers use financial bonuses to reward good performance or withhold payment to penalize bad performance (Fraser and others 1999). Financial incentives for quality can be incorporated into any type of payment system—salary, budget, per case, or per unit. Or employers may reward good performance by using nonfinancial incentives such as exemptions from certain administratively burdensome requirements such as drug formulary compliance (Bailit Health Purchasing 2002). In the words of Newhouse

TABLE 22.1   Framework for Conceptualizing Employer Quality-Based Purchasing Strategies

Generic employer strategies

1. Identify good and bad quality, a prerequisite to all other strategies (2 and 3, below).

2. Focus on supply side and seek to directly influence quality attributes of plans and providers available to employees.
   - Reward good quality and penalize bad quality such as by selective contracting, varying payment according to performance, offering nonfinancial incentives for high-quality care, dropping poor performers.
   - Make resources available explicitly for quality improvement (that is, apart from care-payment scheme) such as grants, technical assistance, training funds.

3. Focus on demand side by encouraging, enabling, and empowering employees—through the provision of comparative performance data—to become quality-based purchasers of health care.

Source: Author.

(2002, p. 21), "if purchasers do not reward higher quality . . . we should not be surprised to see quality problems." Employer attempts to promote provider quality can fall outside the traditional conception of a "purchase transaction." For example, an employer could develop a provider-specific profiling system that tells providers how their performance compares with others—the hallmark of the CFHCC's effort—or provide funds for a provider training program.

Strategies that focus on the demand side seek to enable and empower employees in their own health care decisionmaking. These efforts aim to make plan or provider-specific data available to employees and educate them about markers of good quality. Some employers even offer their employees financial incentives to encourage selection of high-quality plans and providers.

Some employers pursue multiple strategies. Leapfrog Group activities, for example, span both supply- and demand-directed strategies (table 22.2).

TABLE 22.2   Leapfrog Group Strategies

Generic employer strategies	Leapfrog group strategies
1. Identify good and bad quality, a prerequisite to all other strategies (2 and 3, below).	All U.S. hospitals are asked how they fare on Leapfrog's three criteria [that is, (1) install computer system linked to software designed to prevent prescribing errors by physicians entering medication orders; (2) staff intensive care units with physicians who have credentials in critical care medicine; and (3) perform certain complex medical procedures (for example, cardiac artery bypass graft) only if it performs a threshold number of the procedure], and the responses—and nonresponses—are available to the public on the Leapfrog Group's website.
	The National Business Coalition for Health, influenced in part by overlapping membership with the Leapfrog Group, solicits plan-specific information related to the three criteria in the "common request for information" and incorporates the responses into its computer-based clearinghouse of plan attributes.
2. Focus on supply side and seek to directly influence quality attributes of plans and providers available to employees. • Reward good quality and penalize bad quality. • Make resources available explicitly for quality improvement (that is, apart from care-reimbursement scheme).	Some participating employers pay bonuses to hospitals that employ intensivists in their intensive care units and have installed, or begun to install, a computerized prescribing system.
3. Focus on demand side by encouraging, enabling, and empowering employees—through the provision of comparative performance data—to become quality-based purchasers of health care.	Some participating members of the Leapfrog Group work with their employees and others in their geographic area to spread the word about their three criteria and encourage use of the website, which presents hospital-specific information.

Source: Author.

IMPACT OF EMPLOYER STRATEGIES ON QUALITY

While there is some evidence about the extent of quality-based purchasing, we know little about the effectiveness of specific purchasing strategies—what works and under what circumstances it works—and what the unintended consequences are. We know even less about the overall feasibility of relying on purchasers as a force for quality improvement (Fraser and McNamara 2000; Goldfarb and others 2002; Kindig 2001).

From a few employer self-evaluations, we know that some of their efforts seem to be having a positive impact. PBGH found that cervical cancer screening rates increased by 3 percentage points over a two-year period after implementing clinical targets. Testing rates (hemoglobin A1c) for patients with diabetes increased by 3 percentage points over a one-year period (Bailit Health Purchasing 2002). The CFHCC found that cesarean sections went from 36 percent of deliveries in 1989 to 18 percent by 1998 after its provider profiling system was put into place (Bailit Health Purchasing 2002). Though helpful, these descriptive statistics do not consider other causal factors that may be at work and do not allow for generalizing the findings to other employers that reside in different markets, each with its own particular dynamic.

There is additional evidence that provider profiling and public disclosure influence quality. Although the following effort was not created at the instigation of employers, it easily could have been. New York State developed a cardiac surgery reporting system in 1989, publishing annually hospital-specific and surgeon-specific data on risk-adjusted mortality following CABG surgery. The initial report showed wide variation in mortality rates. Poorly performing hospitals responded constructively and improved their cardiac surgery programs; statewide mortality fell substantially as a result. One of the poorest performing hospitals responded by recruiting its first full-time cardiac surgery chief, concentrating cardiac surgery on a single floor of the hospital, hiring nurse specialists, and installing a dedicated cardiac anesthesia service. This hospital now has the lowest risk-adjusted mortality of any hospital in the state. Overall, risk-adjusted CABG mortality fell 41 percent statewide in the first three years of the reporting system. Interestingly, while hospitals and physicians paid close attention to the ratings, health plans and consumers did not. Health plans in New York State did not use data from the statewide cardiac surgery reporting system to direct their enrollees or otherwise reward higher-performing providers, nor did patients avoid high-mortality hospitals (Chassin 2002).

These findings of consumer lack of interest in, and provider responsiveness to, quality measures seem to resonate. According to a recent national poll, ratings and rankings that purport to measure the quality of care provided by individual hospitals, physicians, and health plans have almost no impact on the choices consumers make.[5] Researchers other than Chassin have noted that provider profiling does have a direct impact on provider performance. Hibbard (2002) tracks hospital quality-improvement activities across three scenarios: hospitals whose performance is profiled and publicly reported; hospitals whose performance is profiled but not publicly reported; and hospitals that are not part of any externally generated profiling or public reporting effort. Preliminary findings suggest that hospital quality-improvement activities are most frequent among hospitals whose performance is publicly reported and least frequent among those that are not part of any profiling or public reporting effort.

Until now, the research community has given scant attention to the subject of quality-based purchasing by employers, but that is starting to change. The U.S. Agency for Healthcare Research and Quality (AHRQ) convened a meeting in 2001 of purchasers, researchers, and private foundations to develop an agenda related to value-based purchasing. Subsequent to this meeting, AHRQ incorporated part of the agenda into one of its 2001 program announcements, which is how agency priorities are communicated to the research community (AHRQ 2003).

Private foundations also responded to the need for evidence on quality-based purchasing strategies. The Commonwealth Fund announced in 2002 that it is funding an evaluation of the Leapfrog Group's initiative to encourage use of physicians who have credentials in critical care medicine to staff ICUs. The research project will survey top management in 105 hospitals along with health plans to determine the financial and nonfinancial factors that influence a hospital's decision to adopt the Leapfrog ICU staffing standard (Commonwealth Fund 2002). The Commonwealth Fund also has funded a study on reducing the barriers to value-based purchasing.[6]

The Robert Wood Johnson Foundation (RWJF) is funding an evaluation of a hospital report card initiative under way by the Employer Health Care Alliance Cooperative, a local employer coalition that represents employers in south-central Wisconsin (Hibbard 2002). RWJF also has funded a study of employers' quality interventions to see if they are having an impact.[7]

The RWJF, the California HealthCare Foundation, and the AHRQ are supporting a multimillion dollar, multisite demonstration and evaluation project on "rewarding quality." Grants and technical assistance will be offered to employers and other payers to design, implement, and evaluate alternative payment innovations and nonfinancial incentives for physicians and hospitals to improve the quality of care (National Health Care Purchasing Institute 2002).

CONCLUSIONS

Given the dearth of evidence about the effectiveness of U.S. employers' quality-based purchasing strategies, few lessons can be drawn for other U.S. employers let alone for purchasers in other countries. As is the case for low- and middle-income countries (Dixon, Langenbrunner, and Mossialos 2002; Gauri 2001; Mills 1998; Palmer 2000), the U.S.-specific body of research is especially lacking in the area of purchasing strategies' impact on health gains. Until the next wave of research is completed, we are left mainly with a sense of the prevalence of quality-based purchasing, a small but growing set of frameworks to help organize the component strategies, and a rough understanding of barriers that might impede a quality-based purchasing agenda.

We are also left with a small body of evidence to suggest that providers, when presented with credible information about their performance relative to their peers, do in fact make improvements—particularly when this information is made available to the public (Chassin 2002; Hibbard 2002; Newhouse 2002). Perhaps that is because previously—in the absence of comparative data to the contrary—providers presumed that their performance was state of the art. Or perhaps they instituted quality-improvement initiatives out of fear of losing patients. Regardless, purchaser efforts to collect and disseminate comparative performance data on hospitals and physicians seem to have promise as a quality-improvement strategy and may well have applications to purchasing in lower- and middle-income countries.

Although the findings on impact are relatively recent, the concept of provider-specific reports has been around for a while.

> I am fain to sum up with an urgent appeal for adopting this or some uniform system of publishing the statistical records of hospitals. If they could be obtained . . . they would show subscribers how their money was being spent, what amount of good was really being done with it, or whether the money was doing mischief rather than good. (Florence Nightingale, 1863)

As governments, social insurance funds, community-based insurance organizations, and employers consider their own paths to improve the quality of care, broadening the context beyond purchasing might be helpful. Informed purchasing is one societal approach to pursuing quality of care. The Institute of Medicine (Donaldson 1998) identifies two other broad policy strategies to address health care quality apart from the purchasing or market-based strategy. One rests on voluntary, self-regulated relationships among physician and other provider groups, based on ethical and professional norms. An example of this is the development and sponsorship of practice guidelines by a national professional society. The second approach relies on a government or regulatory remedy, for example, a legal requirement that physicians be licensed in order to practice.

Each of the three approaches stems from a different philosophical premise and relies on a different set of system stakeholders. And each can be—and often is—used in combination with the other two. The actual as well as optimal balance among the three approaches varies over time, however, and is influenced by contextual factors. These factors, all in a constant state of change, include the political environment, economic circumstances, health care market attributes, cultural characteristics (including literacy rates, corruption indices), and the extent of unison or discord among the lender and donor community. The dynamic nature of these contextual factors suggests that there is no such thing as a generic template for improving quality.

We look to the research community to embrace a broad research agenda[8] that ultimately will provide guidance to a wide range of countries, each characterized by its own unique set of contextual factors, on how best to craft an effective, synergistic mix of purchasing, professional development, and regulatory approaches in the pursuit of quality.

NOTES

1. Access safeguards are generally commonplace in U.S. coverage policies and are not considered, for the purpose of this chapter, to be within the scope of quality-based purchasing. These safeguards include employer efforts to define benefit packages (covered services) and require health plans to operate grievance and appeal programs (to arbitrate when care is denied). Developing countries lacking such safeguards, however, may wish to require them as part of a strategic purchasing effort.

2. Though not necessarily representative of contracts in use nationwide, 116 standard contracts, on file in nine U.S. states, were reviewed.

3. J. Bennet, "Insurers Push Higher Co-Payments for Treatment at Pricey Hospitals." *Wall Street Journal*. June 6, 2002, p. D3.

4. M. Freudenheim, "Quality Goals in Incentives for Hospitals." New York Times, June 26, 2002.

5. *Wall Street Journal,* "Most Consumers Ignore Health Ratings," October 11, 2002. p. B2.

6. Goldfarb, N. I. 2003. Email correspondence to P. McNamara., January 30, 2003.

7. Scanlon, D. P. 2003. Email correspondence to P. McNamara, January 30, 2003.

8. In 2003 the Center for Health Affairs at Project Hope, with support from the AHRQ, convened a small group of experts to develop a detailed research agenda to guide future research investments (for example, surveys, case studies, demonstration evaluations) that would improve our collective understanding of the current and potential role of purchasers in improving the quality of health care services *specifically in developing countries*. For further information, contact Project Hope investigators Janet Sutton and Gail Wilensky or visit www.projecthope.org.

REFERENCES

AHRQ (Agency for Healthcare Research and Quality). 2000. *Program Announcement: Impact of Payment and Organization on Cost, Quality and Equity.* http://www.ahrq.gov.

Bailit Health Purchasing, LLC. 2002. "Profiles of Organizations Using Quality Incentives." National Health Care Purchasing Institute. Available at http://www.nhcpi.net/profiles .cfm.

Bergthold, L. A., and L. S. Solomon. 1997. "Group Purchasing in the Managed Care Marketplace." In J. D. Wilkerson, K. J. Devers, and R. S. Given, eds., *Competitive Managed Care: The Emerging Health Care System.* San Francisco, Calif.: Jossey-Bass Inc.

Chassin, M. R. 2002. "Achieving and Sustaining Improved Quality: Lessons from New York State and Cardiac Surgery." *Health Affairs* 21(4): 40–51.

Committee on Quality of Health Care in America, Institute of Medicine. 2001. *Crossing the Quality Chasm: A New Health System for the 21st Century.* Washington, D.C.: National Academy Press.

Commonwealth Fund. 2002. *Recent Grants Awarded by the Board of Directors.* New York, N.Y.: Commonwealth Fund.

Dixon, A., J. Langenbrunner, and E. Mossialos. 2002. "Facing the Challenges of Health Care Financing." Paper commissioned by U.S. Agency for International Development for meeting "Ten Years of Health Systems Transition in Central and Eastern Europe and Eurasia," July 29–31, 2002, Washington, D.C.

Donaldson, M. 1998. "Accountability for Quality in Managed Care." *Journal on Quality Improvement* 24(12): 711–25.

Fraser, I., and P. McNamara. 2000. "Employers: Quality Takers or Quality Makers?" *Medical Care Research and Review* 57(suppl 2): 33–52.

Fraser, I., P. McNamara, G. Lehman, S. Isaacson, and K. Moler. 1999. "The Pursuit of Quality by Business Coalitions: A National Survey." *Health Affairs* 18(6): 158–65.

Gabel, J. 2001. "Employers' Views on Patient Safety and Quality of Care." Report of findings from focus group discussion of D.C. employers, supported by the U.S. Agency for Healthcare Research and Quality, October 7, 2001, Washington, D.C.

Gauri, V. 2001. "Are Incentives Everything? Payment Mechanisms for Health Care Providers in Developing Countries." Policy Research Working Paper. World Bank, Development Research Group, Washington, D.C.

Gold, M., L. Nelson, T. Lake, R. Hurley, and R. Berenson. 1998. "Behind the Curve: A Critical Assessment of How Little is Known about Arrangements between Managed Care Plans and Physicians." In M. Gold, ed., *Contemporary Managed Care: Readings in Structure, Operations and Public Policy.* Chicago, Ill.: Health Administration Press.

Goldfarb, N. I., V. Maio, C. Carter, L. Pizzi, and D. B. Nash. 2002. "How Does Quality Enter into Health Insurance Purchasing Decisions: Final Report to the Commonwealth Fund." Commonwealth Fund, New York, N.Y.

Hibbard, J. H. 2002. "Making Healthcare Quality Information Useful to Consumers." Presentation at annual meeting of National Quality Forum, October 1, 2002, Washington, D.C.

Hibbard, J. H., J. J. Jewett, M. W. Legnini, and M. Tusler. 1997. "Choosing a Health Plan: Do Large Employers Use the Data?" *Health Affairs* 16(6): 172–80.

Kindig, D. A. 2001. "Value Purchasers in Health Care: Pioneers or Don Quixotes?" In *Value Purchasers in Health Care: Seven Case Studies.* New York, N.Y.: Milbank Memorial Fund.

Kohn, L. T., J. M. Corrigan, and M. S. Donaldson, eds. 2000. *To Err Is Human: Building a Safer Health System.* Washington, D.C.: National Academy Press.

Leapfrog Group. 2002. Available at http://www.leapfroggroup.org.

McLaughlin, C. G., and T. Bernard Gibson. 2001. "Employer Incentives and Disincentives to Promote Quality: What Can Economic Theory and Evidence Tell Us?" Paper commissioned by Agency for Healthcare Research and Quality for meeting "Understanding How Employers Can Be Catalysts for Quality: Insights for a Research Agenda," April 4, 2001, Washington, D.C.

Midwest Business Group on Health in conjunction with the Juran Institute, Inc. and the Severyn Group, Inc. 2003. "Reducing the Costs of Poor Quality Health Care through Responsible Purchasing Leadership." http://www.mbgh.org

Milbank Memorial Fund. 2001. *Value Purchasers in Health Care: Seven Case Studies.* New York, N.Y.

Mills, A. 1998. "To Contract or Not to Contract? Issues for Low and Middle Income Countries." *Health Policy and Planning* 13(1): 32–40.

National Health Care Purchasing Institute. 2002. http://www.nhcpi.net.

National Business Coalition for Health. 2002. http://www.nbch.org.

Newhouse, J. P. 2002. "Why Is There a Quality Chasm?" *Health Affairs* 21(4): 13–25.

Nightingale, F. 1863. "Notes on Hospitals" [microform]. 3rd ed. London: Longman, Green, Longman, Roberts, and Green. Available at Annals of Internal Medicine website http://www.annals.org.

Palmer, N. 2000. "The Use of Private-Sector Contracts for Primary Health Care: Theory, Evidence and Lessons for Low- and Middle-Income Countries." *Bulletin of the World Health Organization* 78(6): 821–29.

Scanlon, D. P., E. Rolph, C. Darby, and H. E. Doty. 2000. "Are Managed Care Plans Organizing for Quality?" *Medical Care Research and Review* 57 (suppl 2): 9–32.

Sutton, J. P., and M. Milet. 2002. "Quality-Related Provisions in Plan-Provider Contracts." Final report to the U.S. Agency for Healthcare Research and Quality. Unpublished.

U.S. Bureau of the Census. 2001. http://www.census.gov/prod/2001pubs/p60–215.pdf.

Zelman, W.A. 1996. *The Changing Health Care Marketplace.* San Francisco, Calif.: Jossey-Bass.

About the Coeditors and Contributors

THE COEDITORS

Alexander S. Preker, lead economist and editor of HNP Publication Series, oversees the World Bank's analytical work on public policy in the health sector, market dynamics, health financing, service delivery, pharmaceuticals, and health labor markets, focusing on ways to help developing countries accelerate progress toward achieving the Millennium Development Goals (MDGs) by 2015. He is a member of a team of researchers currently undertaking a major review of disease control priorities in developing countries, with support from the Gates Foundation and the Fogarthy International Center of the U.S. National Institutes of Health (NIH). Recently he has worked closely on a number of projects with the World Health Organization (WHO), the International Labour Organisation (ILO), the Rockefeller Foundation, the International Federation of Pharmaceutical Manufacturers Associations, the International Hospital Federation, the International Federation of Health Plans, and several leading academic centers involved in health and financial protection in developing countries.

Mr. Preker has published extensively and is a frequent speaker at major international events. He coordinated the World Bank team that prepared the World Bank's Sector Strategy for Health, Nutrition and Population in 1997. While working with WHO in 1999-2000, he was one of the coauthors of the *World Health Report 2000: Health Systems: Measuring Performance*. From 2000 to 2001 he was a member of Working Group 3 of the WHO Commission on Macroeconomics and Health, chaired by Jeffrey Sachs. Jointly with the ILO, Mr. Preker won a Development Marketplace Award, which led to a publication *Social Re Insurance: A New Approach to Sustainable Community Health Financing*. His other major recent publications include: *Innovations in Health Service Delivery: The Corporatization of Public Hospitals* (2003); *Private Participation in Health Services* (2003); and *Costing the Millennium Development Goals: Expenditure Gaps and Development Traps* (2003).

Mr. Preker is on the Editorial Committee of the Bank's Publications Department. He is the chief editor of its HNP publications and is a member of the editorial committees of several international journals. He is on the scientific committee of several upcoming international conferences, notably the European Health Economics Association Conference in London (2004) and the International Health Economics Association Congress in Barcelona (2005). He is on the

External Advisory Board of the London School of Economics Health Group and is a member of the teaching faculty for the Harvard/World Bank Institute Flagship Course on Health Sector Reform and Sustainable Financing. He has an appointment as Adjunct Associate Professor at the George Washington University School of Public Health.

His training includes a PhD in Economics from the London School of Economics and Political Science, a fellowship in Medicine from University College London, a Diploma in Medical Law and Ethics from King's College London, and an MD from the University of British Columbia/McGill.

John C. Langenbrunner is a senior health economist with both research and operations experience. He is currently working in the Europe and Central Asia region and has worked on health financing issues in Russia, Poland, Croatia, Azerbaijan, Kyrgyzstan, Kazakhstan, and Uzbekistan. He has worked as well in selected countries in the Middle East and North Africa region (Arab Republic of Egypt, Bahrain, and Saudi Arabia). Before joining the Bank, he worked in selected countries in South Asia and the East Asia/Pacific region. He is currently based in Moscow. In addition to his work on purchasing, he led the Bank's work on a manual for National Health Accounts (NHA) for low- and middle-income countries. This "NHA Producers Guide" was published in 2003.

OTHER CONTRIBUTING AUTHORS

Orvill Adams has worked in the area of health systems development for more than 20 years, in both the public and private sector. He is the director of the Department of Human Resources for Health in the Cluster of Evidence and Information for Policy in World Health Organization Headquarters in Geneva. He began his career in the health sector in 1978 as a district planning and research officer with the Ottawa Carleton District Health Council. He was appointed acting director of research with the Association of Canadian Medical Schools from 1979 to 1980. From 1980 to 1990, he was director of the Department of Medical Economics at the Canadian Medical Association. He was responsible for guiding the work on policy formulation and policy analysis, forecasting of health economic conditions, analysis of constitutional matters pertaining to health care, the study of health care expenditures, workforce policy, and the organization of the health services delivery system. From 1990 to 1994, he was principal in his own company, Curry Adams & Associates Inc., committed to the development and practice of effective and efficient management in the public and private sectors of health, education, and social services. In this capacity he had many and varied international assignments for agencies such as the World Health Organization (WHO), the U.S. Agency for International Development, and The Canadian International Development Corporation. He joined WHO in 1995 in the Division of Human Resources for Health and worked in the area of human resources development and health sector reform. His primary interest is in understanding the management and organization of health systems and their impact on the delivery of health interventions. His postgraduate degrees are in Economics and in International Affairs.

Anita Alban has been a health economist for more than 25 years with expertise in economic analysis including priority setting, outcome measurement, sustainable financing, financing and organization of health care, HIV and economics, and the economics of vaccine. She has worked extensively in Europe including countries in economic transition and a range of countries in Africa and Asia. Her employment record includes director of research in the Danish Institute of Health Services Research and Development, 1986-1997; senior economist, Joint United Nations Programme on HIV/AIDS (UNAIDS), 1997-2000; and director of EASE International, Copenhagen, 2000 to the present. She has published widely in books and scientific journals within her areas of expertise-in recent years mainly on strategic health plans, HIV/AIDS, and access to health services for poor people. She works for Danida, the U.K. Department for International Development, the World Bank, United Nations Development Programme, UNAIDS, and the World Health Organization.

Gerard F. Anderson, MD, is the national program director for the Robert Wood Johnson Foundation-sponsored program "Partnership for Solutions: Better Lives for People with Chronic Conditions." Dr. Anderson is a professor of health policy and management and international health at the Johns Hopkins University Bloomberg School of Public Health, professor of medicine at the Johns Hopkins University School of Medicine, associate chair for health services research in the Department of Health Policy and Management, director of the Johns Hopkins Center for Hospital Finance and Management, and co-director of the Johns Hopkins Program for Medical Technology and Practice Assessment. Prior to his arrival at Johns Hopkins in 1983, Dr. Anderson held various positions in the Office of the Secretary, U.S. Department of Health and Human Services, where he helped to develop Medicare prospective payment legislation.

Dr. Anderson is currently conducting research on a variety of health care financing issues, including international comparisons of spending, utilization, and outcomes in countries in the Organisation for Economic Co-operation and Development, health insurance systems in developing countries, care for chronically ill individuals, medical education, hospital payment reform, and technology diffusion in capitated systems. He has written two books on health care payment policy, published more than 160 peer-reviewed articles, testified in Congress more than 25 times as an individual witness, and serves on multiple editorial committees.

Anders Anell is director of the Swedish Institute for Health for Health Economics, associate professor at the School of Economics and Management, Lund University, Sweden, and a member of the Advisory Board of the Swedish Council on Technology Assessment in Health Care.

Cristian Baeza, MD, is a senior health specialist at the World Bank, Latin America and the Caribbean Region in Washington, D.C. His main area of work and research is on health financing and health systems and their contribution to social protection and poverty alleviation.

Previously, he was senior health systems specialist for social security policy and development at the International Labour Organisation; founder and chief executive officer of the Latin American Center for Health Systems Research (CLAISS), in Santiago, Chile; director of the Chilean National Health Fund (FONASA); health systems specialist at the World Bank, in Washington D.C.; and chief of the International Financing Division and of the Health Sector Reform Project at the Chilean Ministry of Health. He is a visiting associate professor of international health at the Johns Hopkins School of Public Health.

Dr. Baeza has written and lectured extensively on health care financing and health systems in Latin America and has been a contributing member to a number of multilateral initiatives on health systems and health financing. He participated in the core writing team of the *World Health Report 2000*, the World Commission on Macroeconomics and Health (Working Group 2), and the Global Forum for Health Sector Reform. He also has extensive consulting experience in Latin America and in some countries in Eastern Europe and Asia. He has an M.D. from the University of Chile and holds a Master of Public Health from Johns Hopkins University. He also completed a Master in Sciences and a Specialty Program in Neurology from the University of Chile, the Social and Economic Policy Program from ILADES, and the Strategic Management Program from REDCOM.

Paolo Carlo Belli is a health economist in the World Bank's Human Development Unit. His main research interests are health financing, incentives, and health systems reforms. He has explored health insurance issues, the impact of informal out-of-pocket payments, the impact of different payment systems and regulatory regimes for health providers, the potential for engaging public private providers in the provision of essential services, and the impact of child health investments on economic development. He has extensive operations experience with the World Bank in East Timor, Georgia, Poland, and India, and, with the International Health System Group at the Harvard School of Public Health, in Uganda, Romania, Hungary, Czech Republic, and Turkey.

Stephanie Cooper, BA, P.G. Diploma, works in the Centre for Health Economics, University of York, United Kingdom, on the implementation research work-program of the Initiative for Maternal Mortality Programme Assessment run by the University of Aberdeen. She is active in the development community and is currently completing a Master's dissertation.

Finn Diderichsen, MD, PhD, is currently a professor at the University of Copenhagen and was previously a professor at Karolinska Institute in Stockholm in social epidemiology and health policy research. His research is mainly on causes of inequalities in health. He is responsible for the resource allocation formulas developed and used in the health services of Stockholm County.

Ulrika Enemark, MSc (Economics), PhD, is an independent consultant with expertise in health economics and health policy and an associate professor in health economics at the Institute of Social Medicine and Epidemiology, Aarhus University, Denmark. Her employment record includes research positions at the universities of Copenhagen (1989-93), Lund (1993), and Southern Denmark (1993-99). She worked as health economics adviser to the Ministry of Health and Education, Bhutan (1999-2001). She has participated as an independent consultant in task forces, appraisals, reviews, and studies of health sector programs within the framework of health sector reform in a number of countries, including Africa and Asia on assignment for Danida, the U.K. Department for International Development, the World Bank, and the European Union. Her main areas of interest are health care planning and sustainable financing, health sector reform, access of the poor, health-seeking behavior, incentive structures, and monitoring and evaluation.

Tim Ensor is a principal economist with Oxford Policy Management and a senior research fellow in the Dugald Baird Centre for Reproductive Health, University of Aberdeen. He undertook this work while at the University of York where he has taught and done research on health financing issues in low- and middle-income countries for the past 10 years. Much of his work has been in Asia, first in Central Asia and Indochina and, more recently, in South Asia. Between 1999 and 2001 he was senior economist in the Ministry of Health and Family Welfare, Bangladesh. Mr. Ensor trained as an economist first at the London School of Economics (BSc) then at Sussex (MA, Development Economics), and York (PhD, Economics).

Frank G. Feeley is clinical associate professor at the Boston University School of Public Health. He is a graduate of Princeton University (Woodrow Wilson School of Public and International Affairs) and the Yale Law School. From 1996 to 2001, he directed a project funded by the U.S. Agency for International Development providing technical assistance to the Russian Federation in the drafting of new health laws and regulations; as part of this effort, he directed an extensive survey of out-of-pocket health care expenditures in Russia. Much of his current research assesses the role played by the private sector in preventing and treating HIV/AIDS in a number of African countries. Earlier in his career, he was assistant commissioner for regulation in the Massachusetts Department of Public Health and spent several years in the administration of the Medicaid (government-funded medical insurance for the poor) program.

Maria Goddard is assistant director at the Centre for Health Economics, University of York, England, where she also leads a program of health policy research. She has previously worked for the English department of health as an economic adviser. Recent research interests relate to performance measurement and the organization and regulation of health services.

Davidson R. Gwatkin, since his official retirement in March 2003, has served as a consultant to the World Bank and the Rockefeller Foundation on health and poverty. Before that, he had been the Bank's principal health and poverty specialist. Among his principal recent health and poverty activities has been the organization of a set of case studies and a global conference on how well health interventions reach disadvantaged groups, and production of 56 country reports on socioeconomic inequalities in health status and service use.

April Harding is a senior economist in the Health, Nutrition and Population Department of the World Bank. Since coming to the World Bank, Ms. Harding has provided technical assistance and advice to governments in more than 14 countries, primarily on issues related to private sector development and privatization. She manages the analytical work and training related to private participation in the health sector and manages several activities related to health systems development and service delivery more broadly. She speaks and publishes in numerous forums on private participation, privatization, and reform of health services, including a volume reviewing hospital reforms in developing and industrial countries, *Innovations in Health Care Delivery: Organizational Reforms of Public Hospitals*. She recently co-edited, with Alexander S. Preker, *Private Participation in Health Services*, which presents the critical operational issues related to improving public policy toward the private health sector in developing countries.

Prior to joining the World Bank, Ms. Harding was a research fellow in economic studies at the Brookings Institution. From 1987 to 1993, Ms. Harding was a fellow of the Russian and East European Center at the University of Pennsylvania, where she also received a PhD in Economics, with a concentration in Comparative Economic Systems and Public Finance.

Katharina Hauck is a PhD student and research fellow at the Centre for Health Economics, University of York, England. She previously worked for the World Health Organization in Geneva. Her research interests relate to performance assessment, health inequalities, and health econometrics.

Peter Sotir Hussey is a doctoral candidate in health services research in the Department of Health Policy and Management of the Johns Hopkins Bloomberg School of Public Health. He has also worked as a consultant at the Organisation for Economic Co-operation and Development, comparing health care quality indicators in 21 countries. Mr. Hussey has published research articles and book chapters on topics including international comparisons of health spending, prices, and utilization, quality of care, the supply and international migration patterns of health professionals, and population aging.

Dean T. Jamison is a professor of education and of public health at the University of California, Los Angeles. Before joining the UCLA faculty in 1988, Jamison spent many years at the World Bank where he was a senior economist in the research department, task manager for projects and sector work in China and Gambia, division chief for education policy, and division chief for population, health, and nutrition. In 1992-93, he temporarily rejoined the World Bank to serve as lead author for the Bank's 1993 World Development Report, *Investing in Health*. Dr. Jamison studied at Stanford (AB, Philosophy; MS, Engineering Sciences) and at Harvard (PhD, Economics, under K. J. Arrow). In 1994 he was elected to membership in the Institute of Medicine of the U.S. National Academy of Sciences, and he currently chairs the Institute's Board on Global Health.

Xingzhu Liu is a health economist at Abt Associates Inc. He has more than 17 years of experience in health economics and public health issues. Initially he trained in Medicine (MD) and Public Health (MPH, Epidemiology, Statistics, Demographic Study), and then in Health Economics and Policy (PhD). His work experience includes cost-effectiveness and cost-benefit analysis, monitoring and evaluation of public health programs, costing health interventions, health care financing and payment systems, and health care quality and outcomes research. His field research includes survey research design, implementation, and supervision. His quantitative skills include data management and advanced statistical analysis.

Benjamin Loevinsohn, M.D. MPH, is a senior public health specialist at the World Bank, which he joined in 1999. He is the task team leader for health sector activities in Afghanistan and Pakistan. He is also the focal point for the Bank's work on immunization in South Asia and has done extensive work on contracting with nongovernmental organizations to deliver health services.

Before joining the World Bank, Dr. Loevinsohn was senior health specialist at the Asian Development Bank (ADB) (1993-99), where he was a task manager who helped develop and implement five successful investment operations in Bangladesh, Bhutan, Cambodia, and Lao People's Democratic Republic. He led the team that revised the ADB's overall health sector policy and was the task manager for a large study of health sector reform options for policymakers.

His other positions have included founder and chair, ADB Staff Community Fund (1996-99); adviser to the Philippine Department of Health (1990-93); technical officer, UNICEF, Sudan (1987-89); and primary care physician, Government of Nicaragua (1984-85). Dr. Loevinsohn has published many articles in leading scholarly journals, including the *Lancet, Bulletin of the World Health Organization, American Journal of Public Health, International Journal of Epidemiology,* and *Health Policy and Planning.*

Peggy McNamara, MSPH, is a senior policy analyst at the Agency for Healthcare Research and Quality, a U.S. government agency that supports, conducts, and disseminates research on health care quality, access, and costing in order to support evidence-based health care delivery. Ms. McNamara's research portfolio includes a special focus on quality-based purchasing in industrial and developing countries. Previous work experience includes consulting with the World Health Organization and serving on the management team for the Partnerships for Health Reform Plus project funded by the U.S. Agency for International Development. Previously, Ms. McNamara was a fellow at the Eastern Health Board in Dublin, Ireland. Ms. McNamara earned her Master's in Public Health from the University of North Carolina at Chapel Hill, where she was awarded a U.S. Public Health Service Traineeship. She is currently a doctoral candidate at the University of Michigan's School of Public Health, where she was awarded a Pew Fellowship.

Fernando Montenegro Torres has worked on various topics related to health economics, health financing, and health insurance for several public and private, governmental and international organizations, including the World Bank, Inter-American Development Bank, International Labour Organisation, Pan American Health Organization, Instituto Mexicano de Seguridad Social of Mexico, Bloomberg School of Public Health at Johns Hopkins University, and Défense des Enfants International. Dr. Montenegro Torres earned an MD from the Universidad Central of Quito, Ecuador, an MSc in Health Management for Developing Countries from the Karl Ruprecht Universität of Heidelberg, Germany, an MA in Economics and Development from the School of Advanced International Studies at Johns Hopkins University in Washington, D.C., and a PhD from the Bloomberg School of Public Health at The Johns Hopkins University.

Dr. Montenegro Torres has contributed research papers and coauthored book chapters for several institutions and publications, including the World Bank, Inter-American Development Bank, Pan American Health Organization, and *Health Affairs.*

Sheila O'Dougherty is a health financing and health care reform expert with 20 years of experience, including 7 years in central Asia directing the Zdrav Project funded by the U.S. Agency for International Development. She possesses an exceptional blend of policy, technical, and management skills, which are augmented by her extensive experience directing large, field-based projects. After obtaining a Master's in Hospital Administration, she spent four years working with the Health Care Financing Administration in the U.S. Department of Health and Human Services, gaining experience in health policy research, health delivery systems, health financing, health insurance, provider payment systems, and health information systems. Her health policy skills were strengthened at the Senate Finance Committee during President Clinton's attempt to reform the U.S. health system.

Enrique C. Seoane Vazquez, BS (Economics), PhD, has been an assistant professor in pharmaceutical economics and drug policy at Ohio State University, College of Pharmacy, since 2002. His previous work experience includes positions as a hospital chief executive officer in the Spanish National Health System (1989-94) and as a research fellow in pharmaceutical economics and drug policy at the PRIME Institute, University of Minnesota (1995-2002). He has a PhD in Social and Administrative Pharmacy from the University of Minnesota, College of Pharmacy (2002). Dr. Seoane's main areas of interest are drug policy and pharmaceutical economics, pharmaceutical care, and economic evaluation applied to pharmaceuticals. His recent research focuses on pharmaceutical policy and economics in the Americas, Medicare and Medicaid drug benefits, drug financing in developing countries, the role of generic drugs in the health care system, and people's access to pharmaceuticals. His research sponsors include the World Bank, the World Health Organization, Pan American Health Organization, the Inter-American Development Bank, Henry Kaiser Family Foundation, the pharmaceutical industry, and pharmacy associations.

Eric de Roodenbeke is a hospital manager (Hospital Administration Diploma-ENSPRennes) and health economist (Doctorate-Paris 1). He joined the

World Bank in 2004 as a senior health specialist, bringing support on hospital policy issues both for West Africa and for the World Bank Institute. His working experience has been in hospital management and policy support to the health sector in developing counties.

Previously, he was director of the Finance and Purchasing Department of EPINAL, a general hospital; deputy director of the Hotel-Dieu de Nantes and of Bretonneau-Tours, both university hospitals. On both assignments, he did general management and project leadership related to the opening of new facilities. More recently, he led the reorganization of psychiatry in a catchment area of 600,000.

His experience in developing countries has been varied, including a field assignment as leader of a pilot hospital project in Burkina Faso (1989-94) and headquarters responsibilities for hospital policy and health care financing for five years in the French Ministry of Foreign Affairs (1996- 2001). He has monitored projects on hospital policy and health care financing and has undertaken support missions in French-speaking African countries and in Southeast Asia.

He has edited books on hospital management and financing (documentation française and Karthala) in low-income countries and has taught postgraduate courses in health economics for developing countries (CERDI).

Andreas Seiter, MD, is the current global pharmaceutical industry fellow at the World Bank. The main role of this fellowship is to facilitate the exchange of know-how between the World Bank and industry. He joined the World Bank in January 2004 and worked in the areas of HIV/AIDS, IP/innovation, and purchasing of pharmaceuticals (in a country-specific project for Ghana). Dr. Seiter is a physician by training and practiced medicine for four years before joining the pharmaceutical industry in 1984. He held various positions in medical operations, product management, and communications. Prior to joining the World Bank, he was head of Stakeholder Relations at Novartis AG in Switzerland. In this function he was a spokesperson for the pharmaceutical industry on national and international platforms. He helped implement the Corporate Citizenship strategy at Novartis and promoted the concept of open stakeholder dialogue on controversial issues related to the business model of the industry. Multistakeholder events organized by Novartis have found wide appreciation as a platform for constructive debate, attracting high-level speakers such as the former German President Roman Herzog.

Peter C. Smith is professor of economics in the Centre for Health Economics at the University of York, United Kingdom. His research interests include public finance, health care finance, and public service regulation, topics on which he has published widely. He has advised numerous national and international agencies, including the Organisation for Economic Co-operation and Development, the World Health Organization, and government ministries. He is a commissioner at the U.K. Audit Commission.

Sandra Sosa-Rubi has worked in the Ministry of Health and the National Health Institute in Mexico. She has a Master's degree in Health Economics from the CIDE in Mexico. She has worked on topics related to health care reform and its impact on the use of health services; health care utilization patterns in developing countries; and demand for maternal health care. She is a PhD student in Health Economics at the University of York, United Kingdom.

Jon Sussex is associate director of the Office of Health Economics(OHE), London. The OHE is a not-for-profit research and consultancy organization focused on the policy and economics of health care internationally. Mr. Sussex is an honorary visiting fellow at the Department of Economics and Related Studies, University of York, United Kingdom; an expert adviser to the Parliament's Select Committee on Health; and was formerly economic adviser on health and personal social services to Her Majesty's Treasury. His research interests are in the financing and organization of health care systems. His focus is specifically on the role of the private sector in publicly funded health care and on the scope for competition and contestability in health care provision.

Hugh Waters, MD, is a health economist with 15 years' experience working with public health programs. He is currently assistant professor in the International Health Department of the Johns Hopkins Bloomberg School of Public Health. Dr. Waters' areas of expertise are design and evaluation of health insurance programs; evaluation of the effects of health financing mechanisms on access to health care and equity; and costing interventions. He has long-term experience working in Kenya, Cameroon, and Peru and has worked as a consultant with the World Bank, World Health Organization, and several health care projects funded by the U.S. Agency for International Development.

Sophie N. Witter is a development policy analyst and health economist. She is a research fellow at the University of York but is currently based in Uganda. Her recent work has included an evaluation of 45 years of work in Uganda by Save the Children (U.K.) and a study on child poverty. With colleagues at York, she has written textbooks on health economics for developing countries and also for transitional countries. She studied politics, philosophy, and economics at Oxford University and did a Master's in Economics at Leeds University. In addition to her teaching, writing, research, and consultancy experience, she has worked as a program manager for Save the Children in Vietnam and Uganda.

Pascal Zurn is a health economist with a Master's degree in Health Economics from the University of York, United Kingdom and a PhD in Economics from the University of Lausanne, Switzerland. He worked for six years at the Institute of Health Economics and Management in Lausanne. His area of work included health planning, assessment of social cost of AIDS, and cost-effectiveness analyses. Other positions included consultant with the Swiss Tropical Institute for a project in Tanzania and a position in private banking in Geneva. He was a member of the board of directors of Médecins sans Frontières-Switzerland from 1996 to 2000. He joined the Human Resources for Health team at the World Health Organization in August 2001. His areas of work include analysis regarding the issues of imbalance, migration, as well as data collection and monitoring activities.

Peter Zweifel, a Swiss native born in 1946, is a professor of economics at the University of Zurich and director of the Socioeconomic Institute. Together with Friedrich Breyer, he is the author of *Health Economics* (Oxford University Press, 1997); other texts (*An Economic Model of Physician Behavior, Insurance Economics, International Economics*) are available in German only. Besides health economics, his research interests include insurance economics, energy economics, and law and economics. His work has been published by the *American Economic Review, Antitrust Bulletin, European Economic Review, Health Economics, Journal of Risk and Insurance,* and *Public Choice,* among others. Together with Mark Pauly of the University of Pennsylvania, he is the editor of the *International Journal of Health Finance and Economics* (Kluwer). He also serves as a member of the Competition Commission, the Swiss antitrust authority.

Index